The Care of the Older Person

The fifth edition of this widely used book by caregivers brings to you updated and revised content, built on the basic understanding that medicine does not work in a vacuum, but rather alongside other disciplines to provide the environment for a healthy and fulfilling long life. Edited by alumni and senior faculty at McGill University, with international contributions, this book advocates the achievement of better, longer, satisfying, and more productive lives for older persons. It is a helpful resource for physicians, professional caregivers, therapists, students, and residents in medical and nursing disciplines who care for our burgeoning older population and need to know what to look for and when to consult specialists.

Key features:

- Follows a uniform structure with many chapters having a hypothetical vignette for instructional purposes and with the clinical chapters detailing the features and diagnosis of given conditions, along with possible management protocols specific to afflicted older individuals.

- Builds on the success of the previous four editions to provide high-quality content from international experts for physicians and other caregivers in the field.

- Provides possible management protocols to pressing problems, including the nursing home challenge, pandemics such as COVID, and precision therapy for cancer.

THE
CARE
OF THE
OLDER
PERSON

5th Edition

EDITED BY:
RONALD CAPLAN

CO-EDITORS:
JOSÉ A. MORAIS | ABRAHAM FUKS | SERGE GAUTHIER
PHIL GOLD | OLIVIER BEAUCHET | HOWARD BERGMAN

CRC Press
Taylor & Francis Group
Boca Raton London New York

CRC Press is an imprint of the
Taylor & Francis Group, an **informa** business

Fifth edition published 2023
by CRC Press
6000 Broken Sound Parkway NW, Suite 300, Boca Raton, FL 33487-2742

and by CRC Press
4 Park Square, Milton Park, Abingdon, Oxon, OX14 4RN

CRC Press is an imprint of Taylor & Francis Group, LLC

Fourth edition published by RMC Publishing, LLC. 2021

ISBN: 978-1-032-38318-7 (hbk)
ISBN: 978-1-032-38317-0 (pbk)
ISBN: 978-1-003-34447-6 (ebk)

DOI: 10.1201/9781003344476

Typeset in Palatino
by Apex CoVantage, LLC

Contents

Part VI: Understanding, Protecting

Part VII: Medical Terms

Disclaimer

The contents of this book and e-book and all materials contained in this book and e-book are for informational purposes only. The materials and information contained in this book and e-book are not intended to be a substitute for professional medical advice, diagnosis, or treatment. You should always seek the advice of your physician or other qualified health provider if you have questions regarding a medical condition. Never disregard professional medical advice or delay in seeking it because of something you may have read in this book and e-book. Medical professionals should not rely on any drug, drug dosage, or other information in this e-book and book, which is for informational purposes only.

If you think you may have a medical emergency, call your doctor or 911 immediately. The authors do not recommend or endorse any specific tests, physicians, products, procedures, opinions, or other information that may be mentioned in this book and e-book. Reliance on any information provided in this book and e-book is solely at your own risk.

This book and e-book and its contents are provided on an "as is" basis.

About the Editor

Ronald M. Caplan, MD, CM, FACS, FACOG, FRCS(C), Clinical Associate Professor Emeritus Obstetrics and Gynecology, Weill Medical College of Cornell University

Ronald M. Caplan, MD, is an obstetrician gynecologist and medical author. He is a founding editor of *The Care of the Older Person*, along with distinguished McGill Faculty members Olivier Beauchet, MD; Howard Bergman, MD; Abraham Fuks, MD; Serge Gauthier, MD, Phil Gold, MD and Jose Morais, MD.

He did his medical and postgraduate training at McGill University, where his interest in renal disease in pregnancy and homotransplantation culminated in the very first delivery of a baby from a mother who had received a deceased donor kidney transplant.

Dr. Caplan's work goes back more than 50 years to the World's Fair EXPO67 Meditheatre, Miracles in Modern Medicine, where the opening sequence of his delivery of a healthy Rh Positive baby by an Rh Negative mother, an event never seen before by a large lay audience, was viewed by 2.5 million people.

After serving on the Faculty of McGill University, he transferred to New York City and had a long career at the Joan and Sanford I. Weill Medical College of Cornell University, where he became one of the early proponents of minimally invasive surgery, and where he is now Clinical Associate Professor Emeritus of Obstetrics and Gynecology.

He is a Fellow of the American College of Surgeons, the American College of Obstetrics and Gynecology, and the Royal College of Surgeons (Canada).

He previously edited the textbooks *Principles of Obstetrics*, which was translated into both Spanish and Portuguese, and *Advances in Obstetrics and Gynecology*, which was translated into Spanish. He authored another five mass market medical books in multiple editions. Prestigious medical and comprehensive libraries around the world hold copies of his work. He has recently published *Long Life Strategy*, available as an audiobook as well as in paperback and as an ebook via Amazon, Audible and other book sellers.

For all other Editor and Contributor Biographies, please go to our website.
www.careoftheolderperson.com

Editors/Contributors

Olivier Beauchet, MD, PhD, Professor of Geriatrics, Dr. Joseph Kaufmann Chair in Geriatric Medicine, Director of Centre of Excellence on Aging and Chronic Diseases, McGill University

Howard Bergman, MD, FCFP, FRCP(C), Chair, Department of Family Medicine, Professor, Departments of Family Medicine, Medicine, and Oncology, McGill University

Ronald M. Caplan, MD, CM, FACS, FACOG, FRCS(C), Clinical Associate Professor Emeritus Obstetrics and Gynecology, Weill Medical College of Cornell University

Abraham Fuks, MD, CM, FRCP(C), Professor, Department of Medicine, McGill University

Serge Gauthier, CM, CQ, MD, FRCP(C), Director, Alzheimer Disease Research Unit, McGill Center for Studies in Aging, Professor, Departments of Neurology and Neurosurgery, Psychiatry, Medicine, McGill University

Phil Gold, CC, OQ, MD, PhD, FRSC, DSc (Hon), MACP, FRCP(C), Douglas G. Cameron Professor of Medicine, Professor of Physiology and Oncology, McGill University, Executive Director Clinical Research Center (MGH) McGill University Health Centre

José A. Morais, MD, FRCP(C), Professor, Faculty of Medicine, Director, Division of Geriatric Medicine, Lead, Dementia Education Program, McGill University, Co-Director, Quebec Network for Research on Aging

Contributors

Karen C. Altfest, PhD, CFP®
Executive Vice President and Principal Advisor
Altfest Personal Wealth Management
New York City

Paulina Bajsarowicz, MD, FRCPC
Geriatric Psychiatrist
Douglas Mental Health University Institute
Assistant Professor McGill University

Jean Bourbeau, MD, MSc, FRCPC, FCAHS
Respiratory Epidemiology and Clinical
    Research Unit, Montreal Chest Institute
Research Institute of the McGill University
    Health Centre
Department of Medicine
Division of Respiratory Medicine
McGill University

Guy Hajj Boutros, MSc
Kinesiologist and Research Assistant
Research Institute of McGill University
    Health Centre

Lysanne Campeau, MDCM, PhD, FRCS(C)
Assistant Professor of Surgery
Division of Urology
McGill University

Julia Chabot, MDCM, FRCPC, MSc
Assistant Professor
Faculty of Medicine
McGill University

A. Mark Clarfield, MD, FRCPC
Professor Emeritus of Geriatrics
Ben-Gurion University
Medical School for International Health
Faculty of Health Sciences
Ben-Gurion University of the Negev

Anne Croudass, RN MSc
Cancer Research UK, London, UK

Philippe Desmarais, MD, FRCPC, MHSc
Assistant Clinical Professor
Faculty of Medicine
Université de Montréal

Antonio di Carlo, MD, CM, FRCSC, FACS
Professor and Chief
Abdominal Organ Transplantation
Department of Surgery
Lewis Katz School of Medicine at Temple
    University

Liam Durcan, MD, FRCPC
Assistant Professor
Department of Neurology and
    Neurosurgery
McGill University
Consultant Neurologist, Stroke Service
McGill University Health Centre

Hao Feng, MD, MHS
Assistant Professor
Director of Laser Surgery and Cosmetic
    Dermatology
Department of Dermatology
University of Connecticut Health Centre

Catherine Ferrier, MD
Assistant Professor
Department of Family Medicine
Faculty of Medicine
McGill University

Jess Friedland, MD, FRCPC
Geriatric Psychiatrist
Douglas Mental Health University Institute
Program Director
Geriatric Psychiatry Sub-Specialty Residency
    Program
McGill University

Julia Gersovitz, O.C. OAQ, QAA AANB
    FIRAC/FRAIC, FAPT, CAHP
Professor of Practice
Peter Guo-hua Fu School of Architecture
McGill University
Professeure associée
Université de Montréal

Subhas Gupta, MD, CM, PhD, FRCSC, FACS
Chairman of the Department of Plastic
    Surgery
Professor of the Reginald R. Sherrill Endowed
    Chair in Plastic Surgery
Loma Linda University

Eric T. Hedge, MSc
Schlegel-University of Waterloo Research
    Institute for Aging, and Department of
    Kinesiology and Health Sciences
University of Waterloo

Catalina Hernandez Torres, MD, FRCPC
Medical Oncologist
NW Permanente
Portland, Oregon

Jessica Holland, MD, FRCSC
Department of Surgery
McGill University

Tina Hsu, MD, FRCP(C)
Assistant Professor
Division of Medical Oncology
University of Ottawa

Antony D. Karelis, PhD
Professor, Department of Exercise Science
Université du Québec à Montreal

Sunil Karhadkar, MBBS, FACS
Associate Professor of Surgery
Department of Surgery
Lewis Katz School of Medicine at Temple
    University

Sathya Karunananthan, PhD
Postdoctoral Fellow
Ottawa Hospital Research Institute

Aziz Khan, MD
Assistant Professor
Department of Internal Medicine
University of Connecticut Health Center

Young-Sang Kim, MD, PhD
Associate Professor
Department of Family Medicine
CHA Bundang Medical Center
CHA University

Anna Eva Kinio, MD, MSc, PGY-4
Division of Vascular Surgery
McGill University

Heather C. Lambert, PhD, erg, OT(C)
Assistant Professor
School of Physical and Occupational Therapy
McGill University

Cyrille Launay, MD, PhD
Department of Medicine
Division of Geriatrics
University Hospital of Lausanne

Artin Mahdanian, MD, MSc
Assistant Professor and Attending CL
    Psychiatrist
Johns Hopkins University School of Medicine
Suburban Hospital

Louise Mallet, B.Sc.Pharm., Pharm.D., BCGP,
    FESCP, FOPQ
Professor in Clinical Pharmacy
Faculty of Pharmacy
University of Montreal

Pharmacist in Geriatrics
McGill University Health Center

Joseph A. Markenson, MD
Attending Physician
Hospital for Special Surgery
Professor of Clinical Medicine
Weill Cornell Medical College
Attending Physician
Department of Medicine
Memorial Sloan-Kettering Cancer Center

Carmelo Mastrandrea, MD, PhD
Schlegel-University of Waterloo Research
    Institute for Aging, and Department of
    Kinesiology and Health Sciences
University of Waterloo

Joseph J. Montano, Ed.D
Professor of Audiology in Clinical
    Otolaryngology, Director, Audiology and
    Speech Language Pathology
Weill Cornell Medicine
Otolaryngology, Head and Neck Surgery

Silvia Monti De Flores, MD, FRCPC, DFAPA,
    Department of Psychiatry
McGill University

Boris Morin-Defoy, M.Arch, B.Sc. Arch
Lecturer McGill Peter Guo-hua Fu School of
    Architecture
Ecole de Design de l'Université du Québec à
    Montreal

P. David Myerowitz, MD, FACS, FACC
Former Karl P. Klassen Professor and
    Chairman Thoracic and Cardiovascular
    Surgery
The Ohio State University

Peter M. Odell, MD, FACS
Clinical Professor of Ophthalmology Weill
    Cornell Medical College
Attending Ophthalmologist New York
    Presbyterian Hospital

Erin O'Rorke, MD, PGY-1 Resident
Plastic Surgery
Department of Plastic Surgery
Loma Linda University

Randy S. Perskin, Esq., JD
Elder Law Attorney
New York

Astrid F. Pilgrim, MD, MS, Fellow
Critical Care Medicine
University of Pittsburgh Medical School

Michael R. Pinsky, MD, CM, Dr hc, FCCP, MCCM, FAPS
Professor of Critical Care Medicine
Cardiovascular Disease
Anesthesiology, Clinical and Translational Sciences, Bioengineering
University of Pittsburgh Medical School

Bryan Ross, MD, MSc, FRCPC
Respiratory Epidemiology and Clinical Research Unit
Montreal Chest Institute
Department of Medicine
Division of Respiratory Medicine
McGill University Health Centre

Erica C. Roth, MD
Department of Surgery
Lewis Katz School of Medicine at Temple University

Samer Shamout, MD, MSc, Fellow
Division of Urology
McGill University

Barry L. Stein, MDCM, FRCSC, FACS, FASCRS
Director Center for Colon and Rectal Surgery
McGill University Health Center
Assistant Professor of Surgery and Oncology McGill University

Oren K. Steinmetz, MDCM, FRCSC, FACS
Associate Professor
Division of Vascular Surgery
McGill University Health Centre

Michael Stiffel, MD, FRCPC
Assistant Clinical Professor
Faculty of Medicine
Université de Sherbrooke

Norman Straker, MD, DLFAPA
Clinical Professor Weill Cornell Department of Psychiatry
Consultant, Sloan Kettering Cancer Center
Division of Behavioral Science

Dominique Tessier, MD, CCFP, FCFP, FISTM
Clinical Instructor
Family Medicine Department
University of Montreal
Medical Director
Travel Health Group
Montreal

Shachi Tyagi, MD, MS
Assistant Professor of Medicine
Geriatrics, University of Pittsburgh Medical School

Doreen Wan-Chow-Wah, MD, FRCPC
Assistant Professor
Faculty of Medicine
Division of Geriatric Medicine
McGill University Health Centre

Claire Webster, PAC, CPCA, Founder
McGill University Dementia Education Program

Donald White, PhD
Cancer Research UK
London, UK

Michael Wiseman, DDS
Associate Professor
Faculty of Dentistry
McGill University

Mark J. Yaffe, MDCM
Professor of Family Medicine
Department of Family Medicine
St Mary's Hospital Centre and McGill University

Haibin Yin, MD, CCFP (COE)
Assistant Professor
Director of Undergraduate Medical Education
Division of Geriatric Medicine
McGill University

Kevin Yip, MD, Fellow
Rheumatology
Hospital for Special Surgery
Weill Cornell Medical College

Linda Yue, MD, Fellow
Rheumatology
Hospital for Special Surgery
Weill Cornell Medical College

PART I
HELPING

1 Introduction

José A. Morais, MD, FRCP(C)

CONTENTS

It is a well-recognized fact that our society is growing older. This aging of the population is observed in developed as well as in developing countries, albeit at a faster pace in the latter. From the days of the Roman Empire to the early 19th century, average life expectancy at birth remained stable at about 45 years. Since then, there has been a progressive increase in life expectancy with the introduction of improved hygiene and availability of food. The improvement in medical care also contributed to improved survival, especially in older individuals with chronic conditions. Nowadays, a cohort of newborns is expected to live an average of 80 years, with an excess of three–four years for baby girls compared with boys. The net effect of this increased longevity combined with the decline of birth rates is practically a doubling of the percentage of older adults, to reach about 25% of the population by 2030 in most developed countries. The prevalence of those above 85 years, the so-called "old-old," will in fact triple to attain 8% of the population. According to the World Health Organization, the aging of the population is an unprecedented phenomenon in human history. Although many anticipate this demographic revolution with apprehension, it is in fact a triumph of humankind over the adversities of the environment. Among many societal challenges posed by the aging of the population is a growing prevalence of multiple chronic diseases and functional impairments of older adults, giving rise to the geriatric syndromes, especially in those above 85 years of age. The shift in the prevalence from acute and communicable diseases to multiple chronic diseases calls for a realignment of the healthcare system that was previously organized to treat acute conditions. The solution resides in an integrated and coordinated system that is more expensive than one dealing with short-term interventions, although many inefficiencies in care delivery and inappropriate interventions contribute to heighten the cost.

WHY DO WE AGE?

Aging is a universal phenomenon defined as a progressive decline in the functional reserves of many body systems and organs once an individual has reached maturity, which in humans occurs between 20 and 30 years of age. These degenerative changes in organs are responsible for the loss of adaptive responses to stress and an increased risk for age-related illness and death. The theory of evolution proposes that the natural forces that shaped life allowed aging to occur because it would be better to perpetuate the species by investing in mechanisms promoting a high reproductive capacity in young individuals rather than in bodily mechanisms that would maintain individuals indefinitely but at greater risk of dying in a hostile environment. There are a number of theories of aging organized in several categories, but those gaining in popularity among scientists fall under the mechanistic theories of aging, grouped as the somatic mutation theory and the free radical theory. Both of these mechanisms are likely to be involved in aging as they implicate basic cellular processes and can explain other derangements at more complex levels of bodily organization such as dysfunction of neuro-endocrine and immune systems. The somatic mutation theory suggests that most somatic cells undergo replication and in this process, acquire damage by spontaneous mutations or by exposure to toxic products. The accumulation of damage will degrade cell function, leading to senescence. The telomere shortening theory can be considered as a special case of the mutation theory. The free radical theory explains that life is a dynamic process requiring metabolized energy that generates free radicals as by-products of normal redox reactions, (e.g., reactive oxygen species). Such free radicals are the cause of oxidative damage to cell structures and impair their functions. The mitochondrial theory is considered a subcategory of the free radical theory. Although the body possesses many enzymes and surveillance systems to prevent cellular damage and mutations, it is not a foolproof defense mechanism, which is in keeping with the theory of evolution.

DOI: 10.1201/9781003344476-2

WHAT IS GERIATRICS?

The term "geriatric" refers to old age that in most advanced societies has been set arbitrarily at 65 years. It is of interest that this age limit was proposed more than a century and a half ago by a German statesman, Baron Otto von Bismarck, based on the observations that at that time, life expectancy of civil servants aged 65 was on average only two years. He calculated that it would be more profitable for the state to offer them a retirement pension and to hire new, more productive young people. Since then, however, life expectancy at age 65 has steadily increased in most developed countries to reach current levels of about 20 years for women and 15 years for men. Thus, even at age 65, there is opportunity to introduce preventive medicine and to educate people to adopt healthy and active lifestyles. At the same time, the prevalence of chronic diseases increases steadily with age, giving rise to co-morbidities and functional decline. Among older adults, 40–50% have arthritis, hypertension and hearing deficiencies; 20–30% suffer from cardiovascular diseases, dementia, cancer, diabetes, chronic respiratory conditions, lack of teeth and impaired vision; and another 5–10% have strokes, Parkinson's disease and asthma. Hence, concomitant conditions, known as multimorbidity, are highly prevalent as are impairments in activities of daily living. For the age group between 70–85 years of age, 25% have five or more diseases, another 25% will experience disabilities in basic activities of daily living, while 50% will be deficient in the instrumental activities of daily living. Geriatrics refers to the practice of medicine caring for older adults afflicted with many diseases and functional impairments. Geriatricians and family physicians with experience in the field know that a care plan needs to address not only a specific condition but also the interaction that results from all of them and their combined impact on the patient's autonomy. Fortunately, there is recent evidence from scientific literature that we are aging better compared with the previous generation with a decline in the incidence of dementia and disability. For many years, there was debate about the different rates at which the decrease in morbidity and mortality would progress. If lower morbidity would outpace mortality, then we would age better and into older years whereas the converse would have the opposite effect. These recent findings are optimistic, in that if further confirmed, persons can expect to live longer with less disability.

ACTIVE AGING

Aging is a heterogeneous phenomenon that is the result of the interaction between the individual genetic background and environmental factors, not the least of which is the adoption of a healthy lifestyle. Certain families are more prone to develop specific diseases but the appearance of many of them can be delayed or even averted by the adoption of healthy habits. For example, onset of type 2 diabetes can be delayed or prevented by regular physical activity and heathy eating habits. There are also several social and psychological determinants of health, including education, income, social status, social participation, perceived control over one's life, positive attitude, to name but a few. With so many factors at play, it is little wonder that each individual ages at his or her own pace. Gerontology has classified aging into three main categories: active aging (previously called healthy aging or successful aging), normal aging and frail aging. The distribution of these different types of aging varies according to different criteria but the majority falls within the active and normal aging categories with 15–25% considered to be frail. According to WHO (2002), active aging is the process of optimizing opportunities for health, participation and security in order to enhance quality of life as people age. The word "active" refers to continuing participation in social, economic, cultural, spiritual and civic affairs, not just the ability to be physically active or to participate in the labor force. Older people who retire from work, those who are ill or live with disabilities can still remain active contributors to their families, peers, communities and society.

CONTRIBUTION OF OLDER ADULTS TO SOCIETY

Contrary to common beliefs, many older adults are in good health, enjoying life and contributing to society. Such contributions extend to practically all domains of social life despite the challenge of ageism. At the familial level, older persons through their experience of life are of great support to their middle-age children, in counseling on many matters and in the upbringing of the grandchildren. In many instances, they provide financial support to them. At the community level, other than assisting a friend or a neighbor, they participate in organizing cultural and social events, thus enriching their communities. Volunteering is definitely another non-negligible contribution of unremunerated work of older people for the wider community. We all have had the experience of receiving information at the entrance of the hospital by an older person who is volunteering, but they also participate actively on boards of museums, art centers or charitable agencies, or in directly providing services to youth organizations and to more dependent older adults. By so doing, those engaged in volunteering also benefit from being socially active, since outreach and engagement enhance their own well-being and happiness. Finally, remaining part of the work-force is another way of contributing as well as of maintaining physical, cognitive and mental capacities. Society will need to continue its efforts to allow older adults to maintain their societal role as all derive benefits. The change in policies to make retirement age non-compulsory is a first step since we all age differently. Furthermore, facilitating different types of work and adjustments of schedules will permit older people to remain active and to contribute to society.

RESOURCES OR ADDITIONAL READING

United Population World Ageing 1950–2050, Population division, DESA, United Nations, 2002, http://www.un.org/esa/population/publications/worldageing19502050.

Brian T. Weinert and Poala S. Timiras. Invited Review: Theories of Aging. J Appl Physiol 95: 1706–1716, 2003.

Marti G. Parker and Mats Thorslund. Health Trends in the Elderly Population: Getting Better and Getting Worse. Gerontologist 47: 150–158, 2007.

World Report on Aging and Health, http://www.who.int/ageing/publications/world-report-2015/en/.

The Chief Public Health Officer's Report on the State of Public Health in Canada, 2010: Growing Older—Adding Life to Years, http://publichealth.gc.ca/CPHOreport.

2 Caring for the Older Person

Abraham Fuks, MD, CM, FRCP(C)

CONTENTS

"[T]he secret of the care of the patient is in caring for the patient."

The epigraph is a phrase from a talk by Dr. Francis W. Peabody to medical students at Harvard and published in *JAMA* in 1927 under the title, "The Care of The Patient." It has been cited countless times over the past century by those describing a mode of medical practice that is desired, yet too often lacking. The idea has been repeated and promulgated by many speakers at medical school convocations and graduations and remarkably, Peabody's observations and admonitions remain vibrant and cogent today, and, I shall argue, are especially germane to the care of the elderly. The phrase served as an inspiration for the title of this book and certainly for this chapter whose objective is to examine the implications of the concept for contemporary practice and education.

We can better discern the intent of Peabody's comment by examining the words and syntax of his distinction. To be entrusted with the "care of the patient" is to receive a mandate to fulfill a duty. This is an obligation for a caregiver in any domain of medicine and is never taken lightly. Indeed, it is helpful to appreciate that clinical care is a duty of physicians, rather than a right that accrues to patients. That does not detract from a societal obligation to provide health care as a right that is owed to all persons rather than a transactional process. However, provision of care is the responsibility of the physician, though of course, the patient must provide consent. Peabody teaches us that care has additional dimensions and desiderata beyond the simple mandate or duty. "Caring for" a person refers to someone who is important or valued, often in a relationship, and for whose well-being one's concern may extend beyond the requirements and duty of care. The distinction can also be applied to objects, as care of a car indicates a need for maintenance and function while care for a new automobile suggests a deeper connection than with a simple mode of transport.

Peabody explains the relational aspect implicit in "caring for the patient" as follows:

> The significance of the intimate personal relationship between physician and patient cannot be too strongly emphasized, for in an extraordinarily large number of cases both diagnosis and treatment are directly dependent on it, and the failure of the young physician to establish this relationship accounts for much of his ineffectiveness in the care of patients.

This description is important in that Peabody's reason for stressing the imperative for a relationship is not one of warmth or friendship or even a moral obligation. Rather, the clinical relationship is valuable in leading to accurate diagnoses and effective treatments. He provides a helpful exposition:

> What is spoken of as a 'clinical picture' is not just a photograph of a man sick in bed; it is an impressionistic painting of the patient surrounded by his home, his work, his relations, his friends, his joys, sorrows, hopes and fears.

This is a simple but wonderful description of the clinical method that chooses to understand the patient as a person embedded in a family, community and possessing an emotional inner life. It also notes that clinical observations are shaped by the observer who gathers meaningful impressions of an ill person and not simple black and white photos of a diseased patient. I should hasten to add two glosses: Peabody today might have referred to both male and female patients rather than "a man sick in bed." Second, when he speaks of the "ineffectiveness" of young trainees, Peabody does not attribute this to ignorance or apathy but simply to the need for clinical experience accrued over time with strong role models.

Peabody tells us that clinical work is painstaking and demands time and effort. Yet, the human relationships so constructed are rewards in themselves. Finally, he concludes that an appreciation and regard for persons in their full humanity is both necessary for good clinical work and is also the source of its deep satisfaction:

DOI: 10.1201/9781003344476-3

5

The good physician knows his patients through and through, and his knowledge is bought dearly. Time, sympathy and understanding must be lavishly dispensed, but the reward is to be found in that personal bond which forms the greatest satisfaction of the practice of medicine. One of the essential qualities of the clinician is interest in humanity, for the secret of the care of the patient is in caring for the patient.

OLDER PERSONS

The use of the word older, rather than old, indicates that there is no clear line of division between those who are old and those who are not. We live on a functional continuum and each person's trajectory depends on the individual's sense of self, functional capacity, physical capability, and ability to accomplish those aspects of life that bring satisfaction and a lived sense of well-being and purpose. The use of the word person, rather than patient, notes that care for the elderly is not primarily an activity that takes place in a hospital or even a clinic, but enfolds the older person in all aspects of daily life. Clearly, the caregiver must be concerned not simply with the intercurrent episodes of acute illness that readily come to medical attention but the demands of daily living and the impositions on the person by chronic maladies that may not be cured but whose burdens may be lessened.

The misplaced emphasis of care on acute illnesses and the hegemony of diagnosis that afflicts most systems of health care are articulately described by Dr. Jason Mutter in an article titled, "Neglected in the House of Medicine" that appeared in the *Hedgehog Review* in a special issue whose theme was "The Evening of Life." These entrenched elements of the US health care system have an especially deleterious effect on care for the elderly. The author states that the "American health care system that, despite its remarkable technological capacities, achieves poor outcomes for older adults." He attributes this failure to several factors including an emphasis on acute care, urgent care, trauma, and high-tech interventions. While these are certainly necessary, such spheres of medical care have displaced attention to chronic illnesses and the needs of the older person whose ailments need a more deliberate, longer-term horizon with different goals and aspirations. Dr. Mutter goes on to note that a person "becomes visible to the health care system when diagnosed with an acute ailment but then returns to invisibility once that episode has been managed." This stems from a model of care that is focused on diseases, the ICD classification, and supported by payments based on DRGs, complex diagnostic tests and expensive atomized interventions. Lastly, he draws a sharp contrast between two rather different visions of care:

If diagnosis asks, "What does this person have?" then prognosis asks something quite different: "In view of the whole person—health, illness, vulnerabilities, and social supports—how is this person doing, what is their probable course, and how can we alter that course for the better?"

This proactive and expansive vision of health care is appropriate for all but especially germane to care for older persons. Individuals are complex systems with a biopsychosocial nexus within which multiple functions are interconnected and socially embedded. Many components may each function at the limit of capacity yet the whole works in a set of precarious balances. Intervention in one may disrupt the efficacy of another, seemingly unrelated organ system and upset the fragile functional web. In that sense, 'care of' may permit an adjustment of a single anti-hypertensive medication in response to blood pressure readings whereas 'care for' insists on a concern with a broader assessment of risks and benefits to daily function. Thus, Peabody's call to care for the patient entails an integrative, holistic perspective of clinical practice.

THE CURRENT STATE OF CARE

Both basic research on aging and clinical research to improve the management and support for the frail elderly have advanced significantly over the past three decades. Peabody's plea has been echoed over the past hundred years and calls for holistic models of care are heard regularly at conferences and in articles and editorials. Why then is the state of care for the elderly still a poor relation and a neglected domain in health care systems throughout the Western world? Part of the explanation lies in the stigmas associated with aging that are evident in our culture and reflected in our language and behaviors. We have become accustomed to phrases such as silver tsunami, gray plague, and impending demographic disaster that consider the aging of the population in the same urgent terms used to address climate change. The descriptions of dementia and memory loss in apocalyptic terms evoke fear and dread amongst those who wish to grow old, namely, virtually all of us. We now launch wars against amyloid as a newfound enemy and bemoan the failures of such heroic interventions as intrathecal monoclonal antibodies. In brief, the barriers to improving care for the elderly may lie not in a lack of innovative concepts for support, care, and the amelioration of the quality of life, but rather in our entrenched attitudes to those who grow old. This bias, often referred to as ageism, is reminiscent of ancient stigmas associated with mental illness and creates perceptions of aging as a period of decline and dependence and the elderly as the corresponding bookend to infancy and its need for constant support. Other societies and cultures appreciate the later years of life as a period of continuing growth with new opportunities but that is hardly the case in Western society. It is little wonder then that health policies favor the young and those with acute conditions—these reflect superficial considerations but stem from deeply embedded biases. This was sadly evident in the enormous rates of mortality in residences for the elderly and related health care facilities during the COVID pandemic and in the results of subsequent investigations that uncovered the poor care and inappropriate living conditions in many such institutions. A society's interests and concerns can be assessed in part on how it rewards various occupations: perhaps it is not by accident that we underpay teachers and caregivers while concurrently trumpeting our commitment to growing children and aging adults. In reality, we may have simply decided that the tough challenges of both public education and health care are too complex and difficult to repair; we now simply ignore them, hoping they will somehow disappear while placing our societal investments in other domains, for example, space travel and military technology. Nonetheless, we continue to pay the enormous costs for our biases and consequent neglect. Becca Levy and colleagues examined the economic consequences of ageism that they described as "discrimination aimed at older persons, negative age stereotypes, and negative self-perceptions of aging." They found that "the 1-year cost of ageism was $63 billion . . . and ageism resulted in 17.04 million cases" of eight expensive health conditions in those aged 60 or above. They conclude that reducing bias would result in major economic gains and concurrently improve the lives of the elderly by decreasing the risk of major illnesses. A win-win for all!

Care for the older person cannot be provided in models used to look after younger patients who often need management for acute illnesses or those in middle age who may require intensive high-tech but short-term interventions. While such transactional systems are not ideal, they work to provide care in well-developed societies and for patients with significant personal resources and independence. However, staccato care from referral networks of specialists cannot be expected to offer the requisite quality of care for the elderly. Older persons require and respond well to relational models of caregiving, in which attention is continual and anticipatory rather than stroboscopic and reactive. Support and trust are the results of a personal bond with a clinician who is willing and able to listen and who is able to enjoy the anecdotes and reminiscences of older patients and consider these as benefits, not burdens, of caring for those with a wealth of instructive experiences of long and rich lives. Thus, it helps to genuinely care for such individuals since that will motivate clinicians to provide the attention required to nurture and maintain the sense of well-being that enriches daily life—for both parties.

LANGUAGE AND RHETORIC

As noted, the words we use may reveal our biases and perceptions of aging. Moreover, and perhaps more powerfully, language may shape our thinking and our consequent behaviors. A very instructive example was presented in an experimental study of the effects of 'elderspeak' in a facility caring for patients with dementia. Elderspeak describes a mode of infantilizing speech sometimes used by caregivers working with elderly persons that uses syntax and words more commonly heard in addressing the very young. For example, "How are we doing today, my dearie?" couched in a singsong prosody, or, "Are we ready for some treats?" The research compared the behaviors of elderly subjects addressed in one of three registers, elderspeak, normal adult speech, or silence. The highest incidence of aggressive behaviors, such as resisting care by kicking or biting was displayed by persons addressed in elderspeak and the lowest in those spoken to in a normal voice. Silence led to an intermediate level of resistance. It is quite remarkable that in patients with dementia for whom the words themselves may have lost clear meaning, the sensitivity to the disrespect and perhaps degradation of infantilizing speech is retained and is robust.

A counterexample of the benefit of careful linguistic choices was provided by Daniel Busso and colleagues who examined the effect of different framing interventions on implicit age bias in a large sample of American adults. They found that messages that describe aging as "building momentum" and "The energy that we build up as we get older is what powers us to take up new ideas, advance toward new goals, and continue to move our communities forward," reduce bias against aging. A similar effect was noted after messages that speak of intergenerational communities: "By providing opportunities for older people to participate in and contribute to their communities, intergenerational community centers provide benefits for older people and strengthen the whole community." Thus, just as language can reflect and elicit inappropriate behaviors, thoughtful framings and an attention to different tropes may help ameliorate the problem. Judy Segal, a scholar of rhetoric, noted that simply convincing the elderly that aging can be "successful" and "healthy" runs the risk of blaming the older persons when growing old proves difficult. Rather, she recommends that understanding aging as a normal phase of life, and an identity that we all will share, shifts the discourse from a rhetoric of classification and hierarchy to a rhetoric of identification. As Segal notes, "Becoming old is not simply a matter of waning health or waxing decline; becoming old is growing into a person as complex as, arguably more complex than, that person when they were young." This is an optimism worth understanding and sharing as we continue to learn how to care for the older persons in our midst, and for our future selves.

ADDITIONAL READING

Busso, Daniel, Volmert, Andrew, and Kendall-Taylor, Nathaniel (2019). Reframing Aging: Effect of a Short-Term Framing Intervention on Implicit Measures of Age Bias. *J Gerontol B Psychol Sci Soc Sci* 74:4:559.

Levy, Becca, Slade, Martin, Chang, E-Shien et al. (2020) Ageism Amplifies Cost and Prevalence of Health Conditions. *Gerontologist* 60:1:174.

Mutter, Jason (2018). Neglected in the House of Medicine. *Hedgehog Rev* 20:3.

Peabody, Francis (1927). The Care of the Patient. *JAMA* 88:12:877.

Segal, Judy Z. (2020). Ageism and Rhetoric. In *Routledge Handbook of the Medical Humanities*, ed. Bleakley, Alan. Routledge, Oxford.

Williams, Kristine, Herman, Ruth, Gajewski, Byron, and Wilson, Kristel. (2009). Elderspeak Communication: Impact on Dementia Care. *Am J Alzheimers Dis Other Demen* 24:1:11.

3 Frailty

Sathya Karunananthan, PhD, and Howard Bergman, MD, FCFP, FRCPC

CONTENTS

Mrs. Black is a 71-year-old widow with four adult children. Her medical history includes mild osteoarthritis and diabetes, for which she takes acetaminophen as required. She lives alone, tends to be socially isolated, and has mild depressive symptoms. She walks without aids but seems to have slowed down lately. Her cognition is normal, and she is completely independent for all instrumental (IADLs) and basic activities of daily living (ADLs).

Is she frail? What is frailty, and can it be identified in the clinical setting? Are there interventions that effectively delay the onset of frailty or prevent adverse outcomes?

Most geriatricians affirm that they can identify frailty in patients when they see it.[1, 2] Experts generally agree that frailty in older persons refers to a state of vulnerability to adverse health outcomes. It is considered different from aging per se, since some individuals live to an old age without becoming frail. Furthermore, individuals of the same age can be quite different in terms of how frail they are. Frailty would be the opposite of what many consider successful aging.[3]

However, after three decades of research, there remains considerable uncertainty around the concept of frailty and its clinical usefulness. Conflicting ideas abound on the definition of frailty, what criteria should be used for its recognition, and its relationships with aging, disability, and chronic disease.[3-6]

DEFINITIONS AND CONCEPTUALIZATIONS OF FRAILTY

Most experts agree that frailty is the manifestation of impairments in multiple organ systems that results in increased susceptibility to poor health outcomes.[2] The specific characteristics of frailty, however, remain an important point of contention.

Some have proposed that frailty fits the model of a medical syndrome, whereby all of its symptoms are linked through a single underlying biological mechanism. The most widely used definition of frailty fitting that approach includes five criteria:

1. Shrinking (i.e., weight loss).

2. Weakness (i.e., loss of muscle strength).

3. Exhaustion.

4. Slowness (i.e., decreased walking speed).

5. Low levels of physical activity.

An individual with any three or more of these five criteria is classified as frail.[2]

Another widely applied approach is to define frailty as an indicator of global health status, whereby an individual's level of frailty is ascertained through a wide range of factors that may contribute to their well-being. A definition fitting this approach may pull together up to a hundred different characteristics ranging from visual impairment to poor social conditions, chronic diseases, and disability, into a single index of frailty.[7] For each characteristic, an individual is rated as either having a deficit or not. The frailty index is calculated as a proportion representing the number of deficits over the total number of characteristics assessed. By this approach, the more individuals have wrong with them, the more likely they are to be frail.

These approaches represent very different notions of what it is to be frail. The choice of approach has important implications for clinical applicability as well as the potential interventions and prevention of frailty. The number of frailty scores related to these and other approaches is constantly growing. A recent study identified 67 frailty scores with important heterogeneity across scores in the identification of individuals as frail.[5]

DOI: 10.1201/9781003344476-4

WHAT CAN BE DONE ABOUT FRAILTY?

Interventions to prevent or reduce frailty have included physical activity, nutrition, memory training, and individually tailored geriatric care models.[8, 9] Effectiveness of these interventions has been mixed and the body of evidence is limited, given that the definition of frailty is not consistent across studies. Furthermore, these interventions largely overlap with those recommended for prevention or management of chronic diseases related to aging. Researchers have yet to establish whether targeting these interventions to frail individuals has added value.

Thus far, research has provided substantial evidence that frailty, however it may be defined, is a risk factor for various poor health outcomes. Individuals identified as frail are more likely to experience medical complications, disability, institutionalization, or even death, compared to their non-frail counterparts, especially when exposed to stressors such as surgery, chemotherapy, or falls. Based on this, many experts are advocating screening for frailty in all older patients. It has been shown, however, that risk factors that demonstrate high statistical significance may not be good predictors at the patient level. In fact, very little is known about the contribution of frailty in improving patient-level prediction.[10] This needs to be investigated much further in order to justify the adoption of frailty as a clinical tool.

WHAT FRAILTY MEANS TO OLDER PERSONS

Older persons themselves may have their own perspectives of what it means to be frail. For example, factors such as mood have been cited as important to patients and their families; often these are overlooked by clinicians and researchers.[3, 11] Psychological health plays an important role in older persons' beliefs about aging successfully. In a study of older persons where only 15% experienced absence of physical illness, 92% reported feeling like they were aging successfully.[12]

The research evidence has demonstrated that stereotypes of aging, both positive and negative, are internalized by older persons. This can have both short- and long-term effects on their health.[13] For example, when older adults are exposed to negative aging stereotypes, performance on memory tasks, handwriting, and walking speed, as well as physiological measures such as blood pressure, pulse rate, and skin conductance become worse. In fact, in one study, the research showed that an increase in walking speed for those exposed to positive aging stereotypes was comparable to that seen with several weeks of rigorous exercise. Negative stereotypes act as cardiovascular stressors while positive stereotypes reduce evidence of cardiovascular stress. Positive perceptions about aging have impressive long-term effects as well. Individuals with positive self-perceptions of aging have been found to have better functional abilities over a period of 18 years. These findings should serve as a caution about a potential self-fulfilling prophecy when labeling older persons as "frail".

CONCLUSION

Frailty is believed to be an early sign of declining health. As such, it may serve as a "red flag" prior to the occurrence of more severe or irreversible conditions, such as disability. In the example of Mrs. Black, the family and doctors would want to identify any factors that are contributing to her declining health and then attempt to address these. The goal is to prevent or at least slow down her decline.

However, after decades of research and discussion among experts, we are still far from a unified definition or diagnostic criteria for frailty. At this time, there is still very limited evidence on the added clinical value of frailty, and currently no evidence-based guidance on how to manage, treat, or reverse frailty.[9]

For Mrs. Black, better management of her chronic diseases and interventions to improve her social isolation can contribute to slowing down her decline. A diagnosis of frailty, however it is defined, is not likely to have an impact on the clinical care she receives and may only cause harm related to labeling.

REFERENCES

1. Kaethler Y et al. Defining the concept of frailty: a survey of multi-disciplinary health professionals. Geriatric Today: J Can Geriatr Soc. 6: 26–31 (2003).
2. Fried LP et al. Frailty in older adults: evidence for a phenotype. J Gerontol A Biol Sci Med Sci 56: M146–156 (2001).
3. Bergman H et al. Frailty: an emerging research and clinical paradigm—issues and controversies. J Gerontol A Biol Sci Med Sci 62: 731–737 (2007).

4. Hogan DB, MacKnight C, Bergman H. Models, definitions, and criteria of frailty. Aging Clin Exp Res 15(Suppl 3): 1–29 (2003).
5. Aguayo GA et al. Agreement between 35 published frailty scores in the general population. Am J Epidemiol 186(4): 420–434 (2017).
6. Sternberg SA, Wershof Schwartz A, Karunananthan S, Bergman H, Clarfield AM. The identification of frailty: a systematic literature review. J Am Geriatr Soc 59: 2129–2138 (2011).
7. Rockwood K, Mitnitski A. Frailty in relation to the accumulation of deficits. J Gerontol A Biol Sci Med Sci 62: 722–727 (2007).
8. Puts MT et al. Interventions to prevent or reduce the level of frailty in community-dwelling older adults: a scoping review of the literature and international policies. Age Ageing 46(3): 383–392 (2017).
9. Walston J, Buta B, Xue QL. Frailty screening and interventions: considerations for clinical practice. Clin Geriatr Med 34(1): 25–38 (2018).
10. Sourial N et al. Implementing frailty into clinical practice: a cautionary tale. J Gerontol A Biol Sci Med Sci 68: 1505–1511 (2013).
11. Grenier A, Hanley J. Older women and 'frailty' aged, gendered and embodied resistance. Curr Sociol 55: 211–228 (2007).
12. Montross LP et al. Correlates of self-rated successful aging among community-dwelling older adults. Am J Geriatr Psychiatry Off J Am Assoc Geriatr Psychiatry 14: 43–51 (2006).
13. Richardson S, Karunananthan S, Bergman H. I may be frail but I ain't no failure. Can Geriatr J CGJ 14: 24–28 (2011).

4 Physical Activity as a Countermeasure to Frailty

Guy Hajj Boutros, MSc and Antony D. Karelis, PhD

CONTENTS

CLINICAL VIGNETTE

A 78-year-old Caucasian man has difficulty standing up. His body mass index (BMI) is 20 kg/m²
and he has lost more than 7 lbs in the last three months. He has been diagnosed with type 2
diabetes and suffers from hypertension. He fell a few years ago and uses a walker for indoor
mobility. Since then, his mobility has been reduced, and he walks less than 1000 steps per day and
fears walking outside. He started to suffer from low back pain and needs assistance to accomplish
instrumental activities of daily living such as going to the grocery store and visiting friends and
family. He spends most of his time alone watching television and waiting for someone to visit him.

The reduction of physical capacity in performing activities of daily living affects many older adults
and should be taken seriously. There is a need to establish the presence of frailty, determine its risk
factors and propose a plan for assessment and management in which exercise has an essential role.

WHY IS BEING SEDENTARY AN IMPORTANT CLINICAL PROBLEM?

Sedentary behavior may be defined as adopting a sitting or lying posture where little energy is
being expended. In older individuals, there is evidence to suggest that most of their time is spent
in a sedentary state (e.g. sitting) during the day. Almost 60% of older adults reported sitting for
more than 4 h per day. Accordingly, 65% of older adults sit in front of a screen for more than 3 h
daily and over 55% report watching more than 2 h of TV. However, when energy expenditure was
measured objectively in a small study, it was found that 67% of the older population was sedentary
for more than 8.5 h daily. Several studies have shown that long periods of sedentary behavior, such
as sitting, may be associated with negative clinical outcomes including metabolic complications
(i.e. insulin resistance, dyslipidemia), hypertension, cognitive impairments, functional incapacities,
and a decrease in muscle mass and strength as well as an increase in fat mass. Interestingly, there
is evidence to suggest that obese individuals sit 2 h longer than lean subjects.

One could argue that sedentary behavior decreases cumulative energy expenditure due to the
loss of a large amount of muscle contractions that could occur throughout the waking day. This
quantity of energy expenditure has been coined as non-exercise activity. Evidence has shown that
the energy expenditure from non-exercise activity is higher than structured exercise such as walking for 30 min a day 5 times per week or running 35 miles a week, a confirmation of sedentary time.
Health professionals should not neglect this type of energy expenditure. It should be noted that
sedentary behavior for prolonged periods in physically active individuals has been explored. For
example, there is evidence to suggest that high sedentary time may be associated with chronic diseases independent from overall physical activity. Thus, sedentary behavior appears to be an important predictor of health outcomes that goes beyond the level of physical activity of an individual.

WHAT ARE THE RISKS RELATED TO A SEDENTARY STATE?

Prolonged sedentary behavior seems to be associated with an increased risk of all-cause mortality, cardiovascular diseases, type 2 diabetes, Alzheimer's, depression and cancer. In addition, high
sitting time has been reported to increase cardiovascular disease mortality 2.7-fold compared to
those in the elderly population who spend less time sitting. Moreover, higher amounts of sedentary behavior, such as sitting, have been shown to be associated with a 73% increase in the risk of

DOI: 10.1201/9781003344476-5

metabolic complications. As mentioned earlier, older individuals are associated with a decrease in muscle mass and strength, which has been termed sarcopenia. The loss of muscle mass could lead to an increased risk of falls, fractures and being hospitalized for prolonged periods.

Frailty is another common complication that appears in this population. Interestingly, a stressful event in the older individual's life seems to precede frailty. This condition is the consequence of a cumulative decline in many systems (physiological, neurological and musculoskeletal) over one's lifespan. Often a minor infection or a fall results in a dramatic and disproportionate change in health state and the patient goes from being independent to being dependent on another person. Frailty can commonly precede death (27.9%), and be associated with organ failure (21.4%), cancer (19.3%), dementia (13.8%) and other conditions (14.9%). Frailty is more prevalent in women (9.9%) than men (5.1%) and increases with age: 65–69 years: 4%; 70–74 years: 7%; 75–79 years: 9%; 80–84 years: 16%; >85 years: 26%. Frailty is not entirely caused by physical inactivity and sedentary behavior. Other factors that are associated with frailty are:

- Lower educational level.

- Current smoker.

- Current use of postmenopausal hormone therapy.

- Depression or use of antidepressants.

- Intellectual disability.

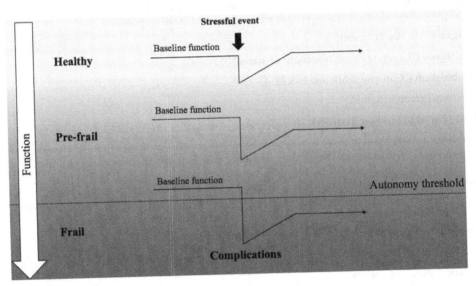

Figure 4.1 How a certain stress can lead to a higher risk of frailty.

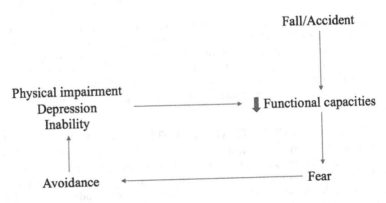

Figure 4.2 Consequences of a fall.

Kinesiophobia (the fear of walking) is another problem that usually appears in the older population, often following a previous fall. Kinesiophobia may decrease mobility, which could lead to isolation, dementia, sarcopenia, cardiovascular disease and mortality.

HOW IS FRAILTY DIAGNOSED?

The prevalence of frailty varies depending on the tool used to define frailty. The studies performed in the United States found that the percentage of frail individuals ranges from 4% to 16% in men and women aged 65 years and older. Injuries and diseases, such as cancer, increase the prevalence of frailty to 43%. Patients with pre-frailty also exist. Pre-frail patients fulfill some of but not all the criteria and represent 28% to 44% in several studies. A variety of frailty measures have been performed in many epidemiologic studies. However, the most common cited frailty tool is the Physical Frailty Phenotype, also known as the Fried criteria, as discussed in the chapter dedicated specifically to frailty. This evaluation was developed based on progressive weakness and declines in the quality of life of older adults that usually follow an accident or diseases that decrease muscle mass and increase cardiovascular risk.

Frailty is not only based on the physical ability of the patient. The accumulation of illnesses, functional and cognitive declines and social situations must be taken into consideration by the clinician. A questionnaire with 10 or more medical and functional related questions could be used by the clinician during the screening as in the frailty index (see Chapter 3). The higher the number of deficits, the greater the patient is considered as frail. Today, finding a fast and quick tool to examine frailty is important because clinicians have limited time with their patients. A tool that takes only few minutes to perform and can be incorporated into history-taking is the FRAIL scale. The component questions listed next define if the patient is frail or pre-frail.

- **F**atigue ("Are you fatigued?").
- **R**esistance ("Can you climb one flight of stairs?").
- **A**mbulation ("Can you walk one block?").
- **I**llnesses (greater than 5).
- **L**oss of weight (greater than 5%).

If patients answer 'Yes' to three or more of the questions, this indicates that they are frail. If patients answer 'Yes' to one or two of the questions, this indicates that they are pre-frail.

Another simple questionnaire that is used in many clinical settings is 'The Study of Osteoporotic Fractures' (SOF) frailty tool. A positive answer to the first question, and negative answers to the next two indicate frailty. The patient is considered frail if two of the three questions are responded to in this way.

- Did you lose more than 5% of your weight during the last year?
- Are you able to rise from a chair five times without the use of your arms?
- Do you feel full of energy?

The clinical frailty scale is a rapid screening questionnaire based on self-reported comorbidities and the need of assistance in activities of self-care and daily living. It is scored between 1 (very fit) and 7 (severely frail).

Many studies used several tools to identify frailty. The most commonly utilized screening tools were comparable in predicting health risks leading to mortality. Unfortunately, the presence of cognitive impairment increases the risk of frailty and deteriorates general health even further. Patients who meet criteria for physical frailty combined with cognitive problems must be considered more at risk than patients without cognitive impairment. Some clinicians use scales that define cognitive status to further refine their judgment and to prescribe assistance in case the patient is in need.

WHAT ARE THE INTERVENTIONS THAT CAN POTENTIALLY REVERSE FRAILTY?

Prevention is a better intervention than waiting until the patient is frail. For this reason, it is very important to explain and clarify at a young age the importance of a healthy lifestyle. Fortunately, the beneficial effects of physical activity can be observed at any age. Current recommendations of physical activity by the American College of Sports Medicine in older adults are a minimum of 30 min of moderate intensity endurance physical activity 5 days per week or 20 min of vigorous intensity 3 times per week during non-consecutive days. In addition, the guidelines recommend performing muscle-strengthening activities at least twice a week during non-consecutive days. A single set of 8–10 exercises with 10–15 repetitions should be performed for each exercise at a moderate to high level of effort using the major muscles of the body to maintain or increase muscle strength and endurance. Unfortunately, only 12% of the elderly population in Canada follow these recommendations. It is important to note that somewhat active older adults who do not achieve these numbers still have better health benefits when compared to inactive older adults. Health professionals could encourage different options/activities to older adults that may limit sitting time such as stand-up desks for computers, interactive video games, standing when using public transportation, devices that vibrate when one is sitting too long and the use of stairs. Specifically decreasing the amount of sitting time in future physical activity guidelines, especially in frail and pre-frail patients, should be considered.

An important question that remains unsolved is whether standing for long periods throughout the day is enough to minimize the risk of disease and decrease the risk of falls. A potential method that could counteract the negative health effects of prolonged sedentary behavior is increasing the number of break-up times. Accordingly, breaking up sedentary time (3–5 min walks every 30 min) appears to have positive effects on multiple metabolic risk factors. In addition, for the pre-frail and frail populations, it is important to practice resistance training to increase muscle strength and bone mineral density. Resistance training is a form of exercise that has been recommended as a safe, feasible, effective and preferred strategy in preventing the loss of muscle strength and increasing muscle mass in older adults. This type of exercise performed two to three times per week appears to have a positive impact on muscle mass, gait speed and strength.

EXERCISES FOR VERY FRAIL PATIENTS

Unfortunately, many frail and pre-frail persons cannot achieve these recommendations for resistance training due to muscle weakness and movement limitation. Some patient cannot even walk a distance of 10 m without a pause, stand up from a chair without help or even perform their everyday self-care. For this type of population, it is recommended to start with seated exercises such as knee extension, arm raise, hip flexion and standing up from the seated position with or without the assistance of their arms. Before starting the exercises, it is crucial to provide a steady base, so the patient will be safe and secure while she/he moves the body during the workout. Once the patient is able to perform 10 to 12 repetitions of these exercises, it is recommended to add a level of difficulty by asking the patient to stand up and to perform the same exercises while holding on to a counter or other stable surface. In addition, it is possible to add more exercises such as hip abduction, hip extension and calf raises. These movements could help to strengthen their lower limb muscles and eventually lead to improved balance. It takes balance to have a safe gait and to prevent falls. To ameliorate balance, a few specific exercises (see Figure 4.3) such as semi-tandem position (one foot ahead of the other as if taking a step) and full tandem (heel of one foot directly in front of the toes of the other foot) are required. Once these exercises are well performed by maintaining the position for 20 to 30 seconds, it is possible to try the one-foot balance but always within reach of a stable support. Frail patients must be supervised by a kinesiologist or a physiotherapist during the first few sessions, and the evolution of the exercises (number of repetition and intensity) must be slower than in healthy aging patients.

AEROBIC TRAINING

Aerobic training is another alternative to improve health outcomes in the elderly. Using equipment that has a lower impact on joints is important, especially in frail patients. Elliptical machines and seated ergocycles are preferred over treadmills because they increase stability and reduce the risk of falls. Some participants must start with exercises in the pool (aqua gym) to prevent negative impacts on joints.

Lately, high intensity interval training (HIIT) has been used to counteract physical, cognitive and metabolic declines. HIIT consists of repeated alternating short bouts of high intensity exercise with recovery periods of low intensity exercise. Different types of exercise equipment can be used to perform this kind of training such as the treadmill, ergocycle and elliptical. Several studies have shown that this kind of exercise decreases cardiovascular risk and improves muscle mass and gait speed more than continuous moderate intensity aerobic exercise. HIIT training sessions are shorter than aerobic continuous moderate intensity exercise sessions. Thus, interval training has become an interesting and a more time-efficient option for exercise training protocols since it can help to break the barrier to engaging in physical activity due to a lack of time. Furthermore, some studies reported that this type of training is not only time efficient, but even more enjoyable than other forms of exercise.

Nutrition, as mentioned in another chapter of this book, is another alternative to counteract frailty in the elderly population. The combination of a proper amount of protein intake (1.0 to 1.2 g/kg of weight) with physical activity has been found to improve muscle mass, functional capacities and the metabolic profile, which in turn improves frailty.

RESOLUTION OF THE CLINICAL VIGNETTE

The patient in our case study has several medical issues. Unfortunately, many older adults of the same age suffer from several conditions as described in the present case. First, a weight loss of more than 7 lbs in the last three months, the low number of steps taken daily and the reduced mobility all establish that he is frail. Second, the metabolic complication of type 2 diabetes with hypertension worsens the situation since diabetes is associated with a lower gait speed. Further,

Warm up:

Neck Flexion   Neck Rotation   Ankle rotation

Strength and balance:

Sit and stand   Heels raise   Knee flexion   Hip abduction

Balance:

Feet together   Semi tandem   Tandem   1leg balance

Upper limb: Aerobic:

Elbow flexion   Elbow extension   Ergocycle

Figure 4.3 Example of an exercise session.

social isolation by spending days alone increases the risk of dementia and depression. The fear of going outdoors is making the patient even more sedentary. The assistance of a physiotherapist or a kinesiologist is vital to counteract the fears and to improve self-confidence. The therapist must start the interventions at a place familiar to the patient, usually his or her home. This decreases the risk of falls.

The intervention must start with a warmup seated on a chair with neck rotations followed by ankle rotations 10 times each. To improve lower muscle strength and balance, the participant is asked to go from a seated position to standing tall (with or without help) for 10 repetitions. This exercise is functional and used in daily life. Once the patient is standing still and holding to a stable counter, he is asked to raise his heels and his toes 10 times each. To improve balance, semi-tandem and tandem exercises are performed for 20 to 30 seconds and for standing on each foot. This workout could be performed 3 to 4 times a week with a day off between the sessions. After a few weeks, the therapist can take the patient outside or to an exercise facility for training. Moreover, since the goal of a training program is to improve the quality of life of the patient, the therapist must provide the patient with some exercises to do by themselves, which allows them to become more autonomous. Once the patient is comfortable in performing the exercises such as stand up from a chair, calf raises and tandem with 8 to 12 repetitions, the addition of an external force will help the patient to have greater improvement in muscle mass. Exercises for upper limb muscle strength are important too. Seated shoulder press and seated biceps curls using lightweight dumb-bells, bottles of water or a resistance elastic band could help the patient in performing activities of daily living such as opening doors and storing personal effects in cabinets. To raise the degree of difficulty, all exercises mentioned could be done when the patient is standing. It is very impor-tant to ensure that the patient is 100% able to perform these exercises by himself especially when the level of difficulty is increased. Aerobic exercise is essential to improve cardiovascular health. Starting the exercises using an ergocycle or an elliptical machine could help to reduce the impact on joints, especially because this population has a high prevalence of arthritis. Depending on the capacity of the patient to perform exercises, aerobic workout could last 5 to 10 min with a very low intensity. Combined exercises (resistance and endurance) could have a better impact on the general health of the patient since our goal is to increase muscle mass and strength and cardiovascular fit-ness levels. After several weeks, this exercise program at a frequency of 2 to 3 times a week should overcome the sedentary habit and allow the patient to feel the difference and look for other kinds of workouts. Overall, being more active will help the patient to reduce many impairments and prevent health-related complications related to being sedentary, especially in older adults.

ADDITIONAL READING

Bonnefoy M, Boutitie F, Mercier C, Gueyffier F, Carre C, Guetemme G, et al. Efficacy of a home-based intervention programme on the physical activity level and functional ability of older people using domestic services: a randomised study. J Nutr Health Aging 2012; 16(4):370–377.

Cesari M, Vellas B, Hsu F-C, Newman AB, Doss H, King AC, et al. A physical activity intervention to treat the frailty syndrome in older persons—results from the LIFE-P study. J Gerontol A Biol Sci Med Sci 2015; 70(2):216–222.

Fried LP, Ferrucci L, Darer J, Williamson JD, Anderson G. Untangling the concepts of disability, frailty, and comorbidity: implications for improved targeting and care. J Gerontol A Biol Sci Med Sci 2004; 59(3):255–263.

Lin F, Roiland R, Chen DG, Qiu C. Linking cognition and frailty in middle and old age: metabolic syndrome matters. Int J Geriatr Psychiatry 2015; 30(1):64–71.

Rockwood K, Mitnitski A. Frailty in relation to the accumulation of deficits. J Gerontol A Biol Sci Med Sci 2007; 62(7):722–727.

Romero-Ortuno R, Walsh C, Lawlor BA, Kenny RA. A frailty instrument for primary care: find-ings from the survey of health, ageing and retirement in Europe (SHARE). BMC Geriatr 2010; 10:57.

5 Doctor, My Spouse Is Getting Forgetful

Serge Gauthier, CM, CQ, MD, FRCPC

CONTENTS

EXEMPLARY CASE

A 78-year-old lady is accompanied by her husband and daughter. The family is concerned about a memory decline over the past two years, worse during the past six months. For example, she forgets conversations, is losing interest in going out, and was twice late paying some household bills. She does not appear concerned about any of this. The family wants to know if this is early dementia and what can be done about it.

On further questioning she has forgotten some of the grandchildren's birthdays in the past year, is looking for things in the house and gets upset about it. She cooks only simple meals and gets flustered when her daughter's family is visiting. She drives in familiar areas, mostly to visit her daughter. The husband has taken over most of the household finances through their common bank account. There is no advance power of attorney for medical and financial decisions. She is independent for self-care. Her medical history is of mild labile arterial hypertension, controlled by a diuretic. She takes vitamin D supplements on a weekly basis. Her mother died of Alzheimer's at age 85.

The physical examination showed a pleasant and healthy looking elderly woman. Her Mini Mental State Examination (MMSE) is 21/30, with wrong day, date, month, year, name of the clinic, forgetting three words after distraction, unable to copy the drawing. She is unable to complete the short version of Trial B found in the Montreal Cognitive Assessment (MoCA), and to set the time at 11:10 on her clock.

The initial clinical impression is of a dementia due to Alzheimer's disease (AD). An un-infused ("plain") head computer tomography showed generalized atrophy compatible with the age of the patient.

At the follow-up visit the MMSE score was 20, and the diagnosis of AD was disclosed to the patient and the family. A road test by an occupational therapist and an advance power of attorney to be drawn by a legal professional were recommended. A cholinesterase inhibitor (CI) was prescribed.

GENERAL WORK-UP AND DIAGNOSTIC RECOMMENDATIONS

Screening for cognitive decline in older persons without symptoms using tools such as the MMSE and the MoCA is not recommended in routine clinical practice. When symptoms suggestive of a progressive cognitive decline are spontaneously brought forward by reliable family members, there has to be a systematic assessment. First a semi-structured questionnaire about the types of cognitive symptoms (memory, language, orientation, judgment), how they affect daily life, and if they are accompanied by mood, personality, or behavioral changes, is utilized. Then a general physical examination and a basic neurologic examination are done, looking for evidence of factors that may suggest a vascular etiology to the cognitive decline. For instance, systolic hypertension associated by an asymmetry of deep tendon reflexes and of plantar responses would suggest a silent stroke.

The latest (4th) Canadian Consensus Conference on the Diagnosis and Treatment of Dementia published in 2012 an update of its recommendations reiterating that structural imaging using computer tomography (CT) or magnetic resonance imaging (MRI) is needed in a specific set of circumstances (Table 5.1).

The most common finding on CT or MRI in persons with mild dementia is generalized atrophy, which may be asymmetric, and is compatible with AD. Small (lacunar) infarcts may be found, and are not considered clinically significant towards the cognitive decline unless they are in a strategic area of the brain such as the thalamus or the head of the caudate, in which case a mixed etiology (AD and stroke) dementia is diagnosed.

DOI: 10.1201/9781003344476-6

Table 5.1 Recommendations from the CCCDTD: Need for Structural Imaging

Structural imaging is needed if cognitive decline and:

- Age less than 65.
- Rapid (one or two months) unexplained decline in cognition and function.
- Short duration of symptoms (less than two years).
- Recent and significant head trauma.
- Unexplained neurological symptoms such as headaches or seizures.
- History of cancer.
- Use of anticoagulation or history of bleeding disorder.
- Early urinary incontinence and gait disorder.
- Lateralizing signs (hemiparesis, unilateral grasp, or Babinski).
- Prominent gait disturbance.

The other relatively common type of late-onset dementia is Lewy Body (DLB), a mixture of AD and Parkinsonian features, which translates into visual hallucinations early in the course of the cognitive decline, fluctuations of symptoms from hour to hour, and motor changes such as rigidity with cogwheeling (the ratchet-like feeling when manipulating the neck or arms of a patient).

GENERAL TREATMENT CONSIDERATIONS

An accurate diagnosis of dementia can be made by all clinicians if there is reliable historical information, some basic cognitive tests, and structural brain imaging when appropriate. The etiology of the dementia over age 75 is essentially AD, AD with stroke, AD with some Parkinson features, or DLB.

What is not as easy is the disclosure of the diagnosis which should be as transparent as for someone with cancer. Most patients with dementia have relative indifference (anosognosia) to their symptoms and to their cause, but clinicians should be on the lookout for someone with depressive symptoms. Practically speaking, the accompanying family member should be made aware of the diagnosis and potential consequences on driving and managing finances. If the patient asks, he can be told about being in "early stages of a common brain aging condition", and if he specifically asks about AD, tell the truth about the likelihood of this specific diagnosis (80% accuracy using clinical diagnosis) unless there is concern for a catastrophic reaction, which is very uncommon.

The loss of autonomy for instrumental and basic activities of daily living is progressive over many years, best handled by gradual adjustments of the family, and is facilitated by support groups. There is no need to make a list of all the changes to occur over five years at the time of diagnosis, but it is wise to anticipate losses through the annual or bi-annual follow-ups: driving, banking, cooking, traveling on foot, day programs, long-term care, end-of-life care will be handled over time.

The mood and behavioral symptoms of dementia are often worse than the cognitive decline and the gradual loss of autonomy. Apathy, irritability, and suspiciousness are common in the early stages of AD, and may be helped by antidepressants acting on serotoninergic pathways. Hallucinations in DLB improve with CIs. Aggressive behavior not manageable by environmental non-pharmacological approaches may require an atypical neuroleptic such as risperidone (pay attention to the black box warning about increased risk of stroke and death). Sometimes aggressive behavior is improved by antidepressants and/or the NMDA receptor antagonist memantine, reducing the need or the dose of a neuroleptic.

REFERENCE

1. Gauthier S, Patterson C, Chertkow H et al. 4th Canadian Consensus Conference on the Diagnosis and Treatment of Dementia. Can J Neurol Sci 2012; 39: Suppl 5.

6 Update on Alzheimer's Disease Diagnosis and Management

Serge Gauthier, CM, CQ, MD, FRCPC

CONTENTS

INTRODUCTION

Although there are important changes in the research definition of Alzheimer's disease (AD) using biomarkers for amyloid (A), tau (T) and neurodegeneration (N) (REF), the clinical definition of AD in day-to-day medical practice is still based on a history of cognitive decline affecting daily life, often accompanied by changes in mood and behavior. This chapter will illustrate the various modes of presentation of AD that many clinicians will come across.

In terms of treatment of AD, there will be no magic pill in the near future, so we must treat symptoms as they emerge over time and help both the person with dementia and the caregivers. A stage-by-stage management approach is discussed.

DIAGNOSIS OF AD—INITIAL ASSESSMENT

Most persons with AD have memory complaints for one to three years before the memory lapses start interfering with their daily life. There are some gender and cultural differences in how significant these lapses are: a grandmother forgetting her grandchildren's birthday is more significant than a grandfather. A man who used to drive around without a problem and now needs help for navigation on a regular basis is significantly changed. Less commonly the person has progressive difficulties getting the words out, not just names of people but names of common objects. The handyman is now looking for his tools and taking much more time than before to fix things in the house. The mother who used to regularly invite the family for dinner now finds it too much of a burden because of the need to plan the meal and cook it properly. These are examples of common complaints in early stages of AD, but there can be variations, such as not recognizing people's faces, or being very suspicious about family members or neighbors stealing things, or having visual hallucinations of persons coming to the house.

When meeting a person with cognitive complaints for the first time, the health professional will ask about various symptoms as illustrated earlier and will try to estimate their impact on daily life such as reliability in paying bills, taking medications, planning an outing. If the person is seen alone there is a need to get complementary information by talking with family or friends. It is sometimes necessary to talk to the accompanying person separately from the person with cognitive complaints, since there may be embarrassment about disclosing functional and behavioral changes. Some families will send the clinician a short email ahead of, or right after the first visit.

The history needs to be expanded to general health issues including past or current medical diagnosis such as sleep apnea, depression, alcohol abuse, etc. Medications in use are examined carefully since some of them may interfere with attention and memory, such as anticholinergic drugs prescribed for bladder urgency, or amitriptyline prescribed for headaches.

Screening memory tests are done, including the Mini Mental State Examination (MMSE) and the Montreal Cognitive Assessment (MoCA). They can be supplemented by other cognitive tests if required, such as the Short Version (15 pictures) of the Boston Naming or the Frontal Assessment Battery.

The physical examination is focused on blood pressure and circulation, including listening to the carotid arteries looking for a murmur, evidence of a general medical problem such as an enlarged thyroid, and asymmetry of the motor examination which can suggest a stroke or space occupying lesion.

The blood work is generally the same done on a yearly basis for a general preventive assessment, including AST/ALT, B12, BUN/creatinine, electrolytes, glycemia, TSH levels. A head

DOI: 10.1201/9781003344476-7

computerized scan (CT) is often done but rarely influences the diagnosis when the history of a gradual cognitive decline over at least one year is associated with a normal general physical examination.

When the person is younger than 65, if there are atypical symptoms such as primarily language or visual complaints, asymmetry on the neurologic examination, a history of cancer or taking anticoagulants, a CT scan is indicated, and may be supplemented by other tests such as magnetic resonance imaging (MRI) of the head, or a position emission tomography (PET) of the brain using various radioisotopes, the most common being fluorodeoxyglucose (FDG), or a lumbar puncture (LP). These are usually ordered by a specialist in a "memory clinic" setting.

DIAGNOSIS OF AD—DIFFERENTIAL DIAGNOSIS

Two visits usually six months apart allow to compare the performance on sequential MMSEs (it is preferable not to use the MoCA more often than once a year because of practice effects), and determine if there is improvement or worsening of symptoms. A diagnosis of mild cognitive impairment (MCI) is made if there is evidence of a cognitive decline not interfering with daily life compared to other persons in the same age, education and cultural group. A diagnosis of dementia is made if the cognitive decline is causing a loss of autonomy for some activities of daily living. AD is the most common cause of MCI with memory complaints (amnestic MCI) and of dementia over age 65, but other factors may be at play such as stroke, leading to a diagnosis of "mixed dementia". Less commonly there is a mix of Parkinson and Alzheimer symptoms (dementia with Lewy bodies—DLB) and fronto-temporal dementia (FTD).

The diagnosis of the cause of dementia may change over time. For instance a person with a normal motor examination at the initial assessment suggesting AD may show after two years one-sided Parkinson-like changes, suggesting cortico-basal degeneration (CBD) or start falling backwards with rigidity in the neck muscles, suggesting progressive supra-nuclear palsy (PSP).

Natural History

Knowledge of the natural progression of AD and related disorders will help plan the management over time.

Many but not all persons with MCI will progress to dementia within five years. The general figure is 15% per year for such a progression, which may be delayed by careful attention to risk factors and enhancing protective factors. Some genetic factors such as the apolipoprotein E 4 (ApoE4) genotype are known to accelerate the rate of progression to dementia.

Mild dementia (needs assistance for directions while driving, needs advice for financial decisions) may be already present at the time of diagnosis, and will progress over an average of eight years to moderate stage (needs supervision for grocery shopping, accompaniment to the bank, turning the oven off and using the microwave) to moderate-severe stage (needs assistance for personal care), severe stage (cannot walk safely, incontinence) and terminal stage (difficulty swallowing leading to aspiration pneumonias). A classification from 1 to 7 is often used as a reference for staging the disease.

This pattern of progression is relatively predictable in AD but less so with other types of dementia. Mixed AD-vascular dementia usually shows a slower decline until a heart attack or stroke intervenes, leading to a shorter survival time. Dementias with an early motor component (DLB, CBD, PSP) are associated with falls that can lead to complications such as hip fractures and head injuries.

Some persons with AD have a slow rate of progression, with little functional decline for five years (they are usually older than 85 and in good general health). Other persons have a more rapid decline (they are often younger with higher education). The variability in speed of progression is partly determined by the brain reserve (more highly educated persons start symptoms of AD later than uneducated persons, but show a more rapid decline), co-existing diseases such as heart failure, social isolation and poor nutrition.

Depressive symptoms are common in the MCI and mild dementia stages of AD, since the person is still aware of the cognitive and functional decline. These symptoms tend to improve over time as the person loses awareness of the disease (anosognosia).

Agitation and aggressivity are usually more common in moderate stage dementia, and they often are worse at the end of the day (sundowning). Sleep disturbances with being up at night are more common in moderate to severe stages of dementia.

Physical impairment such as shuffling gait and falls occur usually in the severe stage. Difficulties in swallowing causing aspiration pneumonia usually follow.

Management of AD

Disclosure of the diagnosis of dementia due to AD or another cause is more easily done with the accompanying person, particularly if that person is also the legally designated representative. The person with dementia rarely asks, and there is a risk of catastrophic reaction in some individuals with anxiety about the future or with depression. In doubt, the clinician may state something like, "You were right to come for an assessment of your memory; there is indeed a problem and we will work on it together".

Persons with MCI or with mild dementia are advised to indicate in writing who they trust in case of future needs: "Who can we ask permission if you have a car accident, you are unable to give an answer about your treatment, and bills need to be paid?" The document used is an Advance Directive called a Specific Power of Attorney. It takes effect immediately and allows a representative chosen by the affected person to act on behalf of that person for personal health care and financial issues. In case of incapacity, the document can be filled in at home with two witnesses, or executed at a notary or lawyer's office (which is preferable). It is recommended to designate a principal and a backup legal representative, or to designate one person for personal care issues and one for financial decisions. A General Power of Attorney allows for broader powers to the representative appointed and is a useful complement to the Advance Directive. Advance Directives can only be put in place when the person has capacity to do so.

Incapacity homologation is the process by which a judge signs off on the documents in cases of incapacity. (See Chapter 44, "How Can Older People Be Protected?" by Randy S. Perskin, Esq., JD.)

Improvement of cognitive abilities can be achieved by optimal care of other medical conditions such as sleep apnea, deafness, vitamin or nutritional deficiencies. Participation in social activities and being physically active may help in prevention of cognitive decline but also does help people with MCI or dementia.

Current medications for dementia due to AD, mixed Alzheimer and vascular dementia, Parkinson's disease-associated dementia and DLB are of two classes: one class increases acetylcholine levels in the brain by inhibiting enzymes that break it down (acetylcholinesterase inhibitors: donepezil, rivastigmine, galantamine); the other class decreases the activity of the neurotransmitter glutamate (NMDA receptor blocker: memantine). These medications have been in use for more than a decade and may improve or stabilize symptoms for six to 24 months. Other medications used in managing dementia include antidepressants and low doses of antipsychotics.

Non-pharmacologic interventions include a quiet environment, more lights in the evening, and education of the caregivers about dementia-associated behaviors.

Persons with dementia are usually diagnosed and taken care of by their family doctor and his/her nurse and other community resources. A referral to a neurologist, psychiatrist or geriatrician may be required if there are issues that the local team has difficulty with. There are also persons with MCI or dementia who wish to participate in research, and they can be referred to memory clinics.

REFERENCES USING A CASE-BASED APPROACH

1. Feldman HH, Jacova C, Robillard A et al. Diagnosis and treatment of dementia. 2. Diagnosis CMAJ 2008; 178(7):825–836.
2. Cherkow H, Massoud F, Nasreddine Z et al. Diagnosis and treatment of dementia. 3. Mild cognitive impairment and cognitive impairment without dementia. CMAJ 2008; 178(10):1273–1285.
3. Hogan DB, Bailey P, Black S et al. Diagnosis and treatment of dementia. 4. Approach to management of mild to moderate dementia. CMAJ 2008; 179(8):787–793.
4. Hogan DB, Bailey P, Black S et al. Diagnosis and treatment of dementia. 5. Nonpharmacologic and pharmacologic therapy for mild to moderate dementia. CMAJ 2008; 179(10):1019–1026.
5. Herrmann N, Gauthier S et al. Diagnosis and treatment of dementia. 6. Management of severe Alzheimer disease. CMAJ 2008; 178(12):1279–1287.

REFERENCES ON DIAGNOSIS AND MANAGEMENT USING A CONSENSUS APPROACH

Australia

1. Laver K, Cumming RG, Dyer SM et al. Clinical practice guidelines for dementia in Australia. Med J Australia 2016; 204:1-3. Full guidelines: http://sydney.edu.au/medicine/cdpc/documents/resources/LAVER_Dementia_Guidleines_recommendations_PRVW%20%284%29.pdf

Canada

1. Gauthier S, Patterson C, Chertkow H et al. 4th Canadian consensus conference on the diagnosis and treatment of dementia. Can J Neurol Sci 2012; 39(Suppl 5):S1–S8.
2. Gauthier S, Rosa-Neto P, Morais JA, Webster C. World Alzheimer report 2021: journey through the diagnosis of dementia. London: Alzheimer's Disease International (2021). https://www.alzint.org/world-alzheimer-report-2021/.

France

1. Haute Autorité de Santé. Guide parcours de soins des patients présentant un trouble neurocognitive associé à la maladie d'Alzheimer ou à une maladie apparentée. Les Parcours de Soins, Mai 2018.

Germany

1. Deuschl G, Maier W et al. S3-Leitlinie Demenzen. 2016. In: Deutsche Gesellschaft für Neurologie, Hrsg. Leitlinien für Diagnostik und Therapie in der Neurologie. Online: www.dgn.org/leitlinien

Singapore

1. Nagaendran K, Chen C, Chong MS et al. Ministry of health clinical practice guidelines: dementia. Singapore Med J 2013; 54: 293–299.

UK

1. https://www.guidelines.co.uk/mental-health/nice-dementia-guideline/454244.article

USA

1. Petersen RC, Lopez O, Armstrong MJ et al. Practice guideline update summary: Mild cognitive impairment. Report of the guideline development. Dissemination, and implementation subcommittee of the American academy of neurology. Neurology® 2018; 90: 1–10. doi:10.1212/WNL.0000000000004826.

7 Navigating the Journey of Dementia as a Caregiver

Claire Webster

CONTENTS

PATIENT SCENARIO

Mrs. L is a 74-year-old woman whose daughter brought her to the neurologist after consulting with their family physician about her mother's unusual behaviour and significant change in personality following the recent death of her husband. Mrs. L had been a physically active, independent and outgoing woman, but over the past 18 months had become socially withdrawn and impatient, suffering from severe mood swings ranging from bouts of anger to depression. She had increasing difficulty managing her finances and preparing meals for herself. She developed a fear of stairs and zero tolerance for loud noise, often putting her hands over her ears while rocking back and forth in distress. She was often confused, had difficulty finding her words and started to use odd and inappropriate language. A few symptoms began appearing a year prior to her husband's passing. Mrs. L had become obsessed with the next-door neighbour, who she believed was operating a cocaine lab. Her car had numerous dents and marks indicative of accidents.

When the symptoms began to increase after her father's death, her daughter thought her mother was suffering from post-traumatic caregiver stress and grief, as her mother had been the primary caregiver to the father for over 30 years. Mrs. L began donating money to the same charity multiple times a year and incurring random expenses. Her daughter noticed that she had been hoarding hundreds of empty plastic fruit containers in her kitchen cabinets and keeping expired food in the refrigerator.

Mrs. L's medical history included high cholesterol, and she had suffered a minor transient ischemic attack (TIA) at the age of 68. There was a history of cardiac issues in her family.

Against her mother's will and in full denial of anything being wrong, her daughter made an appointment with a neurologist. The doctor asked the daughter a series of questions about her mother's cognitive and physical well-being while the mother sat beside her, in great frustration, refusing to accept or admit to any of the information that was being shared. The neurologist performed the MoCA (Montreal Cognitive Assessment Test) wherein Mrs. L scored 17/30. The neurologist informed Mrs. L that she had Alzheimer's disease, and upon learning that she was still driving, immediately called the license bureau, and without any warning, cancelled her driver's license.

In shock and completely unfamiliar with dementia, Mrs. L's daughter asked the doctor if he could explain what Alzheimer's disease is, how to manage the disease, what to expect and whether her mother could still live on her own. The doctor answered, "No, she cannot live on her own. There is information about the disease on the Internet, and good luck." Mrs. L and her daughter left the doctor's office without being provided any information on the symptoms of the disease or guidance on how to plan for the future. They were not counselled on the importance of accessing support services or told what the next steps should be.

Mrs. L's 38-year-old daughter was her only child, and she was raising a family of three young children while holding a full-time job managing a company with her husband. Over the next few years, she would get caught up in a cyclone of caregiving that resulted in severe burnout and

DOI: 10.1201/9781003344476-8

post-traumatic stress disorder. The neurologist's inability to provide information and guidance would have a significant impact on the quality of care and safety of Mrs. L in the coming years, as well as a ripple effect on the mental and physical health of her daughter.

WHO ARE CAREGIVERS?

It is important for the physician to know who the primary caregiver is to the Person Living With Dementia (PLWD) as the disease progresses. By asking this question, the physician can help the newly diagnosed patient and their caregiver recognize that their relationship will change as the disease progresses. This is particularly important since many informal caregivers do not recognize themselves as "caregivers", which may also contribute to stress. A caregiver may be the person's spouse or partner, friend, adult child or other family member, and may not realize that their role in their loved one's life will ultimately change. The caregiver may also have health issues of their own that will impact the level of care they are able to provide.

In their report, *Improving the Quality of Life and Care of Persons Living with Dementia and Their Caregivers*, the Canadian Academy of Health Sciences (CAHS, 2019) notes that assessing the needs of caregivers is key to identifying the support that each caregiver is likely to require.

The health and well-being of the caregiver directly affects the care they are able to provide to their loved one. Upon receiving a diagnosis of dementia (or soon thereafter), a needs assessment should be performed for the caregiver using a validated instrument designed to complete a comprehensive psychosocial assessment that identifies caregiver needs and key areas of concern such as the Caregivers' Aspiration, Realities, and Expectations Tool (CARE Tool). This type of assessment has been found to increase the health practitioner's awareness of the caregiver's needs and can help refer them to timely supports and improve access to appropriate services (Keefe et al., 2014). The fact of having participated in such an assessment recognizes and validates the caregiver's role in addition to providing information about services, an opportunity to tell their story and permission to express their feelings (Keefe et al., 2014).

THE RIPPLE EFFECT OF DEMENTIA ON THE CAREGIVER

Understanding and caring for someone with Alzheimer's disease or other dementia-related illnesses is a long, stressful and intensely emotional journey. PLWDs progress along an unpredictable path to complete loss of self and autonomy. The diagnosing physician needs to consider that the person who accompanies the patient is receiving devastating news about their loved one, and it is imperative to provide them with as much information as possible on that first visit and offer the necessary resources to ensure the best quality of care and safety for both the patient as well as the caregiver's physical, mental and financial health and well-being.

A diagnosis of Alzheimer's disease affects all intimate family and friends of the PLWD. Caregivers need support to care for themselves in order to avoid becoming overwhelmed. They are at an increased risk of developing significant health problems as their loved one's cognitive, physical and functional abilities diminish.

THE RISKS OF NOT PROVIDING EDUCATION AND SUPPORT ABOUT DEMENTIA TO CAREGIVERS

A lack of education about dementia will have a significant impact on the quality of care and safety of the individual who has been diagnosed as well as on the caregiver. Unlike other diseases, the patient who is diagnosed with dementia and their caregiver are rarely provided with information on how to navigate the challenges associated with managing and living with this disease. The medical community does not automatically educate individuals about the disease and/or refer them to the available support services or inform them how to access support from the public health care system.

Caring for someone known previously as a vital and independent individual is incredibly stressful. The caregiver is grieving their loss at the same time as they are looking after their loved one, who often may resist and resent their efforts to help and protect them as the disease progresses. As dementia is a disease that is continuously evolving, robbing the PLWD of their cognitive and physical skills throughout the process, it is important to recognize that the care partner is constantly in a state of anticipatory grief as they witness and mourn the evolving loss of independence and skills of their loved one with dementia. There is also an overwhelming sense of responsibility when it comes to making important daily life and end-of-life decisions on behalf of the person they are caring for.

Caregivers depend on the physician's guidance, support and intervention, but that rarely occurs without a direct request for help from the caregiver. In over 40% of all cases of dementia, there will be at least one member of the informal care team whose own emotional and/or physical health deteriorates to a degree that they are unable to continue looking after their loved one and in most cases, only reach out for support when they have reached a crisis point. Inevitably, this results in feelings of helplessness, grief, anger, guilt and terrible sadness which can lead to coping mechanisms involving excessive amounts of alcohol, cigarettes, drugs, food, gambling and/or shopping, turning into addictive behaviours.

Providing care to PLWDs is known to take more time and cause more distress to caregivers than caring for seniors with other issues. On average, caring for a PLWD requires up 26 hours per week of informal care versus 17 hours of care for other seniors, and 45% of caregivers of PLWDs exhibit signs of distress compared to 23% of those caring for seniors without dementia (CIHI, 2018). Logic tells us that a caregiver who is informed about what to expect as the disease progresses and the services available to aid them is more likely to understand what is going on with their loved one and be prepared to access those services. Similarly, a caregiver who is aware of the various safety issues around the home is going to be able to avoid emergencies by making the environment safer for their loved one. Finally, being recognized as a caregiver, and having the difficulties of that role acknowledged, will open the door to asking for and receiving assistance before emotional and/or physical breakdown occur.

WHAT CAREGIVERS NEED TO KNOW

Physicians have a role to play in assisting caregivers to navigate the dementia journey of a loved one. From the moment that an individual is diagnosed with dementia, their care journey will require the assistance of a multidisciplinary team of health care and legal professionals. All physicians who are in a position to be giving a diagnosis of Mild Cognitive Impairment, Alzheimer's disease or other dementia-related disease should have on hand material about the disease and resources to help their patients and caregivers understand what they are facing.

Information helps caregivers and the PLWD ensure the best and most appropriate care possible. This could include: knowing the different types of dementia and how they are likely to progress; understanding and responding to challenging behaviours; various treatments that exist for some of the symptoms; how to plan for the future in terms of financial matters; how to provide assistance and support with activities of daily living (dressing, bathing, grooming, eating, etc.); the types of care available; and end-of-life choices. Caregivers need to understand at the outset that the disease is constantly evolving, that they will need to constantly adapt to a changing situation, and that they will need help along the way if they wish to remain resilient throughout the journey.

Physicians should be prepared for questions such as: how to communicate with a PLWD throughout the various stages of the disease; how to maintain a connection with a PLWD; what types of activities they can do throughout the various stages of the disease; what are the household safety hazards; when to stop driving; the use of medication or non-pharmacological treatments to manage challenging behaviour; what strategies can be employed to prevent falls and injury; when should transition to a residence/long-term care facility be considered. It is also imperative that caregivers know how to access the various public health agencies and resources that are available in their community to assist with home care support, respite and eventual transition to long-term care.

Physicians should remind PLWDs and their caregivers to discuss and make their preferred financial, care and living arrangements as soon as possible, unless this has already been determined prior to diagnosis.

RESOLUTION OF CLINICAL VIGNETTE—A PRESCRIPTION OF CARE FOR INFORMAL CAREGIVERS

When diagnosing patients like Mrs. L, it is recommended that the physician take the time to ensure that the primary caregiver is given the following "Prescription of Care":

1. Education about the Disease and Its Progression

Dementia affects the individual both cognitively as well as physically over a seven- to ten-year period. Knowing as much as possible about the disease, how it will progress, and how to plan for the future prepares caregivers for the journey and provides them with the necessary information and tools to ensure the best care possible.

2. Accept the Diagnosis and Avoid Denial

Accepting the diagnosis and learning how to adapt to the various cognitive and physical changes that the disease will place upon the person will allow for best care practices. It is important to recognize that the person with dementia is doing the best they can, and if something is not working, it's the responsibility of the care partner to change their approach and behaviour towards the person.

3. Plan for the Future

Planning for the future is an important part of the journey as it relates to making decisions concerning health and personal care, living arrangements, finances as well as legal and estate planning. As the disease progresses, it will become difficult to communicate needs and make choices without assistance. While the person with dementia is still able to, it is highly recommended to meet with family members and legal experts in order to arrange for a mandate/notarized power of attorney authorizing someone to legally make decisions on their behalf when they are no longer able.

4. Ensure a Safe Home Environment

As the disease evolves, a person's vision, mobility and cognitive decline will all have a direct impact on their activities of daily living such as cooking, eating, bathing, grooming, dressing, sleeping as well as other facets of their day-to-day life. Keeping the person safe at home thus becomes a priority in order to prevent falls and injuries. Certain rooms in the home such as the kitchen and bathroom, and stairs, have higher risks. Meet with a physical or occupational therapist, recreation therapist or a specialist who can properly assess the home in order to ensure a safe home environment.

5. Identify and Accept as Much Support as Possible

Caring for someone with dementia can be one of the most stressful situations for a family member to be faced with and it is not possible to do it alone. In order to prevent caregiver burnout, it is extremely important to identify additional family members, friends, community and/or private resources that can provide assistance with household chores, caregiving tasks, transportation as well as psychological support and respite care. Seek out the necessary support services immediately upon diagnosis in order to understand the various available options in order to be properly prepared.

6. Understanding and Responding to Challenging Behaviour

Dementia often leads to communication challenges and unexpected behaviours from the individual who has the illness. These behaviours can sometimes be attributed to changes in the brain, other health issues, the environment, relationships with others, how the person is spending his/her time as well as the individual's own personality prior to diagnosis. In order for the caregiver to be able to assess what may be causing the individual to respond in a certain way, it is important to understand their personal history prior to diagnosis. Information about previous occupations, personality traits, fears, likes/dislikes, music preferences, milestones, food preferences, body temperature and activity level can be used to help a caregiver figure out why some behaviours are occurring and ways to address them.

7. The Importance of Self-Care

Caregivers need to preserve as much energy as possible in order to be able to fulfil their daily tasks. It is recommended that they become more protective of personal time and commitments and ensure that they surround themselves as much as possible with people and projects that add positive energy into their lives. Learning to say no and becoming selective of where, how and with whom they invest their time is key. Establishing a regular exercise routine, healthy eating and quality time spent with friends, family and colleagues is important to maintaining a balanced life.

REFERENCES

The Canadian Academy of Health Sciences (CAHS) (2019). *Improving the Quality of Life and Care of Persons Living with Dementia and Their Caregivers.*

Janice Keefe, Nancy Guberman, Pamela Fancey and Lucy Barylak. (2014). *Caregiver Assessment: An Essential Component of Continuing Care Policy.*

Alzheimer Society of Canada, www.alzheimer.ca.

Caregiver Crosswalk (2016). *Claire's Prescription of Care,* www.carecrosswalk.com.

McGill University Dementia Education Program, www.mcgill.ca/dementia.

8 How to Diagnose and Manage Delirium

Haibin Yin, MD, CCFP(COE)

CONTENTS

CLINICAL VIGNETTE

An 84-year-old female living at home with mild mixed dementia and Parkinson's disease was admitted for right intertrochanteric fracture after a fall. Functionally, she required assistance for most instrumental activities of daily living, and could perform most basic activities of daily living. She had 24-hour private help at home.

Her past medical history included congestive heart failure, Parkinson's disease and atrial fibrillation on warfarin. On POD #2, she began to have visual hallucinations and became disoriented. She also had delusion of persecution. Her mental status fluctuated, from trying to get out of bed to sleepiness. She refused to eat and to take her medications.

She was in abdominal restraints. She was alert and calm, but hesitated for 15 seconds or more to answer questions. Her vital signs were normal. There were no additional heart sounds. Her JVP was slightly elevated. Her lung examination revealed decreased air entry bilaterally. Her abdomen was soft and bowel sounds were present. Her wound was clean with no surrounding edema. Both lower extremities were edematous (R>L) but non-tender. There were no neurovascular damages distally. She had bilateral upper extremity resting tremors and cogwheeling rigidity.

Her medications included morphine 1.25 mg SQ q 2 hours PRN (none taken in past 24 hours), haloperidol 0.5 mg IM tid PRN (received 2 doses in past 24 hours), carbidopa/levodopa 100/25 1 PO tid, warfarin 5 mg PO qd with enoxaparin (prophylactic dose) bridging and furosemide 20 mg PO bid. What could be the potential causes of this patient's delirium and how should it be managed?

WHAT IS DELIRIUM? WHY IS IT IMPORTANT TO RECOGNIZE IT?

Delirium is also known as acute brain failure, toxic-metabolic encephalopathy or acute confusional state. DSM-V defines it as acute changes (with fluctuating course) in attention, awareness and cognition that are caused by an underlying medical condition or medication. Different studies show that it affects one-third of patients over 70 years old on general medical units, amongst which half are delirious on admission. Among geriatric patients in the Emergency Room, 15% are delirious. In the ICU, prevalence could reach 70%.

The most useful tool for diagnosing delirium is the Confusion Assessment method (Table 8.1). This systematic-review-validated tool reaches sensitivity and specificity of over 90%. It has also been adapted for patients in the ICU (CAM-ICU). Other tools (Delirium Symptom Index, The 4-AT Test, etc.) could also be used.

The pathophysiology of delirium is poorly understood. Several hypotheses include primary or secondary neuroinflammation and cholinergic deficiency. The predisposing factors of delirium include old age, functional impairment, cognitive deficits, multiple medical comorbidities and sensory impairment. The precipitating factors can include many medical conditions, medications and interventions (restraints, indwelling devices, etc.).

One of the reasons why it is important to recognize and manage delirium is its poor outcome. A meta-analysis which follows 3000 patients for 2 years showed that delirium was associated with a 2-fold increase in death, 2.4-fold in institutionalization and 12.5-fold in new dementia. Despite the traditional view that delirium was a transient and reversible condition, recent evidence has shown that persistence of delirium occurs in many patients, and is associated with poor long-term outcomes.

DOI: 10.1201/9781003344476-9

Table 8.1   Confusion Assessment Method (Positive if Criteria 1, 2, 3 or 1, 2, 4 are Present).

1. Acute change in mental status from baseline and fluctuation in behavior during the day, and
2. Attention impaired, easily distractible, difficulty keeping track of what is being said, and
3. Disorganized/incoherent thinking or illogical conversation, or
4. Altered mental status (hyperalert, lethargic, difficult to arouse).

Unfortunately, despite this, delirium is often underrecognized by physicians. Several factors could explain this reality. First, hyperactive delirium, which is the most noticeable subtype, represents only 25% of the cases. Hypoactively delirious patients attract less attention of the medical team, despite their poorer prognosis. Second, physicians often have a snapshot of their patient once per day; however, by definition, delirium is a fluctuating syndrome. Third, diagnosing delirium could be time-consuming as it often involves detailed interviews with collateral historians as well as chart reviews to identify the acute change and fluctuation. Finally, in some cases, delirium could be difficult to distinguish from other conditions, such as Lewy Body dementia, depression and mania. Therefore, clinicians should always have a high index of suspicion and be diligent in their assessments.

WHAT ARE THE CAUSES (PRECIPITATING FACTORS) OF DELIRIUM? HOW TO INVESTIGATE?

The causes of delirium are vast. Any acute medical illness or medication can precipitate delirium. Infections are the most commonly diagnosed. Any infection has the potential of being the underlying cause. The presence of asymptomatic bacteriuria, however, often leads to a misdiagnosis of UTI causing delirium. Recent studies show that antibiotic therapy in these patients does not change the course of delirium. Electrolyte imbalances, especially of sodium, calcium and glucose, could cause delirium. Cortisol excess or insufficiency could be manifested as hyperactive and hypoactive delirium, respectively. In patients with history of falls presenting with delirium, intracranial bleeding should be considered in the differential diagnosis. In patients with hypoactive delirium, particular attention should be paid to rule out hypoxia and CNS infections. In patients with cirrhosis, hepatic encephalopathy should be ruled out. Hypoxia or shock due to any cause could cause acute confusion due to brain hypoperfusion. In patients who develop delirium days after admission, alcohol or benzodiazepine withdrawal should be considered. Other precipitants include physical restraints, indwelling devices (Foley catheters, central venous catheters, etc.), immobility, urinary retention, fecal impaction and uncontrolled pain.

Many medications can precipitate delirium. Common candidates are benzodiazepines, opioids, anticholinergics, antiparkinsonians, antipsychotics, antidepressants (especially TCAs and MAOIs) and NSAIDs.

In order to summarize these precipitants, the following mnemonics provided by Wise, M.G. (1986) are helpful (Table 8.2).

Taking history of delirium (mostly taken with the collateral historian) should include a detailed timeline of the acute confusion as well as symptoms leading to or co-occurring with the onset of the acute confusion. A detailed review of systems could help diagnose the underlying causes of delirium. A thorough medication review is important not only for deciphering changes that can contribute to the acute confusion, but also for addressing polypharmacy which could potentially prolong and exacerbate delirium. Past medical history can also provide cues because acute exacerbation or decompensation of many chronic medical conditions could lead to delirium.

On physical examination, the general appearance can provide information such as hydration status, nutritional status, attention and sensorium. Special attention should be given to vital signs. For example, hypotension and tachycardia could indicate ischemia, sepsis or severe dehydration. Fever could indicate infection or pulmonary embolism. Desaturation could indicate cardiac and pulmonary causes. A thorough physical examination should be focused on the potential underlying acute medical conditions. A well-documented mental status examination could help clinicians track the evolution of delirium. If possible, a mini-mental status examination could be done to quantify the cognitive changes during delirium, which could serve the purpose of a point of comparison when delirium improves in the future.

Table 8.2   Causes of Delirium—I WATCH DEATH

I – infectious: pneumonia, UTI, CNS infections, abscesses, osteomyelitis, endocarditis, etc.
W – withdrawal: from benzodiazepines, alcohol
A – Acute metabolic changes: acidosis/alkalosis, hypo/hyperNa, hypo/hyper Ca, acute kidney and liver failure
T – Trauma: intracranial bleeding, brain injury
C – CNS pathology: intracranial tumor, post-ictal state
H – Hypoxia: anemia, pulmonary embolism, CHF, myocardial infarctions
D – Deficiencies: vitamin B1, B12
E – Endocrine: hypo/hypercortisol, hypoglycemia
A – Acute vascular: hypertensive emergency, stroke
T – Toxins and drugs: benzodiazepines, opioids, anticholinergics
H – Heavy metals

Table 8.3   Investigations for Delirium

Essential	CBC, SMA-10, Glucose; INR, PTT; TSH; Vitamin B12, LFTs, ECG
May be required	Blood cultures x 2, urinalysis and culture, urine toxicology lactate, venous blood gas, serial troponins, EtOH level
	Post-void residual, tot and conj bilirubin, albumin, amylase CT-head, chest X-ray

WHAT INITIAL INVESTIGATIONS SHOULD BE REQUESTED FOR DELIRIUM?

Investigations should include basic laboratory tests, including complete blood count, bio-chemistry profile (including urea, creatinine, calcium and magnesium), glucose, coagulation profile, TSH, Vitamin B12 and liver function tests. An EKG could be ordered, not only to identify potential cardiac causes if indicated by history, but also to document baseline QTc, as many medications (including antipsychotics and antibiotics) have potential to cause QTc prolongation.

Other investigations may be required depending on the history and examination. If the patient is febrile, septic work-up (blood cultures, urine analysis and culture, CxR, etc.) should be ordered before starting antibiotics. If there is suspicion of meningitis or encephalitis, a lumbar puncture should be done. Urine or serum toxicology should be ordered if there is suspicion of medication, alcohol and drug toxicity. For patients with suspicion of hypoxemia, hypercapnia or shock, arterial blood gas and lactate could be ordered. If cardiac ischemia is suspected, serial troponins should be ordered. For patients with history of falls, CT-head should be considered. For patients with suspicion of urinary retention, a post-void residual should be obtained.

Table 8.3 summarizes initial work-up for patients with delirium.

HOW TO MANAGE DELIRIUM

Most patients with delirium require hospitalization, not only for investigation and medical therapy purposes but also for behavioral management, to manage acute functional deficits, to manage complications and for rehabilitation. For the management of neuropsychiatric symptoms of delirium, a non-pharmacological approach is favored. For aggressive patients, distraction and de-escalation strategies should be adopted. For patients with day-night reversal, it is important to promote good sleep hygiene by ensuring adequate light during the day and darkness at night. For all patients with delirium, physical restraints should be avoided, as they not only prolong delirium and cause immobilization syndrome, but also increase risk of strangulation. Ensuring proper hydration and nutrition could prevent delirium from worsening. It is also important to monitor and prevent the development of pressure ulcers. It is important to compensate for patients' senso-rial deficits, by encouraging uses of glasses and hearing aids. Orientation cues, such as photos of family members and a calendar, should be used if possible. Early mobilization could be helpful to prevent deconditioning and immobilization syndrome. Occupational therapy assessments are helpful for discharge planning purposes when delirium improves.

WHEN AND HOW TO USE MEDICATIONS FOR BEHAVIORAL DISTURBANCES?

Non-pharmacological approaches should almost always be attempted first to curb agitation. One of the only circumstances where pharmacological approaches should be used first is if the patient's agitation poses a risk of self-harm or a threat to others.

Antipsychotics such as haloperidol, quetiapine, risperidone, olanzapine and ziprasidone are first-line pharmacological treatments for agitation in delirium. Haloperidol is the most efficient against aggression; however, high doses of haloperidol (> 4.5 mg per day) are associated with an increase in extrapyramidal side effects. Based on limited evidence, it is recommended that low-dose haloperidol (0.5 mg to 1.0 mg PO or IM) should be used for the control of agitation and psychotic symptoms, up to a maximum of 3 mg per day. Its onset is 30 to 60 minutes after parenteral administration, longer if PO. Please note that IV haloperidol should be avoided due to QTc prolongation. Quetiapine is the most sedating antipsychotic, and causes fewer extrapyramidal signs and symptoms. Its main limitation is that it can only be given per os. Its starting dose is 12.5 mg to 25 mg with a maximum dose of 50 mg per day.

It is worth mentioning that a recent meta-analysis of randomized trials showed that antipsychotics do not alter the duration or severity of delirium, and do not reduce ICU admissions or mortality. Therefore, clinicians should be cautious when prescribing antipsychotics, by weighing apparent benefits with the risks of antipsychotic side effects and complications (i.e. falls, stroke, increased mortality).

Benzodiazepines are second-line agents, due to respiratory depression, paradoxical excitation, fall risk and oversedation. However, benzodiazepines such as lorazepam could be used first-line in specific situations where antipsychotic use should be avoided. These include patients with seizures, in those in alcohol or benzodiazepine withdrawal, and in those with a history of neuroleptic malignant syndrome or Lewy Body dementia (who are very sensitive to antipsychotics).

Diphenhydramine, dimenhydrinate and other medications with significant anticholinergic effects should be avoided, as they may exacerbate and prolong delirium.

All medications for agitation should be discontinued as soon as possible and should usually not be continued beyond the hospitalization for delirium. In the minority of patients who require antipsychotics on discharge, caution needs to be exerted so that the prescription has a finite duration and should be reassessed frequently with appropriate follow-up.

Table 8.4 summarizes these choices of initial pharmacological regimen.

Table 8.4 Pharmacological Management of Hyperactive Delirium—Standard Order

- Risperidone 0.25–0.5 mg PO bid PRN
- Haloperidol 0.5–1 mg PO/IM q1h PRN for severe agitation. Reassess after 3 doses.

If patient has history of Parkinson's disease or Lewy Body dementia:

- Quetiapine 12.5 mg PO bid PRN agitation. Lorazepam 0.5–1 mg IM q1h PRN for severe agitation. Reassess after 3 doses.

CONCLUSION

As the population ages, clinicians will encounter delirium more frequently as more patients have dementia and have multiple comorbidities. Prompt and efficient management of delirium is essential to preserve a patient's cognition and function, and of course, to decrease mortality.

Among non-delirious hospitalized patients who are at risk, prevention techniques such as the HELP (Hospital Elder Life Program) could reduce the incidence of delirium. One area of research also focuses on finding a delirium risk-prediction score. Hospital resources could then be used to provide prevention techniques targeting those patients who are at high risk of developing delirium, with the potential to decrease its sometimes-catastrophic consequences.

THE CLINICAL VIGNETTE REVISITED

Pre-operatively, this patient was already at high risk for delirium, due to her age, dementia, functional impairment and multiple comorbidities. Initial investigations mentioned earlier should be performed. The potential causes and management plan are summarized in the Table 8.5.

Table 8.5   Delirium: Causes and Management

Possible Causes of Patient's Delirium	Management Plan
Opioids (morphine)	Change to hydromorphone and consider regular hydromorphone for 6–12 hours as delirious patients might not ask for pain medications
CHF exacerbation due to overhydration	Chest X-ray; increase furosemide if needed
Anemia due to blood loss	Follow Hb, transfuse if needed
Right lower extremity DVT	Venous duplex
Worsening of Parkinson's disease due to haloperidol and refusal to take carbidopa/levodopa	Change carbidopa/levodopa to equivalent dose per rectum
	Use quetiapine PO or lorazepam IM for agitation if non-pharmacological approaches fail
Uncontrolled pain	Monitor and manage pain
Constipation	Mobilization, laxatives, DRE to R/O impaction
Urinary retention	PVR, in/out if needed
Stroke despite warfarin bridging	Thorough neurological examination, CT/CTA head if high suspicion
Aspiration pneumonia due to Parkinsonism	Chest X-ray

The non-pharmacological management of this patient includes removal of restraints, early mobilization, nutrition and speech-language pathology consult and promotion of night-time sleep.

FURTHER READING

1. Wise, M. G. Delirium. In R. E. Hales & S. C. Yudofsky (Eds.), American Psychiatric Press Textbook of Neuropsychiatry (pp. 89–103). Washington, DC: American Psychiatric Press Inc, 1986.
2. Marcantonio, E. R. Delirium in Hospitalized Older Adults. N Engl J Med 2017; 377:1456–1466. doi: 10.1056/NEJMcp1605501
3. Chew, M. L. Anticholinergic Activity of 107 Medications Commonly Used by Older Adults. J Amer Geri Soc 2008; 56,7:1333–1341. doi: 10.1111/j.1532-5415.2008.01737

9 Why Does My Patient Have Gait and Balance Disorders?

Olivier Beauchet, MD, PhD

CONTENTS

PATIENT SCENARIO

An 87-year-old woman walks into your office unaided, without any noticeable gait abnormality. She reports that she has balance difficulties with fear of falling but denied any fall. The patient's medication list includes amlodipine 5 mg QD, metformin 500 mg BI, aspirin 80 md QD, atorvastatin 10 mg, donepezil 5 mg QD and temazepam as needed for sleep. Her body mass index is 18 kg/m². The daughter hands you an X-ray report indicating that the patient has severe osteoporosis, moderate spinal (cervical and lumbar) osteoarthritis associated with dorsal kyphosis.

Since your patient has a high risk of falls, you would like to determine the reason for balance complaints to decide whether she needs specific interventions.

WHY IS THIS QUESTION IMPORTANT?

Gait—the medical term used to describe human locomotion—and balance disorders are prevalent in older individuals. It is difficult to ascertain prevalence as no accepted definition exists. However, it is estimated that at least 35 percent of individuals 65 and older report difficulty walking three city blocks or climbing one flight of stairs, and approximately 20 percent require the use of a mobility aid to ambulate. The prevalence of gait and balance disorders can reach 80 percent in the oldest-old (i.e., ≥ 85 years) individuals who live in residence.

Gait and balance characteristics change over the individual's lifetime with a decline of performance. Gait and balance disorders are usually defined as a decrease of performance (for instance, a slow gait speed) causing instability and falls. Gait and balance disorders are the most common cause of falls in individuals 65 and older. They are associated with an increased morbidity and mortality, disability, loss of independence, institutionalization and limited quality of life. Early identification and appropriate interventions may prevent gait and balance disorders and their related adverse consequences.

WHICH ARE THE CAUSES OF GAIT AND BALANCE DISORDERS?

Gait and balance disorders are usually multifactorial in origin and require a comprehensive assessment to determine contributing factors and targeted interventions. Most changes in gait and balance that occur in older individuals are related to physiological aging of the sensorimotor system combined with adverse consequences of chronic and acute medical conditions. The causes of gait and balance disorders fall under three categories of factors:

- The predisposing factors which are individually related and result from adverse consequences of physiological aging of the sensorimotor system combined with chronic medical conditions leading to chronic gait and balance instability.

- The precipitating factors which may be separated in two subtypes: those related to individual acute medical conditions and those related to physical activity inducing gait and balance instability.

- The environment combined with the physical activity while falling.

There is a complex synergic interaction between factors provoking gait and balance instability, explaining why gait and balance instability may fluctuate with time.

DOI: 10.1201/9781003344476-10

The main chronic medical conditions which affect gait and balance stability are:

- Visual impairment with abnormal distance vision including low visual acuity and low contrast sensitivity.
- Lower limb proprioception impairment.
- Lower limb poor muscle mass and strength.
- Lower limb joint deformity, podiatric abnormalities and back deformity (e.g., kyphosis, scoliosis) related to osteoarthritis and osteoporosis.
- Obesity.
- Myelopathy.
- Normal-pressure hydrocephalus.
- Parkinson's disease.
- Cerebellar dysfunction or degeneration.
- Vascular brain disease.
- Vestibular disorders.
- Cognitive impairment: from mild cognitive impairment to severe dementia.
- Depression.
- Fear of falling.

Any acute medical condition may increase gait and balance instability within hours and cause a motor deconditioning (i.e., loss of body postural reflexes and inability to stand up and/or walk without assistance) in older individuals with predisposing factors to gait and balance disorders.

WHO SHOULD BE SCREENED FOR GAIT AND BALANCE DISORDERS?

- Adults aged 65 and over should be asked about or examined for gait and balance disorders at least once per year.
- Adults aged 65 and over who report a fall or have an acute medical condition should be asked about difficulties with gait and balance, and should be examined for gait and balance disorders.

WHAT IS THE CLINICAL ASSESSMENT?

Clinical assessment should be separated into two main parts: global and analytic clinical assessment.
The global assessment detecting gait and balance difficulties begins with watching individuals as they rise from a chair or as they walk into the examination room. The use of a walking aide and its nature (i.e., cane, walker, personal assistance and supervision) should be noticed and the individual should be asked about his/her subjective perception of gait and balance difficulties using a single question: "Do you have any difficulty walking?" with a graduated answer (i.e., never, almost never, sometimes, often, and very often).

This visual observation should be completed with three standardized motor tests providing an objective measure of gait and balance performance: The Timed Up & Go (TUG) test, the Five-Times-Sit-to-Stand test and the gait speed (distance divided by ambulation time) when walking a distance of 4 meters at a steady-state pace. The TUG measures in seconds the time it takes an individual to rise from a chair, walk a distance of 3 meters, turn, walk back to the chair and sit down. This test has been used extensively in geriatric medicine to examine balance, gait speed, and functional ability that would be required for the performance of basic activities of daily living in older people. A score ≥ 20 seconds should be considered as an abnormal performance. The Five-Times-Sit-to-Stand test (FTSS) measures in seconds the time it takes an individual to stand up from a chair five times as quickly as possible. This clinical test explores postural control and lower limb muscular strength. A score ≥ 15 seconds should be considered as an abnormal performance. Walking speed is a simple, objective, performance-based measure of lower limb neuromuscular function which not only allows detection of subtle impairments and preclinical diseases but also is a sensitive marker of functional capacity in older adults. A gait speed at usual pace under 1 m/s should also be considered as abnormal.

The analytic clinical assessment includes collection of:

- Demographic (i.e., age in years and sex) and anthropometric items (height in meters [m], weight in kilograms [kg], body mass index [BMI] in kg/m^2), should be systematically assessed because each may influence gait and balance stability. In addition, the place of living should be considered as a binary variable (home versus institution), and an institutionalized individual should be considered to have a higher risk of gait and balance disorders.

- Given that the burden of disease can influence gait and balance performance, it is important to assess this information as well. Different scales have been developed to score morbidity burden, but they remain difficult to use in clinical routine among older adults, especially because of possible recall bias in individuals with cognitive disorders, and lack of feasibility in daily practice. Medication data, including the number of drugs taken daily, provides a global measure of morbidity status, and has been associated with physician-rated disease severity as well as with individual-rated health status. Hence, recording the use of drugs in the clinical assessment is required. Polypharmacy is defined as use of more than four different medications per day. The use of psychoactive drugs (i.e., benzodiazepines, antidepressants, neuroleptics) needs to be specially recorded.

- Information about falls, with a fall being defined as an event resulting in a person coming to rest unintentionally on the ground or at another lower level, not as the result of a major intrinsic event or an overwhelming hazard, in the previous 12 months period before the assessment, should be recorded. Information on recurrence (i.e., > 2 falls) and severity (defined as fractures, cranial trauma, large and/or deep skin lesion, post-fall syndrome (including an association of fear of falling [FOF], postural instability with absence of postural reflexes), inability to get up alone from ground, time on the ground > 1 hour, and hospitalization) are proposed for the data collection.

- FOF using the single question: "Are you afraid of falling?" with a graded answer (i.e., never, almost never, sometimes, often, and very often) should be asked to the patient as FOF is associated with a greater gait and/or balance instability.

- Collecting information on disorders or diseases that directly influence gait performance is also recommended. First, information on neurological disease (limited to the existence or non-existence of dementia) and other diseases (coded as yes or no) should be collected. Information on memory complaints, MCI, nature of dementia (i.e., Alzheimer's disease [AD], non-AD neurodegenerative, non-AD vascular, mixed), Parkinson's disease, idiopathic normal pressure hydrocephalus, cerebellar disease, stroke, myelopathy and peripheral neuropathy should be recorded. A quantification of global cognitive functioning is also recommended, using for example the Mini Mental State Examination (/30) and the Montreal Cognitive Assessment (MoCA) if MMSE score is above 19/30.

- In addition, among the neuropsychiatric disorders, it is important to collect information about depression symptoms because they can lead to gait instability and falls. The 4-item geriatric depression scale should be used as a screening test. A measure of anxiety is also proposed using the 5-item Geriatric Anxiety Inventory.

- Information on major orthopedic diagnoses (e.g., osteoarthritis) involving the lumbar vertebrae, pelvis or lower extremities, coded yes versus no, as well as the use of a walking aid, should also be recorded.

- Information on sensory and motor subsystems such as muscle strength, lower-limb proprioception and vision are required because the age-related impairment in the performance of these subsystems may affect gait performance. First, the maximum isometric voluntary contraction (MVC) of hand grip strength must be measured with a hydraulic dynamometer. The test should be performed three times with the dominant hand. The mean value of MVC over the three trials should be used as the outcome measure. Second, distance binocular vision should be measured at a fixed distance with a standard scale. Vision needs to be assessed with corrective lenses if used regularly. Third, lower-limb proprioception should be evaluated with a graduated tuning fork placed on the tibial tuberosity measuring vibration threshold.

IS THERE A NEED FOR COMPLEMENTARY INVESTIGATIONS?

The role of laboratory testing and diagnostic evaluation for gait and balance disorders has not been well studied.

There is no systematic investigation recommended to perform. The following complementary investigations are recommended:

- Bone radiography in the event of acute pain, joint deformation and/or functional disability.

- Standard 12-lead ECG in case of dizziness.

- Blood glucose level in patients with diabetes.

- Serum 25OHD concentration if there is no vitamin D supplementation.

Cerebral imaging in the absence of specific indication based upon the clinical examination may not be necessary.

WHAT ARE THE POSSIBLE INTERVENTIONS?

It is recommended to suggest to the patient with gait and balance disorders, irrespective of the place of living, an intervention combining several of the following domains:

- When possible, a revision of the medications to ascertain if the patient takes fall-related drugs (please see earlier) and/or the number of drugs is > 5.

- The correction or the treatment of predisposing or modifiable precipitating factors (including environmental risk factors of falls).

- The wearing of shoes with broad, low heels (2 to 3 cm), and firm, thin soles with a high upper.

- The regular practice of walking and/or any other physical activity (the duration of exercise for prevention of recurrent falls remains unclear).

- A dietary calcium intake ranging from 1 to 1.5 grams per day.

- The use of an adapted walking aid.

- The correction of a potential vitamin D deficiency by a daily dose of at least 800 IU.

It is recommended to prescribe physiotherapy, including:

- Working on static and dynamic postural balance.

- Increasing the strength and muscular power of the lower limbs.

- Other techniques, including stimulation of sensory afferents or learning to stand up from the ground, may also be proposed.

Such interventions may involve rehabilitation professionals, such as occupational therapists. A regular physical activity should be performed at low to moderate intensity exercise. It is recommended to perform rehabilitation exercises with a professional, as well as between therapy sessions and after each session, in order to extend rehabilitation benefits to the daily life.

SCENARIO RESOLUTION

Your patient requires a specific gait and balance assessment as she is an oldest-old (i.e., > 85 years) lady who reports balance difficulties.

Based on the information provided by the list of medications and the daughter, you can conclude that she has an objective gait and balance disorder caused by an accumulation of chronic medical conditions, which are:

- A polypharmacy: Six different medications are taken daily.

- A lower limb diabetic polyneuropathy causing proprioceptive impairment.

- An abnormal static posture due to spinal osteoarthritis and osteoporosis deformities.

- A poor muscle mass and strength because of a malnutrition status (body mass index score 18 kg/m²).

- A cognitive impairment due to a dementia because of the prescription of donepezil.

You can confirm your first analysis by performing a TUG test.
You can propose:

- To discontinue the temazepam.

- To continue anti-osteoporotic treatment and vitamin D supplementation.

- To adopt a regular practice of walking and/or any other physical activity.

You can prescribe physiotherapy including:

- Working on static and dynamic postural balance.

- Increasing the strength and muscular power of the lower limbs.

REFERENCES

1. Nutt JG. Classification of gait and balance disorders. Adv Neurol 2001;87:135–141.
2. Seidler RD, Bernard JA, Burutolu TB, Fling BW, Gordon MT, Gwin JT, Kwak Y, Lipps DB. Motor control and aging: links to age-related brain structural, functional, and biochemical effects. Neurosci Biobehav Rev 2010;34:721–733.
3. Beauchet O, Dubost V, Revel Delhom C, Berrut G, Belmin J, French Society of Geriatrics and Gerontology. How to manage recurrent falls in clinical practice: guidelines of the French Society of Geriatrics and Gerontology. J Nutr Health Aging 2011;15:79–84.
4. Panel on Prevention of Falls in Older Persons, American Geriatrics Society and British Geriatrics Society. Summary of the updated American Geriatrics Society/British Geriatrics Society clinical practice guideline for prevention of falls in older persons. J Am Geriatr Soc 2011;59:148–157.
5. Salzman B. Gait and balance disorders in older adults. Am Fam Physician 2010;82:61–68.

10 Could My Patient Be Malnourished?

José A. Morais, MD, FRCP(C)

CONTENTS

CLINICAL VIGNETTE

An 82-year-old widow has a 4.5 kg weight loss over the last 6 months following the death of her beloved husband. Her present BMI is 21 kg/m² and her triceps' skinfold thickness is in the 10th percentile for age. She is known to have diabetes and osteoarthritis of both knees for which she uses a walker for indoor mobility. She denies being depressed, but her family physician prescribed a tricyclic antidepressant medication soon after the death of her spouse. Since then, she complains of dry mouth with difficulty swallowing food and is constipated. Her other medications are metformin 850 mg BID and naproxen 250 mg BID. The pertinent blood tests available disclosed an albumin of 38 g/L, CRP 2 mg/L, A1C 6%, creatinine 98 umol/L.

Since involuntary weight loss in older adults should always be taken seriously, there is a need to ascertain the presence of malnutrition, determine its risk factors, and propose a plan for assessment and management.

WHY IS MALNUTRITION AN IMPORTANT CLINICAL PROBLEM?

Malnutrition is common in older people and in those who are frail and ill. In the healthy community-dwelling older person, its prevalence is about 2–5%, whereas in the frail, dependent elderly, it can reach 20–30%. In those living in nursing homes or in hospital, levels as high as 50–70% have been reported.

Malnutrition or more precisely, undernutrition, is a state of reduced food intake below recommended daily allowances that leads to loss of body mass (weight) and functional impairment. The functional deficiencies comprise physical performance such as grip strength and gait speed, immunocompetence and tissue repair capacity. As a consequence, malnourished older persons have higher risks of falls and fractures, delirium, depression, cognitive deficits, infections, hospitalizations with prolonged stay, decubitus ulcers and death.

Other terminologies are often used in conjunction with malnutrition. These are protein-energy malnutrition (PEM), anorexia, wasting, cachexia and sarcopenia. PEM refers to a global decrease in food intake with its health consequences and is equivalent to undernutrition/malnutrition; anorexia is a lack of appetite and wasting that is synonymous with loss of body mass. Wasting follows a lack of appetite without inflammation, and therefore, a preferential loss of adipose tissue over muscle mass is a predominant feature. Cachexia on the other hand is a catabolic condition often involving a high degree of inflammation from a disease such as cancer or congestive heart failure. Its prominent feature is suppression of appetite with proportionally more muscle loss than adipose tissue and with fatigue. Sarcopenia refers to a selective loss of muscle mass and strength associated with aging that has a large number of factors contributing to its development.

WHAT ARE THE RISK FACTORS FOR MALNUTRITION?

Older adults are predisposed to anorexia due to intrinsic as well as exogenous causes. At the intrinsic physiological level, one needs to consider the adjustment of energy balance that occurs with aging. Aging is associated with loss of lean body mass, especially muscle mass, a metabolically active tissue, and therefore its loss leads to a decrease in the basal metabolic rate (energy spent at rest to maintain bodily functions). Furthermore, since there is also a progressive decline

DOI: 10.1201/9781003344476-11

in physical activity, the total amount of energy ingested needs to be reduced, otherwise the elderly would gain considerable weight over time.

A theoretical model of anorexia of aging proposes a dysregulation of the appetite control center in the hypothalamus. This dysregulation is in part related to changes in brain neurotransmitters, such as NPY and dynorphin, the latter decreasing the pleasure associated with meals. It is also recognized that there is a higher circulating gastrointestinal peptide cholecystokinin (CCK) upon food ingestion, which is a potent central anorexigen. At the fundus of the stomach, there is reduced nitric oxide production with meals which contributes to a lesser relaxation of the stomach, therefore contributing to a precocious sensation of fullness. Older persons have also alterations in their taste perception from changes in the odor and taste capacities. Thirst perception is equally affected with age, which predisposes to dehydration.

Although these factors are present with aging, they are not by themselves responsible for the decrease in food intake of older persons. Multiple other causes contribute as well. These include:

- Uncontrolled medical conditions that predispose to anorexia through the effect of inflammatory mediators (TNF-α and cytokines), pain, distress, lethargy, delirium, etc.

- Social-economic factors including isolation, poverty and institutionalization.

- Masticatory and swallowing difficulties (e.g., poor-fitting dentures and dysphagia).

- Decrease in functional capacity caused by mobility problems, poor endurance and multiple co-morbidities, which affect the capability to purchase food and prepare meals.

- Mental and cognitive disorders (e.g., depression and dementia).

- Peculiar habits such as aversion to certain foods and alcoholism.

- Medications, in particular: digoxin, SSRIs, NSAIDs, metformin, antibiotics and psychoactive drugs.

It is often difficult to distinguish a single factor as responsible in the vast majority of the cases, as more often several factors interact. The aforementioned pathological/physiological/

Factors Contributing to Malnutrition

MEALS ON WHEELS acronym helps to remember the common risk factors and causes of undernutrition in older adults

Medications (polypharmacy, herbal preparations)

Emotional causes (dysphoria, depression, psychosis)

Appetite disorders (anorexia tardive, abnormal eating attitudes)

Late-life paranoia (social isolation)

Swallowing disorders

Oral factors (tooth loss, periodontal infections, gingivitis, poorly fitting dentures)

No money (poverty)

Wandering (dementia)

Hyperactivity/hypermetabolism (tremors, movement disorders, thyrotoxicosis)

Enteral problems (chronic diarrhea, malabsorption syndromes)

Eating problems (altered food preferences, decreased taste and flavor perception)

Low-nutrient diets (low-salt, low-cholesterol, antidiabetic, fad diets)

Shopping and food-preparation problems (impaired mobility, unsafe environment, inadequate transportation)

Figure 10.1 Factors contributing to malnutrition.

Diagnostic evaluation of PEM

Figure 10.2   Diagnostic evaluation of PEM.

environmental changes can be summarized in a mnemonic, MEALS-ON-WHEELS (Figure 10.1), proposed by Morley and Silver.

Figure 10.2 is an algorithm to assist in evaluating causes of PEM. In general it is helpful to determine if the patient is eating well despite losing weight. If it is the case, the patient is either suffering from malabsorption (a relatively easy diagnosis to make because of GI symptoms) or having increased needs for energy in conditions such as hyperthyroidism, diabetes, cancer, chronic infections or advanced COPD or CHF.

On the other hand, if the patient is not eating well, then a first step is to verify accessibility to food (poverty, mobility issues and meal preparation). If these are not factors, then consider masticatory and swallowing difficulties. If these are not an issue, it is likely that we are facing a case of anorexia from medications, depression, dementia or multi-morbidity.

HOW IS THE DIAGNOSIS OF MALNUTRITION MADE?

On history taking, one reliable but often-ignored parameter of malnutrition is weight loss. A history of 5–10% weight loss over 6 months (> 3 kg) or 2–3% in 1–2 months is a significant amount that threatens the general health. Changes in food habits for any reason (difficulty swallowing, poverty) and GI symptoms (nausea, abdominal cramps and diarrhea) are other important items of information. Any new drugs being prescribed? Typically, one eats three meals a day and eating less frequently puts one at risk. Food assessment is done by a registered dietician through different dietary intake assessment methods, each with its own limitations.

On physical examination, in addition to a low weight for height or a low body mass index (BMI; < 22 kg/m²)", signs of ascites/edema or decreased skin turgor are suggestive of malnutrition. Loss of typical roundness of the face, shoulder and buttocks is often encountered as well as muscle loss at the temporal areas, biceps, thigh and calf. Specific vitamin deficiencies leading to angular stomatitis of the mouth and glossitis are late signs. All of these signs become more difficult to assess in the elderly due to lack of specificity and sensitivity. For example, a decrease in skin elasticity with aging and other causes such as venous stasis contribute to peripheral edema. Typically, it is the dietitian who carries out the relevant anthropometric measurements (body and limb circumferences and skinfold thickness). Values below the 15th percentile for sex and age are very suggestive of malnutrition. Physical performance tests such as handgrip strength using a dynamometer may corroborate the diagnosis.

At the laboratory level, the serum albumin level is the most useful parameter. This protein is produced by the hepatocytes when adequate amino acids and energy are available. The total body albumin pool is about 300 g with 1/3 lying in the interstitial space and its half-life is 20 days. The albumin value doesn't need to be at 35 g/L to be considered low. Any value below 40 g/L puts the patient at risk, although typically values < 38 g/L are used as cut-off for malnutrition. If coupled with a low cholesterol value of < 4 mmol/L, the likelihood of malnutrition is greatly augmented. Despite adequate dietary intake of both energy and protein, albumin and pre-albumin are decreased in 1) the presence of inflammation (cancer, immunological disorders, trauma and infections), 2) patients who have received large amounts of intravenous fluids (dilutional), 3) protein-losing enteropathies (losses through the gut) or 4) nephropathies (losses through the kidney). On the other hand, albumin in the interstitial space can be recruited to the circulation during periods of poor intake without inflammation, which is the case in simple anorexia (wasting).

Measurement of pre-albumin values is rarely required, since it is under the same regulatory control as albumin. It may however be useful in monitoring the response to a nutritional intervention due to its half-life of 2 days. Cut-off values for undernutrition are below 180 mg/L.

Low hemoglobin and lymphocyte counts are less specific and are a late manifestation of malnutrition. In the absence of any other cause, a lymphocyte count below 800 cells/mL is however a sign of severe malnutrition. Anergy testing is rarely performed but would likely demonstrate a reduced immune response.

USEFUL TOOLS FOR THE DIAGNOSIS OF MALNUTRITION

There is no single parameter with the requisite sensitivity and specificity; thus, it is recommended that a combination of 3 or 4 indices from different domains (history, physical examination and investigation) be assessed. In this regard, several screening and diagnostic tools are available. Among these, two have received significant attention, the Mini Nutritional Assessment (MNA) and the Subjective Global Assessment (SGA).

The MNA has been validated in many settings, including long-term care and acute care hospital sites and can be used to screen and diagnose early undernutrition in frail persons. It comprises items that are related to cognition, mental and physical function as well as dietary intake and anthropometric measurements. The total possible score is 30—values below 17 are diagnostic of malnutrition, between 17–24 suggest a risk of malnutrition and above 24 signify good nutritional status. A shorter version based on the first 14 points of the MNA exists that is almost as reliable as the full version for screening and has the merit of precluding a full assessment if values are 12 or higher. If score of the shorter version is < 11, one should perform the full MNA. The MNA formula can be downloaded at no cost: http://www.mna-elderly.com/mna_forms.html.

The SGA is a clinical assessment of nutrition status based on history and physical examination. In taking a history, one reviews changes in dietary intake, weight loss, GI symptoms and functional capacity and on physical examination, one should look for signs of undernutrition, including ascites and edema. It requires only minimal training. The rater then classifies patients subjectively as well-nourished, mildly/moderately malnourished or severely malnourished. This tool has been validated with respect to clinical outcomes and has a good inter-observer agreement. The form can be downloaded at no cost: http://nutritioncareincanada.ca/.

WHAT ARE THE INTERVENTIONS TO REVERSE MALNUTRITION?

Before proposing an intervention, it is necessary to determine the factors contributing to undernutrition in the specific case instance (review the mnemonic MEALS-ON-WHEELS). Intervention can be as broad as helping with meal preparation, providing spoon feeding or diagnosing an underlying medical condition.

The first step in the management of undernutrition consists in identifying and treating the underlying causative factors. If the nutrition status does not show improvement in 1 week with this first-line approach, than nutritional support may be necessary. If not done previously, it is recommended at this stage to seek the advice of a dietitian. Figure 10.3 is an algorithm with an approach to treatment of malnutrition.

The dietician will assess in detail the patient's food intake and preferences and will propose a meal plan with more frequent meals and snacks enriched with food additives to enhance energy intake to 30–40 kcal/kg/d and protein to 1.2–1.5 g/kg/d. If this doesn't suffice, an oral formula supplement can be offered together with food additives. It is best to provide such added formula feedings in the evening to avoid interference with meals resulting in meal replacement without higher total energy intakes. A high density formula supplement of 1.5–2 calories/mL can deliver up to 400 calories with as much as 15 g of protein per container.

Whenever possible, combining some degree of physical activity such as frequent short walks with the dietary intervention can ameliorate appetite and food intake. The use of oral orexigenic

Figure 10.3 Management and treatment of PEM.

medications is controversial in older adults, including the new synthetic tetrahydrocannabinol molecule, dronabinol. However, in case of depression, one should consider mirtazapine, a tetra-cyclic antidepressant with appetite stimulating properties. Hormones are useful only in those in whom a deficiency state has been diagnosed.

In cases in which malnutrition progresses rapidly, assessment in an acute care setting may be considered to provide access to the different specialists, investigational platforms and interdisciplinary teams. In certain cases, enteral feeding may be indicated and can be initiated.

RESOLUTION OF THE CLINICAL VIGNETTE

The higher the number of indices of malnutrition, the greater the certainty of its presence. In the case of the person described at the outset of this chapter, the weight loss of more than 3 kg in 6 months, a BMI of less than 22 kg/m² and the low triceps skinfold percentile are very suggestive.

The risk factors comprise isolation (death of husband), recent bereavement, side effects from the medication (dry mouth, constipation), swallowing difficulties, chronic pains from arthritis and reduced mobility to purchase food. Consideration should include metformin due to its propensity to suppress appetite and naproxen which can lead to peptic ulcer disease (nausea).

Serum albumin is often used as one of the criteria to diagnose malnutrition. In the present case, a value of 38 g/L can be misleading since there is mild dehydration (Cr 98 umol/L), that may be responsible for a factitious elevation. Since CRP is in the normal range, it rules out inflammation. The A1C level is also too low for this frail patient, suggesting overly 'tight' control of capillary glucose putting the patient at risk of hypoglycemia.

The amount of weight loss indicates referral to a dietitian, but at this stage, one can emphasize the avoidance of food restriction or a severe diabetic diet, which is often the case in diabetic patients. The dietitian is likely to suggest high density food additives with regular meals and snacks as a first approach. If no change in weight is observed at follow-up in 2 weeks' time, an oral formula supplement should be provided for evening consumption, to avoid interference with regular meals, thus resulting in little gain in total daily calorie intake.

A medication review is mandatory. Metformin should be reduced to 250 mg po BID and naproxen discontinued. For pain management, one can offer acetaminophen. The tricyclic anti-depressant should be stopped and clinical review after 2 weeks can ascertain if symptoms of dry mouth, swallowing difficulties and constipation have disappeared. If not, one would need to consider a GI assessment.

Finally, a functional evaluation should be undertaken and community support offered to this patient to compensate and support her life situation. Above all, we should help overcome her isolation and assess her meal preparation and food purchasing capacities.

REFERENCES

1. Kucukerdonmez O, Navruz Varli S, Koksal E. Comparison of Nutritional Status in the Elderly According to Living Situations. J Nutr Health Aging. 2017;21(1):25–30.
2. Landi F, Calvani R, Tosato M, et al. Anorexia of Aging: Risk Factors, Consequences, and Potential Treatments. Nutrients 2016;8:69. doi:10.3390/nu8020069
3. Stajkovic S, Aitken EM, Holroyd-Leduc J. Unintentional Weight Loss in Older Adults. CMAJ. 2011 Mar 8;183(4):443–449. doi: 10.1503/cmaj.101471
4. Pirlich M, Lochs H. Nutrition in the Elderly. Best Practice & Res Clin Gastroenterol. 2001;15:869–884.
5. Gaddey HL, Holder K. Unintentional Weight Loss in Older Adults. Am Fam Physician. 2014;89:718–722.
6. Morley EJ, Siver AJ. Ann Intern Med. 1995;123:850–859

11 Dental Care in Older Persons

Michael Wiseman, DDS

CONTENTS

THE MOUTH AND BODY CONNECTION

Mrs. Jones is an 87-year-old woman whose daughter requests a full mouth exam from her dentist. Mrs. Jones is taking medications for osteoporosis, dementia, and has a mechanical mitral valve.

Her oral condition includes a partial upper denture that is a little "loose". She has two loose teeth, plaque and food present in her mouth. Her daughter reports that she uses food thickeners and has a little problem with swallowing. She also complains of a missing filling.

HOW IS THE MOUTH IMPORTANT FOR THE WELL-BEING OF MRS. JONES?

Three prominent chronic infections of the elderly are urinary tract infections, intra-abdominal infections, and periodontal disease. Periodontal disease has been suggested to have a link with such medical conditions as diabetes, Alzheimer's disease, osteoporosis, and hypertension. It has been estimated that the incidence of periodontal disease in individuals aged 65 or above is 60% [1].

It has also been demonstrated that oral pathogens and inflammatory mediators do not remain in the ulcerated and inflamed gingival pocket and can travel beyond the *in situ* location to both the central nervous system and systemic circulation [2].

ASSOCIATION OF PERIODONTAL DISEASE AND SYSTEMIC HEALTH: WHAT IS THE EVIDENCE?

1. Diabetes

Diabetes is the most common endocrine problem in older adults. There seems to be a bidirectional relationship between diabetes and periodontal disease. Studies have shown that the typical older person with diabetes has decreased wound healing, taste alterations, and increased oral infections [3]. Diabetes has been shown to increase the effects of periodontal disease. However, studies have demonstrated that treating the periodontitis has led to improved glycemic control [4].

2. Alzheimer's Disease

Alzheimer's disease has been defined as a progressive neurodegenerative disease and is the most common form of dementia. Characteristically, pathological deposition of synaptic β amyloid plaques and intracellular phosphorylated tau protein creating tangles are present. It has been postulated that pro-inflammatory cytokines and lipopolysaccharides from periodontal pathogens travel from the gingival sulcus and cross the blood-brain barrier activating glial cells creating an inflammatory response. Lipopolysaccharides from periodontal pathogens such as *P. gingivalis* and *T. denticola* were detected in post-mortem Alzheimer's disease patients [5].

It is important to note that many of the medications used to treat the anxiety and other neuro-psychological manifestations of patients with dementia have xerostomic side effects making the mouth dryer. Oral hygiene must be enhanced. Using a power brush is suggested.

3. Atherosclerosis

Studies have shown that patients with periodontal disease have a 2.22 times higher risk of developing coronary heart disease independent of confounding factors [6]. Oral bacteria DNA

DOI: 10.1201/9781003344476-12

has been identified in atheromatous plaques suggesting migration from the periodontitis affected oral cavity [7].

WHAT OTHER CONCERNS SHOULD THE DENTIST AND PHYSICIAN BE AWARE OF?

Mrs. Jones' intraoral exam reveals that teeth numbered 31 and 41 (lower central incisors) are mobile and should be extracted. She is taking warfarin (Coumadin) for her mechanical heart valve and alendronate (Fosamax). The possible complications associated with her systemic conditions and tooth extractions are bleeding, bacterial endocarditis, and medication-related osteonecrosis of the jaw.

The dentist asks for an INR and the results are 3.2. The target INR for a patient with a mechanical heart valve is 2.5–3.5 [8]. The dentist wisely decides not to alter or stop the warfarin therapy as there exists a greater potential for a thromboembolic event such as a cerebral vascular accident versus a dental bleed [9]. The dentist used localized hemostatic agents (sutures and Surgicel cellulose) and the patient reported no bleeding.

All patients with replacement heart valves, regardless of their composition, must receive antibiotic premedication prior to extractions, scaling, and root planing, or any dental act which may cause bleeding. The antibiotic of choice follows subacute bacterial endocarditis (SBE) protocols to prevent endocarditis. In a non-penicillin-allergic patient it is amoxicillin 2 grams, 1-hour preop. If the patient has a confirmed penicillin allergy, then another antibiotic of choice would be clindamycin 600 milligrams, 1-hour preop. For patients on concurrent antibiotics such as amoxicillin for another indication an alternative antibiotic from a different class such as clindamycin must be chosen [10]. Please see Table 11.1 for appropriate dosages.

In our scenario, Mrs. Jones was prescribed amoxicillin 500 mg tid for 7 days due to the fact that her lower teeth were moving and a purulent exudate was noted. Due to concurrent antibiotic use, she was prescribed clindamycin 600 mg, 1-hour preop.

The dentist consulted with the patient's rheumatologist who stated that the incidence of medication-induced osteonecrosis with alendronate was low. However, dental extractions should always be done with a complete medical review.

An important consideration is the autonomy of the patient in making decisions. In our scenario, all health providers must obtain consent prior to treatments. As the daughter was the decision maker, the health provider may be prudent to query if there exist any other individuals mandated to accept treatment options.

ORAL CARE AND QUALITY OF LIFE

Mrs. Jones was feeling a little depressed about her denture continuously falling when she was conversing with her friends at the nursing home. She decided to eat her meals in her room instead of the communal dining room.

By listening to the patient, a dentist can recognize her embarrassment and social isolation due to her unstable denture. The dentist repaired her upper denture and made her a lower partial denture after the teeth extractions. This vey simple intervention improved her self-worth and mastication, greatly improving her quality of life.

The patient's daughter questioned the dentist about deciding whether it was more prudent to replace the missing teeth with implants or a fixed bridge. The dentist, being morally correct, chose the treatment options based upon the patient's neurologic and physical status. The dentist chose a simple partial denture.

The success of dental treatment can be predicted by the dental compliance and capability index (Table 11.2) [11]. The scores yielded by the index correspond to the level of dementia. Scores ranging from 0–3 are representative of early dementia. At this level dental treatments should involve a

Table 11.1 Antibiotic Regimens for Prevention of Endocarditis Prior to Dental Procedures

Situation	Agent	Dose
Oral	amoxicillin	2 g
Oral (if allergic to penicillin)	azithromycin/clarithromycin clindamycin	500 mg/500 mg/600 mg
Unable to take oral amoxicillin	ampicillin/cefazolin	2 g/1 g IM or IV
Unable to take oral and allergic to amoxicillin	cefazolin	1 g IV

Table 11.2 Dental Compliance and Capability Index

Question	Score
Can the patient brush their teeth/dentures?	Yes = 0, Needs Assistance = 1, Completely Dependent = 2
Can the patient communicate their chief complaint?	Yes = 0, Partially = 1, No = 2
Can the patient follow simple instructions?	Yes = 0, Occasionally = 1, No = 2
Can the patient hold a radiograph?	Yes = 0, Sometimes = 1, No = 2
Is the patient violent?	Yes = 2, Sometimes = 1, No = 0

strong fluoride prevention program and function could be restored by simple implants or crowns. Scores from 4–7 are commonly found with moderate dementia. The use of fluoride rinses should be used with caution at this stage as many patients within this classification have swallowing problems. Treatments to restore the dentition should not be aggressive. In lieu of crowns, bridges, or implants, partial dentures would be the best choice. Scores from 8–10 correspond to patients with severe dementia. These patients should have only fluoride varnishes, and palliative or emergency treatments only.

The dentist suggested that the patient's daughter purchase a power brush to improve her hygiene, and as well to use a fluoridated toothpaste. The dentist recognized that the patient should limit mouth rinses due to her dysphagia and risk of aspiration. It was decided that a fluoride varnish would be prescribed to prevent caries and due to its adhesive nature, the risk of aspiration would be minimized.

The missing filling was replaced. In this case, as the patient was a little anxious, an anxiolytic was prescribed. Care must be taken in the selection of the appropriate agent as one must not choose an agent with a long half-life. In this case the dentist chose lorazepam (Ativan) 0.5 mg sublingual 1 hour prior to the procedure. An alternative agent could be oxazepam (Serax) 7.5–15 mg orally given 1 hour before the procedure. Diazepam (Valium) should never be prescribed to elderly patients as its half-life is basically equivalent to the age of the patient (i.e., a 90-year-old patient will have a diazepam half-life of 90 hours) [12].

Choosing the correct analgesic is important in the senior patient. The use of an opioid in the elderly is fraught with unwanted side effects. There is an increased rate of falls, possible delirium, and constipation when opioids are used to control pain. A better pain alternative would be to use a combination of an NSAID plus acetaminophen. Acetaminophen and NSAIDS have different pain relief pathways: using the combination provides a synergistic effect. This combination has been found to be superior to opioids and does not have the negative opioid effects [13]. NSAIDS are safe when used for a short period (< 2 weeks) in the absence of chronic renal failure.

DYSPHAGIA AND ASPIRATION PNEUMONIA

A severe consequence of dysphagia is aspiration pneumonia. There is evidence that with developing dementia, the rate of dysphagia increases leading to a high rate of death from aspiration pneumonia [14, 15]. Evaluation of the aspirant associated with aspiration pneumonia shows a high level of oral microorganisms associated with dental plaque [16]. The dentist is an ideal professional for identifying patients with high risk of aspiration if they note the accumulation of food within the oral cavity, decreased salivation, decreased tongue and soft palate motility, high levels of plaque, xerostomia, and decreased cognition. As mentioned within our scenario, Mrs. Jones is noted to have a lot of plaque and residue food debris within her mouth. A consult is made to the occupational therapist/speech pathologist to evaluate her swallowing.

REFERENCES

1. Genco RJ, Sanz M. Clinical and public implications of periodontal disease and systemic disease: An overview. Periodontology 2020, 83:7–13.
2. Winning L, Linden G. Periodontitis and systemic disease. BDJ Team 2015, 2, 15163.
3. Preshaw PM, Alba AL, Herrara D, Jepsen S, Konstantinidis A, Makrilakis K, Taylor R. Periodontitis and diabetes: A two-way relationship. Diabetologia 2011, 55:21–31.
4. Corbella S, Francetti L, Taschieri S, De Siena F, Fabbro MD. Effect of periodontal treatment on glycemic control of patients with diabetes: A systematic review and meta-analysis. J Diabetes Investig 2013, 4:502–509.

5. Poole S, Singhrao SK, Kesvalu L, Curtis MA, Crean S. Determining the presence of periodontopathic virulence factors in short-term postmortem Alzheimer disease brain tissue. J Alzheimer Dis 2013, 36:665–677.
6. Bahekar AA, Singh S, Saha S, Molnar J, Arora R. The prevalence and incidence of coronary heart disease is significantly increased in periodontitis: A meta-analysis. Am Heart J 2007, 154:830–837.
7. Figuerro E, Sanchez-Beltran M, Cuesta-Frechoso S, Tejerina JM, del Castro JA, Gutierrez JM et al. Detection of periodontal bacteria in atheromatous plaque by nested polymerase chain reaction. J Periodontol 2011, 82:1469–1477.
8. ACC/AHA 2006 Guidelines for the management of patients with valvular heart disease: Executive summary. Circulation 2006, 114:450–527.
9. Weltman NJ, Al-Attar Y, Cheung J, Duncan DPB, Azarpazhooh A, Abrahamyan L. Management of dental extractions in patients taking warfarin as anticoagulant treatment: A systematic review. J Can Dent Assoc 2015, 81:f20.
10. Wilson WR, Gewitz M, Lockhart PB, Bolger AF, DeSimone DC, Kazi DS, Couper DJ et al. American heart association young hearts endocarditis, and Kawasaki disease committee of the council on lifelong congenital heart disease and heart health in the young; council on cardiovascular and stroke nursing; and the council on quality of care and outcomes research. Circulation 143:e963–e978, 2021.
11. Niessen LC, Jones JA, Zocchi M et al. Dental care for the patient with Alzheimer's disease. J Am Dent Assoc 1985, 110:207–209.
12. Mandelli M, Tognolli G, Garattinis S. Clinical pharmacokinetics of diazepam. Clin Pharmacokinet 1978, 3:72–91.
13. Moore PA, Hersh EV. Combining ibuprofen and acetaminophen for acute postoperative pain management: translating clinical research to dental practice. J Am Dent Assoc. 2013; 144:898–908.
14. Bosch X, Formiga F, Cuerpo S, et al. Aspiration pneumonia in old patients with dementia. Prognostic factors of mortality. Eur J Intern Med 2012; 23:720–726.
15. Langmore SE, Skarupski KA, Park PS, et al. Predictors of aspiration pneumonia in nursing home residents. Dysphagia 2002; 17(4):298–307.
16. Scannapieco, FA. Role of oral bacteria in respiratory infection. J Periodontol 1999; 70(7):793–802.

12 Eating, Drinking and Swallowing Problems of Vulnerable Older Adults

Heather C. Lambert, PhD, erg., OT(C)

CONTENTS

SCENARIO

Mrs. Gold is an 85-year-old woman who was living alone in her apartment. She developed pneumonia four months ago. Because of the infection she found herself unable to cope with the demands of independent living. Her children helped her to move into a private long-term care facility a month ago; a move that seemed to be very unexpected from Mrs. Gold's point of view. Since her admission, she has lost about 4 kg and complains of a dry mouth and feeling a lump in her throat during meals. She eats very little and becomes upset at mealtimes, reporting a sense of 'something terribly wrong' especially at the end of the meal. She coughs when drinking water.

INGESTIVE SKILL LOSS

The term 'ingestive skill loss' has been used since the early 1990s to denote any difficulty related to mealtimes. The construct of ingestion includes positioning oneself appropriately, using utensils and tableware, cutting or otherwise preparing food for transportation to the mouth, removing food from the utensil or vessel, chewing, preparing the bolus, and swallowing. These actions require the successful integration of a large number of sensory, motor, cognitive, and behavioural tasks; the impairment of any one of these has an effect on the safe consumption of food and drink. As such, when clients complain of difficulty with eating or swallowing, it is important to consider the entire construct of ingestion and not just the swallow. If actions in the chain of events leading to the swallow are not successfully completed in a safe and timely manner, the swallow itself cannot occur safely. It is therefore important to pinpoint all of the problems within the ingestive process that are problematic for the client, especially given that the sequelae of ingestive skill loss include diminished quality of life; social withdrawal; weight loss, malnutrition and dehydration; pulmonary complications such as pneumonia, pneumonitis, or chronic lung changes; asphyxiation; and death.

The sequelae of ingestive skill loss are not only physical. The occurrence of ingestive problems causes significant psychological stress to both clients and caregivers. Providing nourishment is how many cultures show love or support, and an inability to do this can be felt as a betrayal or a negligence of obligations. Indeed, the vast majority of cultural and religious celebrations involve food and drink, and participating is imperative. For some, eating is an important component of lifestyle and identity, and the loss of any aspect of this ability deals a significant blow to their sense of self. The embarrassment that follows publicly drooling, coughing, or choking will lead many to withdraw from social activities involving food and drink, which is the vast majority of such occasions. Finding ways to mitigate or correct ingestive skill loss is thus important to the maintenance of life roles and psychological well-being, which is in turn essential to a person's physical health.

Managing ingestive skill loss generally takes one of two avenues, depending on an individual's physical status and the role food and drink plays in their identity. For individuals who feel that 'food is life', active participation in rehabilitation and the quick resumption of normal eating habits and preferred foods is often the priority, even at the expense of long-term health. For others, eating and drinking are merely necessities for survival, and this relative indifference to food may result in better acceptance of limitations in diet and other compensatory techniques. Furthermore, some

DOI: 10.1201/9781003344476-13

individuals are risk-averse, and will prefer to take a more restrictive approach to managing their feeding issues in order to substantially reduce the risk of aspiration or infection. Those who are relatively risk-tolerant are oftentimes willing to try more liberal management strategies and maintain a relationship with sustenance that is as 'normal' as possible, accepting that if the strategies are insufficient they may develop pulmonary issues or other complications of dysphagia. All of these variables will weigh into the health care professional's approach to management for each client.

CAUSES OF INGESTIVE SKILL LOSS

It is estimated that up to 38% of older adults living in the community and up to 68% in long-term care have loss of skills related to swallowing; it is impossible to estimate the prevalence of difficulty with other tasks related to self-feeding, eating, and drinking. This very high prevalence is due to age-related changes and the prevalence of chronic conditions in this segment of the population.

With aging comes a loss of speed, strength, and coordination that gradually impairs the older person's ability to consume difficult food consistencies in the way they did in younger years. Losses touch upon most of the anatomical structures required to successfully eat and drink; examples of these are presented in Table 12.1. Furthermore, many healthy older adults report

Table 12.1 Examples of Anatomical Changes with Aging Affecting Ingestion

Body Structure	Age-Related Change	Resulting Problem	Effect on Ingestion
Tongue	• Loss of strength.	• Difficulty moving food in the mouth.	• Inability to collect chewed food into bolus. • Inability to move food to the teeth for chewing. • Difficulty moving food from the mouth to the pharynx.
Teeth and oral cavity	• Dentition in poor condition. • Ill-fitting or broken dentures. • Loss of dentition and poor opposition of remaining teeth.	• Difficulty chewing. • Painful chewing. • Inability to chew. • Introduction of oral bacteria into food. • Development of open sores. • Oral infection with thrush or other organisms.	• Asphyxiation risk. • Refusing to eat. • Food residue under and around dental plates. • Aspiration of bacteria- or yeast-laden material.
Salivary glands	• Lack of saliva production.	• Xerostomia.	• Difficulty chewing and swallowing due to lack of lubrication. • Poor intake.
Epiglottis	• Deterioration of cartilage results in curling and shrinkage of epiglottis.	• Food trapped in the valleculae after the swallow. • Difficulty swallowing. • Poor airway protection. • Weak cough.	• Risk of aspiration. • Inability to clear airways of foreign material.
Anterior neck muscles	• Sarcopenia. • Weakness.	• Difficulty elevating laryngo-hyoid complex.	• Poor opposition of epiglottis to trachea. • Poor airway protection. • Difficulty opening cricopharyngeal segment.
Spine	• Arthritis, osteophytes in the cervical region.	• Impingement on the space available for dilation of the pharynx and/or esophagus during the swallow.	• Lump in throat, 'Globus sensation'. • Difficulty moving the bolus through the pharynx or down the esophagus.
Heart	• Decreased cardiac output.	• Fatigue increasing with exertion.	• Deterioration of muscle strength and speed of reflexes with effort. • May begin the meal safely and gradually become unsafe.

Table 12.2 Examples of Age-Associated Sensory Changes Affecting Ingestion

Sense	Example Conditions	Functional Problem	Effect on Ingestion
Vision	• Cataracts. • Glaucoma. • Macular degeneration. • Presbyopia.	• Loss of acuity in the dark. • Central blindness. • Difficulty focusing on close objects.	• Unable to identify food in low light. • Unable to find or identify plated food. • Difficulty cutting and getting food on the utensil for transport to the mouth.
Smell, taste	• Age-related changes. • Neurodegeneration. • Cranial nerve injury. • Brain injury. • CNS disease.	• Decreased perception. • Difficulty identifying foods. • Low salivary production. • Alteration in perception.	• Loss of interest in eating/drinking. • Poor nutrient intake. • Consumption of overcooked or undercooked food. • Consumption of high levels of salt and sugar. • Inability to identify spoiled food, inadequately cooked food, or allergens. • Difficulty chewing and swallowing because of lack of lubrication.
Touch	• Age-related changes. • Neurodegeneration. • Peripheral or cranial nerve injury. • Brain injury. • CNS disease.	• Decreased hot/cold perception. • Decreased light touch. • Decreased firm touch. • Decreased proprioception. • Decreased gnosis.	• Burns. • Inability to detect spilled food on skin. • Inability to detect drooling. • Delayed or absent reflexes (i.e. swallow, cough). • Difficulty judging when food is adequately chewed. • Difficulty collecting food or liquid in a bolus for swallowing. • Difficulty identifying food remaining in mouth or pharynx after swallowing.
Hearing	• Age- or occupation-related loss of acuity. • Tinnitus.	• Decreased ability to understand voices. • Decreased ability to detect or interpret environmental noise. • Decreased ability to discern voices from background noise (or tinnitus). • Perception of noise as too loud or otherwise noxious.	• Difficulty understanding instructions. • Social withdrawal. • Distraction.
Proprioception	• Age-related change.	• Difficulty sitting upright. • Problems with head stability.	• Difficulty maintaining upright position of head and neck necessary for safe feeding and swallowing.

progressive loss in the acuity of the basic senses associated with ingestion (Table 12.2). This loss of movement and sensation places the older individual at high risk of ingestive skill loss.

Remarkably, not all older adults develop ingestive difficulties despite these profound changes, which can be explained by physiologic reserve. A healthy young adult typically possesses all the necessary component skills to successfully consume nutrition and hydration (or indeed, do any task), with a certain 'safety margin' (i.e. their physiologic reserve). This amount of reserve is not measurable and varies between people. As a person ages, the natural damage or deterioration accumulates and diminishes the reserve, but typically not to an extent that causes dysfunction. When an illness occurs, causing significant temporary or permanent anatomical change or physiologic dysfunction, the individual's ability may then fall below the minimum requirement, causing a functional problem. As the person recovers or undergoes rehabilitation, the dysfunction resolves and the person comes closer to—and hopefully surpasses—that minimal threshold. An individual may be able to regain a premorbid level of function; however if there is a lingering component to the illness some functional loss may remain. With the passage of time and the accumulation of these mild impairments of function, any individual may eventually develop permanent difficulties with ingestion.

The acute, chronic, or degenerative illnesses that impact the ingestive skills of older persons most frequently are presented in Table 12.3. However, any condition that affects structures and functions of the head, neck, or torso or has an effect on endurance or respiration may have an impact on ingestion. Moreover, the extent of ingestive skill impairment and the potential for recovery is highly dependent on the exact nature and severity of the underlying condition. It is important to note that the cortical representation of the swallow is bilateral, and so unilateral damage to the brain will cause less impairment and be more amenable to rehabilitation than bilateral damage.

Table 12.3 Common Causes of Ingestive Skill Loss in Elderly Persons

Condition	Symptoms	Possible Effect on Ingestion
Cortical stroke	• Unilateral or bilateral weakness or sensory loss, contralateral to the stroke • Spasticity. • Hyporeflexia.	• Difficulty self-feeding. • Insufficient strength and coordination to chew. • Difficulty moving bolus. • Loss of bolus in oral cavity and pharynx, ipsilateral to weakness. • Swallow reflexes are delayed and/or weak, leading to residue in the pharynx and mouth. • Poor airway protection.
Medullar stroke	• Unilateral or bilateral weakness or sensory loss, ipsilateral to the stroke. • Flaccidity. • Hyperreflexia. • Loss of coordination.	• Difficulty self-feeding. • Insufficient strength and coordination to chew. • Difficulty moving bolus. • Loss of bolus in oral cavity and pharynx, ipsilateral to weakness. • Uncoordinated oral movements and swallow. • Gagging and coughing with little stimulation. • Poor airway protection.
Parkinson's disease	• Tremors. • Bradykinesia. • Rigidity. • 'Freezing'. • Drooling.	• Difficulty moving the bolus in the mouth, characterized by multiple attempts to retract the tongue (i.e. 'pumping'). • Slow and uncoordinated chewing. • Difficulty forming a bolus. • Delayed triggering of the swallow reflex. • Social withdrawal.
Dementia	• Distractibility. • Agnosia. • Anosognosia. • Inappropriate behaviour. • Disorientation. • Inability to interpret physiological signals. • Rigidity. • Areflexia.	• Difficulty orienting to the meal. • Emotional outbursts. • Food stealing. • Difficulty self-feeding, cannot use utensils appropriately. • Consumption of non-food items. • Forgetting to eat or drink. • Eating or drinking too much. • Attempting to eat too-large bite sizes, or uncut items. • Unable to open mouth. • Unable to chew or swallow.
Cardio-respiratory disease	• Fatigue. • Breathlessness. • Discoordination of breathe-swallow.	• Deteriorating function during meal. • Difficulty taking adequate nutrition and hydration. • Airway compromise. • O_2 desaturation during meal. • Aspiration.

Aspiration

The greatest risk to an individual's health and well-being, and the most feared sequela to an ingestive problem, is aspiration. The root cause of aspiration is always a failure of airway protection, caused by dysfunction of sensory or motor components affecting the mouth, pharynx, or esophagus. Aspiration may occur if there is entry of ingesta into the pharynx before a swallow is triggered, if the seal of the airway is insufficient to resist the pressure applied to the bolus during the swallow, if there is residue in the mouth or pharynx after the swallow, or if there is reflux of material from the esophagus into the pharynx. Non-prandial aspiration of saliva is also common, hence individuals who are receiving non-oral feeding with nothing by mouth may still experience aspiration and the associated negative consequences. Furthermore, aspiration may occur constantly or intermittently throughout the meal, only at the end of the meal when the person is fatigued, and/or only with certain foods or drinks. The volume of aspirate is also dependent on the physical properties of the bolus. Careful identification of the timing and conditions of aspiration is necessary to develop an effective intervention plan.

Aspiration can be broadly categorized as silent or non-silent. Non-silent aspiration has the hallmark of the person choking, coughing, or clearing their throat after aspiration. These efforts to clear the airway are indicative that there is food or liquid that has entered the laryngeal vestibule or the trachea. Unless the person has a respiratory condition, there is no reason for a person that is not aspirating to cough or clear their throat during a meal. Therefore, any occurrence of these signs strongly suggests that the person is experiencing some degree of aspiration. In silent aspiration, the individual does not cough or clear when material enters the airway. This can be due to a fault in either the sensory or motor component of the cough reflex arc. However, the astute clinician can occasionally identify when this is occurring by observing other, more subtle signs of airway compromise such as emotional outbursts that occur only during meals, fear, hoarseness when attempting to speak, and noisy or wet-sounding respiration.

Aspiration is a life-threatening complication of ingestive problems due to its association with pneumonia, which can be lethal especially in frail elders or individuals who have underlying conditions. In addition, chronic aspiration, even of minuscule quantities, can cause lung changes and respiratory issues without infection. However, the presence of aspiration does not dictate that the person will develop a respiratory problem; in fact many who aspirate do not experience any negative consequences. The most significant factors contributing to the development of pulmonary complications are oral hygiene and dependence on another person for feeding, even in the absence of clinically identified dysphagia. Therefore, an important consideration in developing an intervention plan for any given client is whether the individual is distressed by the aspiration and the extent to which the aspiration is causing infection or other pulmonary complications. If they are not physically or psychologically affected by the aspiration, less restrictive management with active surveillance for the development of problems may be appropriate.

EVALUATION

The complete evaluation of an older adult with dysphagia can be a complex process, as each of the anatomical structures and physiological events must be assessed in a systematic manner. Oftentimes, various aspects of the assessment process are divided amongst health professionals, or carried out by a dedicated dysphagia team. Most clients are pre-screened by physicians or nurses using criteria related to mental status, understanding of commands, and ability to maintain an appropriate head and trunk position. If the individual is able to complete these tasks, the client's swallowing skills are considered safe to be assessed for oral intake.

In the dysphagia evaluation, the clinician may elect to perform a screening test that includes the timed consumption of measured amounts of cold water, which will not irritate the lungs any more than saliva should it be aspirated. This gives important information regarding the swallow reflex and movement of the pharyngeal structures during the swallow. A physical assessment of oral structures and functions, including testing the gag, palatal, and swallow reflexes, is often performed. It is important to note that approximately 10% of the healthy adult population does not have a gag reflex that can be elicited during such an exam, and the absence of a gag reflex does not preclude oral eating and drinking. The patency of the swallowing and protective reflexes gives the clinician important information regarding the associated sensory and motor pathways.

Arguably the most important component of a thorough evaluation is the observation of a typical meal in the client's usual mealtime setting. This allows the clinician to identify problems arising from the environment including positioning, lighting, utensil use, and environmental distractions; or problems with self-feeding, chewing, swallowing, or respiration. It is crucial that the clinician observe the entire meal to determine if problems are intermittent or if they systematically worsen or improve as the meal progresses.

If the clinician wishes to document the precise physiological events of the swallow, it is possible to perform objective assessment using a videofluoroscopic swallow study (VFSS, also called a modified barium swallow) or a functional endoscopic evaluation of swallowing (FEES). In VFSS, the client consumes a variety of solid and liquid consistencies mixed with barium, and their progress through the oral cavity and pharynx is documented with dynamic radiography. This examination allows the identification of any physiologic abnormality impacting the timing or physiology of the swallow, as well as the presence, timing, and extent of aspiration. In FEES, a fibre optic camera is passed transnasally and positioned above the pharynx, which allows direct visualization of the soft tissues of the pharynx and larynx, as well as the movements of the pharynx and the quality and timing of airway protection during solid and liquid swallows. Both tests have their advantages and disadvantages, which are beyond the scope of this article. However, it is crucial that the clinicians be aware of problems particular to the frail elderly population. Elders tend not to function as well during these assessments as they do in their own environment, due to factors not limited to the unfamiliarity of the testing environment, stress of the test itself, fatigue from transport to the hospital, and the foods used in testing. This drastically increases the risk of a false positive identification of pathology. In addition, neither test lasts long enough to identify an intermittent or fatigue-related problem. Because of the questionable validity of these assessments in this population, it is considered inappropriate to use them with the sole purpose of confirming the presence and extent of aspiration. The appropriate use of these assessments is to quantify parameters such as excursion of certain anatomical structures during the swallow and the relative timing of swallow events, with the goal of developing rigorous physical rehabilitation programs. While this information is valuable for individuals who have dysphagia because of injury or illness, it is seldom needed when intervening with frail elders who have developed ingestive difficulties due to age-associated anatomical and physiological changes with the superposition of a chronic or acute illness. In addition, many elders tend not to be interested in or are unable to follow a rigorous rehabilitation program, which typically involves several sessions of physical exercises daily, and often entails the regular use of electrical stimulation and/or physical manipulation by a specially trained therapist. In deciding whether to refer someone for these tests, it is wise to ask if the results of the test will change the intervention plan, or if management will be the same regardless of the outcome.

INTERVENTION

In the absence of an acute or acquired pathology upon which active rehabilitation efforts may be applied, intervention to improve the safety and efficiency of meals generally focuses on management of the environment, optimizing the position of the client, promoting self-feeding, modifying food textures, carefully timing oral hygiene, and prioritizing those food- and drink-related occasions that are important to the client's well-being. Non-oral feeding may be considered for some individuals.

Modifications to the environment are made to optimize the client's ability to see and smell their meal, focus on the meal without excessive distraction, hear people in their surroundings, organize the utensils and dishes presented to them, interact with others, and move into and out of the dining area as needed or desired. Changes to a dining area need to be planned based on the difficulties experienced by the client and the typical mealtime environment, as the environmental factors that will allow one person to enjoy their meal may be detrimental to others. For example, if a communal dining area is too distracting because of noise and the movement of other people as they socialize, an individual with feeding difficulties may do better when seated in a quiet corner of the dining room, away from the noise and traffic. Some people in communal living situations prefer to eat in their rooms for that reason. However if a roommate is toileting on the other side of the privacy curtain the meal will not be enjoyable. Light levels that are sufficient for someone with cataracts may be too bright for someone who experiences migraines. Dining areas are relatively simple to reorganize in a home environment. However, communal dining in a residential facility may need to be addressed creatively, with areas within the space used for people with varying needs for supervision, lighting, and noise levels. All dining spaces benefit from moderate lighting, unpatterned table coverings, no more decorations or implements on the table than necessary, and no television or music. Modifications for individuals needing more or less stimulation than this can then be applied on a case-by-case basis.

Positioning in a chair or bed will have a direct impact on individuals' ability to feed themselves and swallow safely. Typically, unless there is a medical restriction to transferring to a chair, there is no reason for an individual to take a meal in bed. In bed, it is difficult to position the person so that they are sitting erect enough (a minimum of 60 degrees from horizontal) and with sufficient head support, but not sliding down. The energy expended by a person trying to maintain a good position for eating while in bed is much greater than when a person is seated in an appropriate chair. Furthermore, it is often difficult for a person who is not physically fit to feed themselves effectively from bed, because of the reach required and the suboptimal line of sight to the tray. Therefore, it is strongly recommended that a person with ingestive difficulties be transferred to a well-fitting chair in which their hips are at 60 to 90 degrees of flexion; feet and back supported; arms in a functional position whether on armrests, table, or wheelchair tray; and with a head rest if the person is not able to maintain head control throughout the meal. In addition, ensuring that the person is able to use their hands easily is crucial, and liberating hands from a bib or other protective covering is frequently neglected. Generally speaking, 'geri-chairs', transport chairs, and commodes are not appropriate seating for mealtimes, unless specifically recommended by an occupational therapist.

Self-feeding is important to maintain for as long as possible, given the causative relationship between dependence for feeding and aspiration pneumonia. A wide variety of adaptive utensils, plates, and drinking vessels are available to meet specific needs, and can be selected and furnished through an occupational therapist.

It is important to note that drinking from a straw is contraindicated for any person that has (or is suspected of having) any kind of pharyngeal impairment. Straw drinking does avoid the necessity of lifting the vessel to the mouth and maintaining the liquid in a bolus for swallowing. However, it deposits the bolus at the back of the mouth without allowing any preparatory time for the swallow or airway protection. Hence, if there is difficulty triggering the swallow in a timely manner or protecting the airway, the individual is at much higher risk for aspiration than if they drink from an adapted vessel such as a cup with a cut-out for the nose or with a spout.

If the individual has difficulty with the praxis (ability to interact successfully with the environment) to self-feed, motor memory may be triggered if a carer demonstrates utensil use or provides hand-over-hand assistance. If an individual is completely unable to self-feed, it is crucial that the carer is trained in the task for each client, including any modifications to the usual process that has been recommended by the dysphagia team (Table 12.4). The general guideline is that the client should perform as much of the task as they are able, either independently or with a carer's support, with the carer performing the feeding tasks only when the client is completely unable.

Oral hygiene is an important consideration for the client with ingestive problems. Given that oral bacteria are a causative factor in aspiration pneumonia, oral hygiene should be performed before the meal if the person is at risk for aspiration. The client or carer must ensure that the teeth, dentures, and tongue are thoroughly cleaned. Dentures should be verified on a regular basis to ensure that they are in good repair and fit well, to optimize chewing and prevent mouth and gum sores. If it is impossible for dentures to be fitted optimally, it may be preferable that the client eat without them, although the elimination of hard or fibrous food textures may be needed. Oral hygiene should also be performed after the meal if there is a risk of residue in the mouth which can be later aspirated. Some clients do require oral hygiene both before and after meals to ensure safety; if only one is possible, before the meal is the more critical to long-term maintenance of health.

Adapting the consistency and texture of food and liquid is one of the most common adaptive approaches to an ingestive problem. While there is a movement to apply standard labels to various consistencies of food and liquid, this transition is still in progress and the old terminology will be used here.

Solid foods are often labelled as regular solid, soft solid (pancakes, omelettes, poached fish, dark poultry, canned fruit, cooked vegetables), minced and moist (all food is chopped to 2 mm size pieces and liquid added for ease of processing), and purée (completely smooth). Within each category there can be variability in texture; for example, baby applesauce is completely smooth and regular applesauce is slightly granular and the liquid may separate. The combination of texture and consistency determine the effort that the individual needs to exert in orally preparing the food and moving the bolus to the pharynx, the amount of residue that is likely to be left in the mouth and pharynx after the swallow, and the amount of sensory feedback the food gives. Overall, the softer and smaller the fragments are, the easier they are to handle during oral processing. The decreased sensory input offered by smoother textures can be offset by adding seasoning or changing the temperature of the item.

Liquids can also be modified to decrease the risk of aspiration. Thinner consistencies move faster in the mouth, are more difficult to control during the swallow, and may invade an

Table 12.4 Feeding Techniques for Individuals with Ingestive Skill Loss

Task	Technique
Positioning	• Transfer the client to a suitable chair. • Ensure the client's position is appropriate (feet supported, hips at 90 degrees, back upright, trunk aligned with hips, arms supported but able to move, facing forward, with head support if needed). • Modify positioning according to recommendations from the positioning or swallowing specialist. • Reposition the client as needed during the meal.
Set-up	• Make sure hands are free from bib or other protective garment. • Minimize clutter on the table. • Consider offering one utensil at a time if distractibility or praxis is an issue. • Avoid tablespoons to prevent overfilling of the client's mouth. • Consider offering one plate or one food item at a time if distractibility or behaviour is an issue. • The plate should be within the client's reach if they do not play with the food. If this is a concern, the plate should be within view. • Open containers as necessary. • If cutting food is necessary, cut it all before the meal begins.
Offering solids	• Use a teaspoon to feed safely. Tablespoons are too large if ingestive skills are impaired. • Give verbal prompts: identify the food being offered, cue to open and close mouth, cue to swallow as needed. • Before feeding the person, try verbal prompts and hand-over-hand feeding. • Feed only food consistencies and textures that are on the approved diet.
Offering liquids	• Use a cup, glass, mug, or adapted cup, not a straw. • Offer only one sip at a time. • Offer only liquids that are on the approved diet. • Monitor liquid consumption especially if liquids are thickened.
Feeding	• Sit in front of the client, or if to the side offer the utensil from the front to maintain alignment of head and trunk. • Even if the client is unable to respond, keep talking to keep their focus on the meal. Inform the client what food is on the utensil if you are feeding. • Use a teaspoon to feed, never a tablespoon. • Keep different foods separate. • Allow the client to close lips to spoon to remove food, do not scrape food on the teeth or upper lip. • Watch the person's chest during the meal. After each mouthful, make sure that the person inhales and exhales at least once before offering the next mouthful. • Listen for changes in voice or respiratory sounds.
Warning signs	• If the person is coughing, hoarse, has a 'wet' voice, or sudden emotional upset, stop feeding and ask for assistance. • If a person is unable to breathe, clear the airway. • The client should remain seated in a chair for a minimum of 20 minutes after the meal to prevent reflux. • Food stealing, erratic behaviour, or emotional outbursts during the meal are frequently indicators that a person is uncomfortable or afraid, and the person should be assessed.

incompletely protected airway more easily than thicker consistencies. Liquids may naturally be thin (water, juice, tea, coffee) or nectar-thick (fruit nectar, vegetable juice, Boost). Thickening agents made from modified corn starch or agar can be added to liquids to thicken them to honey or pudding consistency if the individual so requires. In addition, increased sensory feedback offered by cold or hot temperatures, stronger flavours, and carbonation may also improve a client's ability to manage certain liquids.

The challenge with altering textures is ensuring that the individual maintains adequate nutrition and hydration on the modified diet. Any food or liquid that has been modified will lose some sensory appeal and flavour, resulting in decreased intake. It is recommended that additional seasonings be added to solids, and liquids be flavoured and served cold or hot to maximize appeal. Puréed foods that are re-formed to resemble the original item are commercially available and do improve intake because of their visual appeal, but these tend to be prohibitively expensive. Furthermore, thickened liquids are more filling than regular liquids and do not quench thirst, so they tend not to be consumed in sufficient quantities to maintain hydration. Unthickened water can be offered to some individuals needing thickened liquid, but there are specific criteria that the client must meet to be considered safe, and clinical guidelines for the preparation for and timing of water consumption must be strictly followed. Because of these challenges, it is crucial that a client not be forced to accept a diet that is any more restrictive than absolutely necessary, and that a dietitian follows the individual to monitor intake. Some clients elect to live with a certain amount of risk and consume some items that are not within the recommended diet; this can be necessary to the individual's psychological well-being and may contribute to better adherence to a modified diet overall.

REFERRAL TO SPECIALISTS

The optimal assessment and intervention for ingestive skill loss is delivered by an interdisciplinary team, ideally composed of the physician, nurse, occupational therapist, dietitian, and speech-language pathologist; plus other specialists as required. Each rehabilitation profession has its own area of expertise in this domain (Table 12.5); however there is significant overlap in the roles each profession plays in ingestive skill intervention. Because of the lack of resources in the Quebec health care system, it is unusual to find teams that work exclusively with this clientele, and many health care settings do not have all of the central members of such a team on staff. Occupational therapists tend to take the lead in many health care settings in Quebec, as they are more numerous than speech-language pathologists and are likely to be intervening with regard to the clients' safety, positioning, and activities of daily living in a broader context. In other geographic areas, it may be speech-language pathology, dietetics, or nursing that takes the lead.

In the absence of a team, physicians can refer a patient for whom feeding and swallowing is becoming problematic to the local community services centre (CLSC) or to a professional in private practice with expertise in this area. The physician should take a detailed history of the elder's eating and drinking difficulties and assess as needed to rule out pathologies that may be contributing to ingestive difficulties such as arthritis of the cervical spine, reflux, esophageal diverticula, or cricopharyngeal spasm. Medications should also be reviewed for side effects including xerostomia, altered mental status, extrapyramidal movements, and depression of reflexes, and substitutions made where possible. The timing of medications should also be considered, either to ensure that they are having maximal effect (as for anti-Parkinson's medications) or that the secondary effects are minimized at mealtimes (as for benzodiazepines). Conveying this information to the rehabilitation professional at the time of referral will be of great value as they work to uncover the source and possible interventions for the client. Nevertheless, it is important not to delay a referral to a specialist while awaiting the results of these assessments, due to the severe sequelae that may develop if ingestive problems are left unattended.

The physician is also crucial in supporting the client's decision making regarding their care. As previously mentioned, clients may elect to consume foods which put them at risk of aspiration because the occupation of eating is important to them. Others may easily accept a very restricted diet, so that they avoid developing pneumonia. Many people choose to continue consuming certain 'unsafe' foods regardless of the risk because of their personal significance, and the importance of this decision should not be underestimated. Whatever the person's attitudes and beliefs regarding food, it is important to weigh the risks and benefits of interventions with the client, including special accommodations that may be made for celebrations and outings, in order to maximize both safety and quality of life.

EPILOGUE

Mrs. Gold had a fruitful conversation with the physician, dietitian, and occupational therapist at the long-term care facility. The professionals took the time to sit down with her and discuss not only the difficulty she was having, but also her relationship with food. With careful questioning, she realized that not only was she missing home-cooked meals and adjusting to the relatively bland institutional food, but that she was missing some of the comfort foods that she used to make with her children and grandchildren. The physician found that she had been prescribed both a narcotic and a benzodiazepine, both of which can cause swallowing issues; he was able to substitute one of these medications in the hope to optimize her swallowing. The OT and dietitian

Table 12.5 Traditional Roles of Rehabilitation Professionals in Ingestion

Profession	Traditional Role*
Dietetics	• Evaluate the nutritional needs of the client. • Monitor the client's weight and hydration. • Prescribe a diet to manage ingestive skill loss, including food and liquid consistencies. • Balance all of the client's physical and medical needs with respect to diet. This may include regulating calorie intake, ensuring there are sufficient vitamins or minerals, reduction of salt, management of diabetes, and respecting allergies and intolerances, as well as food and liquid consistencies. • Ensure the diet is accepted by the client, and make adjustments as necessary. • Set the facility's menu. • Oversee the production of meals.
Occupational Therapy	• Evaluate ingestive skills. • Oversee and interpret the administration of VFSS and FEES. • Evaluate anatomy and physiology of the head and neck. • Evaluate functional oral motor skills. • Evaluate swallowing. • Assess the client's values and wishes with respect to feeding. • Verify the client is seated in a safe and functional manner and prescribe modifications as necessary. • Optimize self-feeding ability of the client. • Train carers in feeding skills. • Prescribe adaptive equipment including drinking vessels, utensils, and flatware. • Assess overall mealtime performance and behaviour. • Design interventions that are functionally based and take into consideration all aspects of the client's values, interests, strengths, and weaknesses. • Recommend food and liquid textures to the dietitian. • Assist in decision making for interventions.
Speech-Language Pathology	• Oversee and interpret the administration of VFSS and FEES. • Assess anatomy and physiology of the head and neck. • Evaluate functional oral motor skills. • Evaluate swallowing. • Design interventions to rehabilitate oral motor and pharyngeal function. • Design interventions to optimize self-feeding skills. • Recommend food and liquid textures to the dietitian. • Assist in decision making for interventions. • Plan and implement interventions to ensure the client can communicate needs.

* This is a generalization applicable to Quebec; roles may differ significantly among geographic locations and practice settings, and depend on the needs of the institution.

observed Mrs. Gold having a meal and made some suggestions to make mealtimes easier. By adding extra seasoning to food at the table it became more appealing, and Mrs. Gold was able to eat more. The dietitian also suggested that she try a soft diet, so that she didn't have to work as hard during meals. The addition of flavouring to water, as well as the addition of more fruit juices, carbonated water, and sugar-free soft drinks helped to reduce the coughing during meals a little but eventually she admitted that it wasn't quite enough and she accepted trying slightly thickened liquids. The OT helped her decide with her family what foods met her requirements and could be brought in for a special treat. The OT checked that she was sitting properly and that the environment suited her, and suggested that she eat in a quieter area of the dining room so that she could concentrate on her meal. Mrs. Gold decided with her team that they would try these changes for a while, and if she continued having coughing spells or was starting to develop pulmonary complications, she would have a VFSS to evaluate the swallowing mechanism and see if any additional changes needed to be made.

RECOMMENDED SUPPLEMENTARY INFORMATION

1. Groher ME and Crary MA. (2021). Dysphagia: Clinical Management in Adults and Children, 3rd edition. Elsevier.
2. International Dysphagia Diet Standardization Initiative (2019). www.iddsi.org
3. National Foundation of Swallowing Disorders (2022). www.swallowingdisorderfoundation.com
4. National Foundation of Swallowing Disorders (2011). Swallow—A Documentary. https://www.youtube.com/watch?v=MrbEUDO6S5U&t=7s

PART II
VULNERABILITY

13 Architecture and the Aging

Julia Gersovitz O.C. OAQ, QAA, AANB, FIRAC/FRAIC, FAPT,
CAHP and Boris Morin-Defoy, M.Arch, B.Sc.Arch

CONTENTS

INTRODUCTION

To write about architecture in the service of the older person during the COVID-19 pandemic is deeply unsettling. Both the authors of this chapter are practising architects who live in Quebec, Canada, and we are very much aware that as of the end of 2021, as a result of the first wave of the disease, 75% of all Covid-related deaths in the province occurred in nursing homes.[1]

This grim statistic might at first glance be linked to the fact that Quebec has the highest percentage of seniors in long-term care (LTC) in the country. However, the problem seems to be nation-wide:

> While Canada's overall COVID-19 mortality rate was relatively low compared with the rates in other OECD[2] countries, it had the highest proportion of deaths occurring in long-term care. LTC residents accounted for 59% of all reported COVID-19 deaths in Canada, compared with an average of 38% in other OECD countries.[3]

In the United States, as of April 2021, one-third of Covid deaths were linked to nursing homes.[4] Given the ongoing status of the pandemic, these statistics must be viewed as 'live'; however, the snapshot is telling and probably will be little changed by the end of the crisis.

Terms such as 'ageicide' made the headlines in Quebec. "It's as if the human rights charter didn't apply to [long-term care residents]. They let them die", is how one union representative was quoted during testimony before a coroner's inquiry. In the aftermath of the grim revelations of abandonment and the grieving, there is a growing understanding that the serious problems at long-term care facilities need immediate attention. There is chronic understaffing and lack of

DOI: 10.1201/9781003344476-15

coordination of services. Issues relating to conflicts between profit motive and fundamental care are being debated, without clear political action to remedy what has been revealed as a colossal failure of responsibility.

Lest one be lulled into thinking that this catastrophe is the result of a once-in-a-lifetime occurrence, it is interesting to read a critique sponsored by the American Institute of Architects, over six decades ago, in 1959: "The home for the aged, in common with some other institutions, has frequently been characterized by its static quality—an immutable attitude and mode of operation, and an apparent unresponsiveness to the changes taking place around it."[5] It is indeed time for questioning and radical thinking.

In this chapter on architecture and the aging, the authors question the mindset that has too often underpinned conventional architectural models for housing older adults in North America—be it in autonomous living conditions or in nursing homes—and provide brief descriptions of other innovative approaches that have been implemented successfully in Europe.

PRESENT MINDSET

One's Lot in Life

It is interesting to note that when housing for older adults began to be seen as a specific type of architecture in the late 1950s, profit motive was not yet identified as an important driver. Homes were either publicly funded or volunteer-based. The public building was stigmatized, with its historic links to the 'poor farm'. "The negative emotional connotations of being a public charge in a public institution persist to such an extent that the stigma attached is almost as strong as it ever was, and remains difficult to overcome."[6]

It is sadly unclear if the negative connotations identified in this 1959 text have entirely been removed in 2021, despite the creation of patient advocacy groups. There lingers the idea that those who are in the public charge must accept their lot, rather than demanding a better one. For example, in Canada, in order to house the disadvantaged as economically as possible, publicly funded long-term care homes have mixed the cognitively impaired with the physically compromised, such as persons with paraplegia, despite the obvious disparities in their needs and abilities.

This perception of inevitability should be challenged, because it contributes to an ongoing lassitude on the part of the public to demand improvements in the living conditions of the publicly, and to some extent privately, funded homes. The tragic outcomes of the pandemic have exposed, if only briefly, this societal complacency and forced a reckoning.

Need for Diversity

Volunteer-based homes were historically sorted along religious or ethnic associations, much as they are today. It is important to note that groups which have never been specifically identified until recently remain underserved. These groups include the LGTBQ+ and Indigenous peoples.

Cotton-Wool Warehousing

CanAge is Canada's national seniors' advocacy organization. In a recent discussion with Laura Tamblyn Watts, the founder and CEO, and Diana Cable, Director of Policy, the question of risk was raised. Ms. Tamblyn Watts acknowledged that countries have different attitudes to risk management. In North America, the risk (and litigation) adverse mindset leads to a more sheltered approach to the care of the aging person. At its worst, this results in conditions best summed up by the phrase "television and sedation". Too often the resident becomes an unwilling occupant in a cotton-wool warehouse.

Tamblyn Watts' understanding mirrors the findings of the International Psychogeriatric Association: "Health professionals tend to adopt a risk averse approach when assessing older adults, with a focus on weaknesses and inabilities, the primary concern being the prevention of adverse events within the hospital and on discharge."[7] In other words, mitigation of potential dangers outweighs the need to encourage the older adult to go out and about in society. "A commitment to supporting an older adult to make care-related decisions should be demonstrated by encouraging, rather than restricting, their capacities and wellbeing, as well as by taking into account outcomes such as dignity, rights, freedom and privacy."[8]

Care in North America has to be recalibrated to accept greater risk in exchange for the greater enjoyment associated with living. In Holland, patients with dementia can go on supervised bicycle trips to their local shopping centre or around their neighbourhood. The outings are made possible by the use of tandem bikes, designed so that a resident and a worker pedal side by side.[9] This emphasis on physical activity and interaction with the larger community is only achievable if one accepts the risks inherent in having the resident leave the comparative safety and controlled environment of their care home.

GUIDING PRINCIPLES

The authors embrace as a fundamental premise the following statement, first written in 1959 by Ollie A. Randall, Vice Chairman of the National Committee for the Aging:

> The most encouraging trend in congregate living is the recognition that the older person *is* a person, and has desires and yearnings that deserve attention and respect; that life in the home should allow as much gratification of these feelings as possible; and that the home should make the effort to fit its accommodations and services to the individual, rather than insisting as has been done so frequently and uncompromisingly in the past, that the individual be obliged to make a one-sided adjustment to the rules and regulations of the home. . . . [O]lder people do not, just because they are older, lose the need for the very essence and spirit of life.[10]

The text addresses the need to accommodate diversity and individuality and to acknowledge that all humans have the right to age on their own terms. Too often, for reasons of staffing shortages or profit considerations or risk aversion, these fundamental principles have been set aside; instead they should govern all decision-making in architecture for the aging.

It should be noted that the authors have not dealt with income levels in the discussion. It is obvious that the greater the disposable income, the greater the options. However, the European experience demonstrates that creative and innovative ideas can be generated within existing funding parameters.

As well, although technological solutions are expensive when they are first launched into the marketplace, historically, they become more economically viable over time. 'TigerPlace' is a US-based assisted living apartment building that integrates sensor technology into the architecture, in order to respond quickly to crises such as falls and also to facilitate early detection of illnesses. The use of such technology for monitoring and surveillance can result in a loss of privacy, but this trade-off may be entirely palatable to some, for the promise of greater autonomy. Given the speed with which new technologies are being launched on the marketplace, the possibilities for users are in constant evolution.

OPTIONS

Aging in Place

Much has been written about the best place to grow old: one's own home—what the National Institute on Aging terms "aging in place". Fully 96% of Canadians and 77% of Americans over 50[11] would prefer to continue to live out their lives at home. There are many books, articles and websites on how to best manage, if not fully control, the physical environment to accommodate senior living. These range from widening doorways and designing a full bathroom and bedroom suite on the ground floor of a house to more easily implementable changes, such as removing tripping hazards and changing doorknobs to levers.

Successful aging in place does not come only from adapting the physical environment of the home. It also results from creating age-friendly communities, where all age groups in a society can move about their daily activities in a safe and thoughtfully designed urban environment. In 2007, the World Health Organization published a guide to what it termed 'active aging', titled *Global Age-Friendly Cities: A Guide*.[12] The document remains a useful checklist in the design toolbox for planning liveable cities. In the United States, resources on a city-by-city or state-wide level can be found through NORC programs. NORC is an acronym for a naturally occurring retirement community, where a large percentage of the residents are over 60 and living in accommodations that have not been purpose-built for aging. In Canada, the potential of NORCs for aging in place is being explored, but they do not have access to the same federal government funding that Americans have through Title IV of the Older Americans Act of 1965.

The aging-in-place model does not or cannot suit a wide swath of the population. In analyzing how to present other options, we realized that we needed a sorting mechanism; otherwise, the variety of possibilities can be overwhelming. A person's *age* is too arbitrary to be an accurate indicator of one's capacity. A super-ager can flourish in a physical environment that would prove much more daunting or unmanageable to a younger, but more physically or cognitively challenged, peer. This chapter is therefore organized around the authors' intuition that the degree of a person's *autonomy*, both physical and cognitive, will be the key determinant in selecting their housing.

The initial sorting by *autonomy* created four groups: (A) the fully autonomous; (B) the mostly autonomous, who need some support when out and about to continue to live at home; (C) the semi-autonomous, who must rely on support for daily tasks within and without the home; and finally (D) those who have severely compromised autonomy, through physical or cognitive impairment. It is understood that as a person ages, they may move from one group to another, escalating their need for services as they do so.

It is immediately evident that from an architectural perspective, each distinct group can be blended with its neighbour—a construction can accommodate residents from groups A and B or groups B and C. The only limitation is imposed by the goodwill and cooperation of the individuals who constitute the more autonomous group. Group D remains somewhat distinct, because of the elevated level of care demanded by the cognitive impairment and in some cases by physical disability. However, since this chapter has been written to challenge the status quo, alternative solutions to the prevailing care model for Group D are provided for discussion and investigation.

Designing for a Range of Autonomy

The autonomous and the semi-autonomous have an array of options for independent living, aside from staying in their own house. The complexes are marketed under a variety of names: retirement communities, retirement living, active lifestyle, active adult community and senior communities. Information on these types of dwellings is readily available on the internet. A caveat: there tends to be homogeneity in available choices, partially driven by market research. Often, the target demographic is narrow, focused on a single shared culture, rather than accommodating— and therefore having to manage— different desires in activities, holidays, food choices, etc. For example, several developer/operators of senior residences in Quebec offer multiple housing types and care levels. However, the overwhelming majority of their advertisements feature white, conventionally dressed people; there is little to no indication of the diversity in the population that now characterizes both the province and Canada.

These homes, however sorted (public, volunteer or profit) are essentially providers of care. The degree of services depends on the needs required by the aging resident. Care can be 'autonomous', 'personalized', 'semi-autonomous', etc. However, in recent years, there have been some interesting alternatives proposed, which are essentially grassroots activist models. They tend to accept, and perhaps encourage, greater non-conformity than the models described earlier. The first is the cooperative housing model. The second is the 'Baba Yaga' version, which was developed in France for independent single women.

The Cooperative Housing Model

The roots of cooperative housing in the United States run throughout the 19th century, fuelled by socialist and feminist principles of freedom through collaboration. Modern experiments in cohousing in North America have their roots in Danish experiments that date from the 1960s. In Canada, one example is the Prairie Sky Cohousing, advertised as an "intentional community in Calgary, Alberta".[13] Individual dwelling units are small, but community facilities are emphasized. The principles of "community, respect, sustainability and affordability" weathered the Covid lockdown of 2020–2021. Residents spoke of how the community coped during the pandemic by relying in part on intergenerational collaboration. Retired residents volunteered to take care of children when the schools were shut down, allowing their parents and guardians to keep working. Anecdotes are common throughout cohousing websites of 'village' bonds enabling residents to live longer in place because of the help of their neighbours.

In Canada, the Canadian Cohousing Network provides resources to parties who might be interested in setting up a cohousing community; in the United States, the Cohousing Association of the United States is a valuable resource.

The Baba Yaga Model

Brainchild of a French feminist, Thérèse Clerc (1927–2016), the first Maison des Babayagas[14] was established in 2012, to provide a housing alternative for single women, between 60–90, who are committed to maintaining their own sense of self and to community engagement. Clerc wanted to challenge the existing model of senior housing in France, which she saw as isolating, rigid and ultimately demeaning. In the following two quotations from an interview with the RFI radio network that she gave in 2013, we understand both her perspective and her call to arms. "Old age isn't about being shipwrecked. It isn't about illness. It can be beautiful, and I plan to live it that way, with my friends and colleagues here."[15]

The *maison* was purpose-built to accommodate about 21 women and was financed by the French government, when bureaucrats were finally convinced that the model was not a drain on state funds, so much as a different way to allocate the funds.

Residents pool their resources, participate in a regime of chores and provide, if they so desire, services to the larger community. The point is not what the services are; it is that they engage the women with the surrounding society, rather than isolating them from it. "Staying intelligent will keep us healthy. . . . I believe women who are happy, not bored, will live healthier lives", said Clerc.[16] In consequence, the site for the Maison des Babayagas was chosen for its central location within Montreuil, a vibrant inner suburb of Paris. This is an important architectural and urban design decision. In North America, too often sites for old-age homes are either in isolated or unappealing locations such as adjacent to expressways, chosen not for their easy accessibility to the surrounding city, but for the relative cheapness of the land.

A Canadian version, Baba Yaga Place, was established in Toronto, Canada, in 2013 and will begin operation for residents of all genders in 2023.

Private-sector marketing is often an interesting way to observe shifts in the zeitgeist. In late 2021, le Groupe Maurice published a flyer that was striking for its target audience. Instead of a laughing, conventionally garbed older man and woman gazing into each other's eyes, the photograph displays three women, with unruly grey hair and idiosyncratic clothing, one of whom is gripping the handlebars of a bicycle. Thus, we can understand that baba yagas have been identified as a target market within North America.

Designing for Compromised Autonomy

For some aging adults, the previously enumerated living solutions will not meet the demands of their declining autonomy, due to the development of severe and incurable neuro-cognitive disorders. As a result, these seniors and their families will need to consider a transition to a long-term care centre.[17] Although not technically centres for palliative care, long-term care centres are the last place of residence for most of their patients.

As the first wave of the Covid pandemic took centre stage at long-term care centres, the dire living conditions of their residents were laid bare. Although the pandemic catapulted the architectural and organizational problems into the public eye, there is clear evidence that these problems predated the current crisis. As Pat Armstrong and Susan Braedley pointed out in their 2016 book, *Physical Environments for Long-Term Care: Ideas Worth Sharing*: "In most high income countries, there is a new emphasis on home care or on what is often called aging in place. Far less attention is paid to long-term residential care".[18]

The magnitude of the scandal that erupted in the spring of 2020 emphasized the urgent need to re-evaluate these living environments.

The first major shift in the conceptualization of long-term care centres must be in their architectural scale and spatial nature. The typology of the large healthcare institution should be set aside in favour of solutions that are closer to the human scale, closer to residential architecture. Nursing homes commonly borrow their design language and planning principles from outdated hospital models. Long, uniformly lit corridors are lined with undifferentiated doors leading to bleak, antiseptic rooms. The fluorescent lighting is as ubiquitous as the homogeneous materials that cover every surface, despite research that demonstrates that the elderly respond well to different textures and colours.[19] The most striking sensory experience is the cacophony derived from poor acoustic design; it is rivalled only by the olfactory signature that lingers everywhere.

A Proposed Quebec Model

The goal in replacing the hospital model should not be to implement another 'universal' answer, but to seek solutions that respond to different cultural and environmental contexts. Recent innovations can provide interesting directions. In 2019, an initiative led by Quebec's Minister Responsible for Seniors called Maison des aînés—Pavillion alternatif[20] was launched to address the current scale issues in its nursing homes. The cornerstone of the Maison des aînés' design strategy is to limit living units to between 6 and 14 individuals, who share common abilities and interests.[21] It is thought that the smaller units, or 'micro-environments', will have a positive effect on the overall well-being of residents—on their behaviour, their autonomy, their social interaction, as well as their sleeping patterns. These improvements should in turn lower the dependence on prescription drugs.[22]

In order to maintain a certain level of operational efficiency, micro-environments are to be grouped around a common back-of-house for functional and administrative services. This design decision has several advantages. First, the residents' private and shared living spaces feel more 'homey', in part because central nursing stations and other visual cues that define an environment for illness and death—instead of one for living—are visually remote. Second, the centralized back-of-house limits the need for outsourcing of services, such as laundry and catering, which can be dangerous vectors for infectious diseases.

Scale is not the only aspect of nursing homes that should be challenged; autonomy is of equal importance. Although a need for help in daily living tasks is the *raison d'être* for placing an elderly person into a long-term care facility, the organization and design of the home should promote a level of independence for its residents. This autonomy is contingent on the ability of the residents to orient themselves in their environment. In consequence, particular attention should be paid to the design of wayfinding.

The architecture should present choices in an intuitive way. For example, accessible outdoor spaces should be visible from the corridors, shared rooms and private spaces so the residents know they have the option of being outdoors without having to remember the path. Architectural clarity can promote greater freedom of choice for residents.

Autonomy is a complex issue in nursing homes, since wandering is often seen as a problem to be controlled. It is addressed in part with contemporary technological solutions. Wearable devices orchestrate a more fluid access system, better monitoring residents to reduce frustration engendered by locked doors. The Hogeweyk village, discussed later, provides a different approach to controlling wandering.

Design that encourages residents to participate in daily tasks such as caring for houseplants, opening windows or preparation of food stimulates cognition and a consequent sense of autonomy. For example, a small accessible kitchenette, now a requirement in Swedish long-term care facilities, is instrumental in creating a high level of satisfaction for the residents.

Location, Location, Location

The importance of locating nursing homes within urban centres, as opposed to suburban locations, can be extrapolated from the sections of this chapter that target more autonomous sectors of the aging population. Pedestrian access to community life such as markets, shops and cafés is not only instrumental in giving the residents some semblance of belonging in the city, but it also greatly encourages volunteer participation. It incentivizes natural caregivers, such as a family member, to be more present since they can combine a visit to the nursing home with errands or leisure outside the home.

The Natural World

Integrating landscape design into the urban nursing home is fundamentally important. In the present awakening about sustainability principles, we may be seduced into believing that previous generations of architects and landscape architects did not value the benefits of the natural world in the same way that we do now. Nineteenth-century examples of hospitals set amidst greenery are easy to find. In 1956, under the approval of the American Institute of Architects, an international design competition was launched for the design of a home for older people. The chairman of the jury was Pietro Belluschi, Dean of the School of Architecture and Planning at MIT. All of the winning entries are of note for their landscaping design, grouping the residential units around lushly planted exterior courts. Some were for the exclusive use of the residents within the unit; others were larger and designed as common facilities. Some were designed for games, others as 'quiet gardens'. The variety and the proximity of these proposed green spaces to the living quarters is striking, even 65 years later.

As hospitals and care institutions developed through the last quarter of the 20th century, funding favoured the design philosophy of highly efficient, highly technological buildings. The natural world, if not banished, was marginalized from these ultra-modern 'healthcare machines'.[23]

In recent decades, a great deal of research has been funded in part by HMOs to make the proof that gazing at a garden, or being in one, accelerates the healing process, by reducing stress, mental fatigue and even pain.[24] These findings can be of use in discussing environments for those aging. As Susan Rodiek of Texas A&M summarized her research in a *Scientific American* article titled "Nature That Nurtures", "Older people need and benefit from outdoor space and greenery just as much as the young".[25] The enjoyment of plantings does not have to be passive; the opportunity to work in the garden, albeit with modifications for physical limitations, can provide welcome activity and a sense of accomplishment.

Dementia Villages

In 2009, a new nursing home paradigm for seniors with severe neuro-cognitive disorders opened in the town of Weesp, in the Netherlands, outside of Amsterdam. Brainchild of a team of local care administrators, including Jannette Spiering and Yvonne van Amerongen, the 'Hogeweyk' has revolutionized thinking about the care of the older adult with dementia, spawning 'Dementia Villages' across Europe, Britain and North America. Although not the most attractive and positive name for this type of residence, we nevertheless retain it as it is best recognized this way.

The Hogeweyk complex, designed by the Dutch architects Molenaar & Bol & vanDillen,[26] offers the perception of a residential neighbourhood with a grocery store, a pub, restaurant and theatre. Residents are assigned to a specific house, according to their cultural background, interests or religious beliefs. The architecture of each house reflects these differences. Residents each have their own room; they share common cooking and lounging facilities. The interior design is deliberately non-institutional, resembling conventional taste in Holland during the 1950s–1970s.

Access to greenery is close at hand. Each house has access to terraces, courtyards and within easy walking distance, the 'town square', where there is a fountain, as part of the landscape design. The water feature provides cooling in the summer, calming sounds and a focal point for gathering and socializing. Residents are free to roam the site and take advantage of the various services; they just cannot leave the gated confines of the managed reality.

The concept supports unique needs, lifestyles and personal preferences. Living in The Hogeweyk puts boredom, loneliness and hopelessness in another perspective. It focusses on possibilities, not on disabilities. And it goes without saying that this is all supported by trained professionals.[27]

A lynchpin of the Hogeweyk is the use of reminiscence therapy (RT),[28] which seeks to promote an environment that is comforting in its familiarity, thereby both reassuring the resident and providing opportunities to interact through well-remembered tasks or memories. "Reminiscence therapy can be a powerful tool for dementia patients", says Dr. Peter Whitehouse, professor of neurology and neuroscience at Case Western Reserve University and president of the Intergenerational Schools International. "It makes those with Alzheimer's more content and happier because they return to a time in their lives when there was no perceived failure—a time when their memory was intact and they did not feel lost."

While contemporary in its form and materials, the brick architecture is designed to be reassuringly familiar, minimally institutional and at a human scale of two storeys. Food shopping (without payment) encourages a sense of autonomy. Residents can choose when they want to go to the theatre and restaurant. These amenities are also available to patrons from the surrounding residential neighbourhood. The additional income helps to offset the operational costs, which are comparable to other European facilities and are in line with current for-profit North American costs.

Similar to the Maison des aînés described earlier, but at the scale of a neighbourhood, the Dementia Village minimizes its healthcare nature; nurses and other staff are dressed in street clothes, not in hospital uniforms. As noted, residents can roam about the complex. However, there are limitations. Pieter Sijpkes, a professor at the McGill University School of Architecture, is originally from the Netherlands. In speaking of Hogeweyk, where one of his relatives now lives, he was generally enthusiastic. However, he remarked sadly, "As we were leaving, my relative walked us to the gate, and said that we could leave now, but that she could go no further".[29] The purported freedom inevitably confronts certain realities of care.

Dementia Villages are becoming popular, at least in the western hemisphere. If each society builds to reflect its values and interests, it is not surprising that the most surreal examples, where fantasy overtakes reality, are being built in the United States. These designs, where normalization veers towards deception, raise ethical dilemmas for some scholars and researchers. Critiques abound with references to Disneyland or to the movie, *The Truman Show*. Given the level of some critics' disquiet, it is surprising that the British dystopian television show from the 1960s, *The Prisoner*, is not cited as well. Annmarie Adams and Sally Chiver's essay, "Deception and Design: The Rise of the Dementia Village", presents an ambivalent analysis of both Hogeweyk and its imitators.

In its 2009 annual report, the Nuffield Council on Bioethics in London, England, wrote that distracting or at worst deceiving patients with dementia "serves to undermine the remaining grip the person with dementia may have on the everyday world".[30] This concern may be worth considering for some of the destinations marketed as 'dementia villages' in the United States, which have been set up as day centres. In this situation, the patient with dementia is transported back and forth from a recreated past to a very different present, on a possibly daily basis.

However, other experts are much more positive about the use of illusion. Larissa MacFarquhar presents a very nuanced reflection about the dementia village typology in her 2018 *New Yorker* essay, titled "The Comforting Fictions of Dementia Care".[31] Tamblyn Watts reminded us that many types of buildings are designed to fool or deflect or minimize interaction. For example, she said, hotels do not highlight the doors leading to the back-of-house facilities, because the visitor is not allowed access to those rooms. What is the fundamental difference then, in a disguising a door that a resident cannot leave through on their own as a bookcase? Is it better if the door with its locks and institutional hardware is constantly visible but never operable? "The idea is not to fool the resident, but to accommodate them, and to provide them with a sense of control and dignity."[32]

Dementia comes with many faces. If the dementia village provides a sense of comfort and control to some, then it represents a viable typology. Residents seem more engaged and less passive than in more conventional nursing homes. They interact more with their immediate environment and go out with supervision into the larger world. As stated in 1959, "The greatest possible participation in life is important to the well-being of the elderly".[33] That is still true today.

The Maison des aînés is clearly integrating some of the principles of Hogeweyk that relate to de-institutionalizing its architecture and to "building better, not bigger".[34] These are good first steps and ones that bear repeating across North America.

Recommendations

The following recommendations apply to private citizens, to administrators of care homes, to government policy makers, to urban planners and to architects. They are offered in the hope that they can contribute to the transformative change that CanAge is advocating.

National Standards

Implement national standards of care. This seems obvious, but the pandemic has exposed how variable and dangerously idiosyncratic standards of care are.

Tax Incentives

Review taxation programs to facilitate aging in place. As examples, CanAge has advocated for pension program reform; municipalities could review tax-incentive programs to encourage central locations for communal housing; increases in funding of government programs that pay for universal accessibility upgrades should be considered.

Intergenerational Living

Less than 15% of Canadian homes are intergenerational. Be more open to innovations that mix generations within the housing stock and accommodate different needs in the architectural resolution; consider the adoption of Universal Design as a basic standard moving forward.

Zoning

Encourage municipalities to change zoning laws to allow accessory dwelling units (ADUs). ADUs, sometimes called granny flats or lane-way houses, are small dwellings, such as mews or coach-houses, which can be built at the rear of a property or on a lane. They permit the older adult to downsize, freeing up their existing house for the next generation. Sixty percent of Americans would consider moving into ADUs to have better proximity to their family, access to services and reduced costs.[35] Inspiration should be drawn from California Health and Safety Code's new January 2021 legislation that requires that cities and counties develop a plan that incentivizes and promotes the creation of ADUs.[36]

Living Communities

Urban land use planning tools should be used to promote the integration of housing for older adults into the fabric of surrounding neighbourhoods.

New Technologies

Embrace the use of technology in the care of the older person. This does not have to be a passive activity, monitored solely by caregivers. In a 2017 white paper, titled *A Dignified Elderly Care in Denmark*,[37] Healthcare Denmark describes a number of devices that older adults can use to monitor their health and safety. The pandemic highlighted the need to provide high speed and widespread internet connectivity into nursing homes.

Diversity

As noted earlier, the needs of certain groups are not being addressed, although advocacy has been more vocal in recent years. The LGTBQ+ community has raised issues about isolation and discrimination that need to be mitigated. Indigenous populations have histories and experiences that may not dovetail well into conventional approaches. For example, there is concern that Indigenous elders, already suffering from residential school abuse, may be retraumatized by dementia villages that focus on recreating an earlier time in the resident's life, such as their childhood. This is similar to the experiences of some Holocaust survivors.

Staffing and Volunteers

The special report by Quebec's Citizen's Protection Agency highlights the chronic staffing shortages in nursing homes as one of the root causes of the magnitude of the crisis in long-term care homes during the first wave of the pandemic.[38] Nursing homes should be designed to attract and retain qualified professionals. Design decisions should consider not only the needs of the residents, but those of paid and unpaid laborers as well. The forced absence of family caregivers during Spring 2020 proved that the contribution of volunteers is essential; future homes should reflect this reality and plan for their presence.

Sustainability and the Natural World

Embrace design ideas that incorporate sustainability principles and encourage frequent interaction with the natural world. The Hogeweyk commitment to landscape integration is admirable, as are the efforts made to facilitate gardening, through the inclusion of waist-high planters. Franklin, in the *Scientific American* article, provides a checklist of seven design concepts that should be followed for a successful garden for aging adults. They include paying attention to the design of sculptural elements; ensuring that there is a significant percentage of greenery; planting trees that can mature in size, not only to provide shade, but to encourage bird life; and finally designing easy access into the garden and pathways through the garden that accommodate the less mobile and those with lesser vision.

LAST WORDS

Finally, as architects, we leave the last words to two of the authors of *Planning Homes for the Aged*. Edwin B. Morris Jr., Assistant to the Director, AIA, wrote a call to arms that continues to resonate today:

> The architect who enters this new field is faced with a tremendous challenge and a public obligation. An immense amount of research, hard work, common sense, and good thinking must be applied to the job. The home for the aged presents an unparalleled opportunity for architects to do something for the public good, to enhance their own professional stature, and to elevate the architectural profession. But even more important is the contribution they can make to the health, welfare and happiness of older people.[39]

We live in an exciting time, when, confronted by the horrible truths exposed by Covid, there is a palpable desire for change. There are several examples—the Maison des Babayagas, the Dementia Village—that demonstrate that unconventional and rather remarkable responses can be built and supported by the larger community. There are choices now for more dignified, more engaged aging, no matter what the level of autonomy, and we all—architects, administrators, medical practitioners, ethicists, caregivers, politicians and most importantly, older adults—should be collaborating towards innovative designs that challenge the status quo.

However, as we all strive for technological excellence, we must not forget that architectural solutions should also be aesthetically pleasing, worthy of being *homes* in the best sense of the word. As Edward Noakes, AIA, who became a leading proponent of universally accessible architecture, wrote in 1959:

> A well-designed home is a source of pride and affection. A building designed by a mediocre or flashy talent rapidly becomes a source of boredom, if not ridicule. Without beauty, a home for the aged can be no more than an institution for sheltered care; it certainly cannot be a home.[40]

NOTES

1 This statistic is of March 2021. St-Onge, P., & Shaw, M. L. (2021, April 8). *Quebec's Covid-19 LTC disaster: Up to 6,700 lives could have been saved: Montreal Economic Institute.*—IEDM/MEI. Retrieved January 27, 2022, from https://www.iedm.org/quebecs-covid-19-ltc-disaster-up-to-6700-lives-could-have-been-saved/.

2 OECD is an acronym for Organization for Economic Cooperation and Development.

3 CIHI. (2020, June 25). *Long-Term Care and Covid-19: International comparisons.* CIHI. Retrieved January 27, 2022, from https://www.cihi.ca/en/long-term-care-and-covid-19-international-comparisons.

4 McCullough, J. J. (2021, April 6). *Opinion: Canada has failed nursing home residents during the pandemic.* The Washington Post. Retrieved January 27, 2022, from https://www.washingtonpost.com/opinions/2021/04/06/canada-covid-deaths-long-term-care-nursing-homes/.

5 Mathiasen, G., & Noakes, E. H. (1959). In *Planning homes for the aged* (p. 4), F.W. Dodge Corporation.

6 Ibid.

7 Stockwell-Smith, G. (2022). *The role of risk in the acute care of older adults.* IPA. Retrieved January 27, 2022, from https://www.ipa-online.org/news-and-issues/role-of-risk.

8 Ibid.

9 Sagan, A. (2015, May 4). *Dementia villages: Is getting patients to believe a false reality OK?* | *CBC news.* CBCnews. Retrieved January 27, 2022, from https://www.cbc.ca/news/health/canada-s-version-of-hogewey-dementia-village-recreates-normal-life-1.3001258.

10 Mathiasen, G., & Noakes, E. H. (1959). In *Planning homes for the aged* (p. 4), F.W. Dodge Corporation.

11 Davis, M. R. (2021, November 18). *New AARP survey reveals older adults want to age in place.* AARP. Retrieved January 27, 2022, from https://www.aarp.org/home-family/your-home/info-2021/home-and-community-preferences-survey.html.

12 *Global age-friendly cities: A guide.* WHO. (2007). Retrieved January 27, 2022, from https://www.who.int/ageing/publications/Global_age_friendly_cities_Guide_English.pdf?ua=1.

13 Prairie Sky Cohousing. (n.d.). Retrieved January 27, 2022, from https://prairieskycohousing.wordpress.com/.

14 Maison des babayagas translates as House of the Baba Yagas. Baba yaga is an Eastern European term meaning 'witch'. Usually a baba yaga's house is a log structure elevated on 'chicken legs', stilts that the house to relocate at the whim of the baba yaga.

15 Abbit, L. (2016, March 6). *Urban cohousing the babayaga way.* Senior Planet. Retrieved January 27, 2022, from https://seniorplanet.org/senior-housing-alternatives-urban-cohousing-the-babayaga-way/.

16 *Feminist Retirement Home in Paris celebrates aging with the message "Growing old is not an illness".* GirlTalkHQ. (2017, June 21). Retrieved January 27, 2022, from https://www.girltalkhq.com/feminist-retirement-home-in-paris-celebrates-aging-with-the-message-growing-old-is-not-an-illness/.

17 In Quebec, these centres are referred to with the acronym CHSLD, which stands for *centre d'hébergement et de soins de longue durée,* or a long-term care and residential centre. In this text, we refer to long-term care centres; the residential aspect is implied. Another commonly understood term for this typology is nursing home.

18 Armstrong, P., & Braedley, S. (2016). *Physical environments for long-term care: Ideas worth sharing.* Canadian Centre for Policy Alternatives.

19 Feddersen, E., & Lüdtke Insa. (2014). *Lost in Space.* Birkhäuser Basel.

20 The English translation would be: Seniors' Home—Alternative Pavilion.

21 A key departure from the traditional model of the CHSLD is the separation of elders that require long-term assistance due to neuro-cognitive disorders—to reside now in a Maison des aînés—from other residents housed in Pavillons alternatifs.

22 Gouvernement du Québec, Ministère de la santé et des services sociaux. (2019). *Maison des aînés et pavillon alternatif—Document Cadre.* Direction des projets immobiliers.

23 Ulrich, R. S. (2002). *Health benefits of gardens in hospitals.* Green Plants for Green Buildings. Retrieved January 27, 2022, from https://greenplantsforgreenbuildings.org/wp-content/uploads/2014/01/HealthSettingsUlrich.pdf.

24 Franklin, D. (2012, March 1). *How hospital gardens help patients heal.* Scientific American. Retrieved January 27, 2022, from https://www.scientificamerican.com/article/nature-that-nurtures/

25 Ibid, Franklin.

26 Rupprecht, I. (2012, September 9). *Dementia Village 'de hogeweyk' in Weesp.* Detail. Retrieved January 27, 2022, from https://www.detail-online.com/article/dementia-village-de-hogeweyk-in-weesp-16433/.

27 *The Hogeweyk dementia village ~ care concept.* The Hogeweyk Dementia Village ~ Care concept. (n.d.). Retrieved January 27, 2022, from https://hogeweyk.dementiavillage.com/.

28 Reminiscence therapy is also associated with the creation of memory boxes, the construction of memory walls outside patient rooms and the playing of familiar music and songs.

29 Conversation between Pieter Sijpkes and Julia Gersovitz, at his home, 2021.

30 Sagan, A. (2015, May 4). *Dementia villages: Is getting patients to believe a false reality OK? | CBC news.* CBCnews. Retrieved January 27, 2022, from https://www.cbc.ca/news/health/canada-s-version-of-hogewey-dementia-village-recreates-normal-life-1.3001258.

31 MacFarquhar, L. (2018, October 1). *The comforting fictions of dementia care.* The New Yorker. Retrieved January 27, 2022, from https://www.newyorker.com/magazine/2018/10/08/the-comforting-fictions-of-dementia-care.

32 Laura Tamblyn Watts in a Zoom discussion with Julia Gersovitz and Boris Morin-Defoy, October 29, 2021.

33 Mathiasen, G., & Noakes, E. H. (1959). In *Planning homes for the aged* (p. 5), F.W. Dodge Corporation.

34 Laura Tamblyn Watts in a Zoom discussion with Julia Gersovitz and Boris Morin-Defoy, October 29, 2021.

35 *Canada homeShare.* Canada HomeShare. (n.d.). Retrieved January 27, 2022, from https://www.canadahomeshare.com/.

36 California Department of Housing and Community Development—HCD (n.d.). *Accessory dwelling units (ADUs) and junior accessory dwelling units (JADUs).* Accessory Dwelling Units (ADUs). Retrieved January 27, 2022, from https://www.hcd.ca.gov/policy-research/accessorydwellingunits.shtml.

37 *A dignified elderly care in Denmark.* Healthcare Denmark. (2019, September). Retrieved January 27, 2022, from https://www.healthcaredenmark.dk/media/plvbj4yz/elderly-care-v10919.pdf.

38 Rinfret, M. (2021). *Rapport Spécial Du Protecteur Du Citoyen.* Bibliothèque et Archives nationales du Québec.

39 Mathiasen, G., & Noakes, E. H. (1959). In *Planning homes for the aged* (p. 69), F.W. Dodge Corporation.

40 Mathiasen, G., & Noakes, E. H. (1959). In *Planning homes for the aged* (p. 64), F.W. Dodge Corporation.

ADDITIONAL READING

Abbit, L. (2016, March 6). *Urban cohousing the babayaga way.* Senior Planet. Retrieved January 27, 2022, from https://seniorplanet.org/senior-housing-alternatives-urban-cohousing-the-babayaga-way/

Anthes, E. (2021). *The great indoors: The surprising science of how buildings shape our behavior, health, and happiness.* Scientific American/Picador.

Armstrong, P., & Braedley, S. (2016). *Physical Environments for Long-term Care: Ideas Worth Sharing.* Canadian Centre for Policy Alternatives.

Baba Yaga. Foundation for Intentional Community. (2021, April 14). Retrieved January 27, 2022, from https://www.ic.org/directory/baba-yaga/.

California Department of Housing and Community Development—HCD. (n.d.). *Accessory dwelling units (ADUs) and junior accessory dwelling units (JADUs).* Accessory Dwelling Units (ADUs). Retrieved January 27, 2022, from https://www.hcd.ca.gov/policy-research/accessorydwellingunits.shtml.

Canada homeshare. Canada HomeShare. (n.d.). Retrieved January 27, 2022, from https://www.canadahomeshare.com/.

CIHI. (2020, June 25). *Long-Term Care and Covid-19: International comparisons.* CIHI. Retrieved January 27, 2022, from https://www.cihi.ca/en/long-term-care-and-covid-19-international-comparisons.

Davis, M. (2021, November 18). *New AARP survey reveals older adults want to age in place.* AARP. Retrieved January 27, 2022, from https://www.aarp.org/home-family/your-home/info-2021/home-and-community-preferences-survey.html

A dignified elderly care in Denmark. Healthcare Denmark. (2019, September). Retrieved January 27, 2022, from https://www.healthcaredenmark.dk/media/plvbj4yz/elderly-care-v10919.pdf.

Feddersen, E., & Lüdtke Insa. (2014). *Lost in Space.* Birkhäuser Basel.

Feminist Retirement Home in Paris celebrates aging with the message "Growing old is not an illness". GirlTalkHQ. (2017, June 21). Retrieved January 27, 2022, from https://www.girltalkhq.com/feminist-retirement-home-in-paris-celebrates-aging-with-the-message-growing-old-is-not-an-illness/.

Franklin, D. (2012, March 1). *How hospital gardens help patients heal.* Scientific American. Retrieved January 27, 2022, from https://www.scientificamerican.com/article/nature-that-nurtures/.

Global age-friendly cities: A guide. WHO. (2007). Retrieved January 27, 2022, from https://www.who.int/ageing/publications/Global_age_friendly_cities_Guide_English.pdf?ua=1.

Gouvernement du Québec, Ministère de la santé et des services sociaux. (2019). *Maison des aînés et pavillon alternatif—Document Cadre.* Direction des projets immobiliers.

The Hogeweyk dementia village ~ care concept. The Hogeweyk Dementia Village ~ Care concept. (n.d.). Retrieved January 27, 2022, from https://hogeweyk.dementiavillage.com/.

Lange, A. (2018). *The design of childhood: How the material world shapes independent kids.* Bloomsbury Publishing.

MacFarquhar, L. (2018, October 1). *The comforting fictions of dementia care.* The New Yorker. Retrieved January 27, 2022, from https://www.newyorker.com/magazine/2018/10/08/the-comforting-fictions-of-dementia-care.

Mathiasen, G., & Noakes, E. H. (1959). In *Planning homes for the aged* (p. 4). essay, F.W. Dodge Corporation.

McCullough, J. J. (2021, April 6). *Opinion: Canada has failed nursing home residents during the pandemic.* The Washington Post. Retrieved January 27, 2022, from https://www.washingtonpost.com/opinions/2021/04/06/canada-covid-deaths-long-term-care-nursing-homes/.

Prairie Sky Cohousing. (n.d.). Retrieved January 27, 2022, from https://prairieskycohousing.wordpress.com/.

Rinfret, M. (2021). *Rapport Spécial Du Protecteur Du Citoyen.* Bibliothèque et Archives nationales du Québec.

Rupprecht, I. (2012, September 9). *Dementia Village 'de hogeweyk' in Weesp.* Detail. Retrieved January 27, 2022, from https://www.detail-online.com/article/dementia-village-de-hogeweyk-in-weesp-16433/.

Sagan, A. (2015, May 4). *Dementia villages: Is getting patients to believe a false reality OK? | CBC news.* CBCnews. Retrieved January 27, 2022, from https://www.cbc.ca/news/health/canada-s-version-of-hogewey-dementia-village-recreates-normal-life-1.3001258.

St-Onge, P., & Shaw, M. L. (2021, April 8). *Quebec's Covid-19 LTC disaster: Up to 6,700 lives could have been saved: Montreal Economic Institute.—IEDM/MEI.* Retrieved January 27, 2022, from https://www.iedm.org/quebecs-covid-19-ltc-disaster-up-to-6700-lives-could-have-been-saved/.

Stockwell-Smith, G. (2022). *The role of risk in the acute care of older adults.* IPA. Retrieved January 27, 2022, from https://www.ipa-online.org/news-and-issues/role-of-risk.

Ulrich, R. S. (2002). *Health benefits of gardens in hospitals.* Green Plants for Green Buildings. Retrieved January 27, 2022, from https://greenplantsforgreenbuildings.org/wp-content/uploads/2014/01/HealthSettingsUlrich.pdf.

14 Are the Immunizations of My Patient up to Date?

Dominique Tessier, MD, CCFP, FCFP, FISTM

CONTENTS

CLINICAL VIGNETTE

Jeannette and Andrew are both 75 years old. Jeannette is healthy, but her strength has been put to a test in recent months as her husband was hospitalized on several occasions. Andrew was admitted 6 months ago with a diagnosis of myocarditis secondary to acute influenza. He was re-admitted to intensive care after contracting an invasive pneumococcal infection. After weeks of hospitalizations, 10 days after being back home, shingles appeared on his right chest. He still suffers from post-herpetic neuralgia. As he says, "he permanently lost something" and does not feel he will ever be the same. Jeannette would like to know if anything could be done to prevent her from going through what Andrew suffered. She is concerned with the fact she needs to remain healthy to care for her deteriorated husband.

WHY ARE IMMUNIZATIONS IMPORTANT?

Immunization programs are hailed as one of the greatest achievements in medicine. They saved more Canadian lives over the last 50 years than any other health intervention. Still, every year, up to 50,000 people will die in North America alone due to vaccine-preventable diseases. Influenza and invasive Streptococcus pneumoniae are responsible for most of the deaths.

The frequency and severity of infectious diseases increase with old age. Infections carry a substantial risk of illness, loss of independence, disability, and death in elderly persons. Unfortunately, immunization rates are relatively low, rarely above 50% in older adults, including in very high-risk groups. These infections are leading causes of catastrophic disability in older adults. In Canada, there are also significant differences in immunization rates between different ethnic and racial groups.

HIGH-RISK GROUPS

Many risk factors increase the rates and severity of complications and deaths in the older adult. With increasing age, even in people active and fit, the immune system undergoes characteristic changes, termed immunosenescence, which lead to increased incidence and severity of infectious diseases. Unfortunately, it is also responsible for insufficient protection following vaccination. Therefore, some vaccines are specifically designed for older adults and others are contraindicated. Without any other risk factor, this immunosenescence is responsible for hospitalizations with prolonged stay, and death.

Regarding vaccination against the SARS-CoV-2 virus that causes COVID-19 disease, see Chapter 17, COVID-19 in Long-Term Care.

WHAT ARE THE RISK FACTORS THAT SHOULD ALERT YOU TO RECOMMEND IMMUNIZATIONS?

- Travel: influenza with a yearlong risk around the equator line, yellow fever, Japanese encephalitis, typhoid, enterotoxigenic Escherichia coli (ETEC), cholera, etc.

DOI: 10.1201/9781003344476-16

- Cardio-vascular and ischemic diseases.

- Diabetes.

- Immunologic disturbances including HIV and cancer, use of medications affecting the immune system.

- Mobility restrictions and activity limitations in daily life.

- Chronic respiratory conditions.

- Lifestyle: alcoholism, illicit drug use, smoking, inactivity, being homeless.

The combination of chronic medical conditions can significantly affect the risk of complications and deaths related to vaccine preventable diseases.

VACCINE RECOMMENDATIONS

Influenza

Each year influenza is believed to infect 10–20% of the population. The highest risk of mortality occurs in patients > 65 years of age and those with underlying conditions. Annual vaccination is recommended in most provinces and states.

Direct and indirect potential complications of influenza include bronchitis and pneumonia, asthma and COPD exacerbations, ear and sinus complications, acute myocardial infarction, ischemic heart disease and cerebrovascular diseases, and exacerbation of renal disorder and diabetes.

At the individual level, the Centers for Disease Control and Prevention (CDC) and the National Advisory Committee on Immunization—Canada (NACI) recommends that high-dose trivalent influenza vaccine (HD-TIV) should be offered over standard-dose TIV to persons 65 years of age and older. NACI concludes that, given the burden of disease associated with influenza A (H3N2) and the good evidence of better efficacy compared to standard-dose TIV in this age group, HD-TIV should be offered over SD-TIV to persons 65 years of age and older (Grade A). There is insufficient evidence to make comparative recommendations on the use of MF59-adjuvanted TIV and QIV over standard-dose TIV (Grade I). HD-TIV is covered by Public Health programs in some provinces.

Diphtheria-Tetanus-Pertussis

In most provinces and territories in Canada as well as in USA, a tetanus and diphtheria (reduced toxoid) vaccine (TD) is recommended every ten years. Pertussis in adults is not common but complications include sleep disturbance, rib fractures, subconjunctival hemorrhages, rectal prolapse, and urinary incontinence, all from intense and persistent coughing. One booster dose per adult lifetime (and one at each pregnancy) of acellular pertussis-containing vaccines is recommended. In the USA and Canada, pertussis vaccine for adult use is only available as an acellular preparation in a combination vaccine (Adacel®, Boostrix®).

Pneumococcal Infections

Polysaccharides vaccine programs in Canada and USA (PP-23) are targeted at reducing the risk of invasive pneumococcal diseases, not pneumonia. The immune response is very different with the conjugated vaccine (PC-13), which induces a stronger and longer lasting secondary immune response. PC-13 have been demonstrated to prevent community-acquired pneumonia and invasive pneumococcal infection. To allow for the best immune response, PC-13 should be administered 8 weeks prior to PP-23. If PP-23 was administered first, wait one year before administering PC-13.

Shingles

Any person who has had varicella is at risk of developing Herpes Zoster (HZ). However, HZ occurs most frequently among older adults and immunocompromised persons. Age is the most important risk factor with two-thirds of the cases occurring in individuals over 50 years of age. The severity of illness associated with HZ and its complications also increases markedly with age. Up to 10% of persons over 65 years of age will be admitted to hospital with an episode of HZ.

HZ infection is characterized by pain and a unilateral vesicular eruption, usually in a single dermatome. The most frequent complication of acute HZ is post-herpetic neuralgia (PHN) which is characterized by prolonged and often debilitating neurogenic pain that lasts for more than 90 days from the onset of rash. Because treatment options for PHN are of limited effectiveness, PHN often has major adverse impacts on quality of life. Older adults, people living with chronic conditions such as diabetes or autoimmune diseases, and persons who are immunocompromised may be at greater risk of developing PHN. They are also at risk of experiencing longer lasting HZ rash than the general population. Other potential complications of HZ include ophthalmic sequelae (Herpes Zoster ophthalmicus), central nervous system infection, nerve palsies including the Ramsay-Hunt Syndrome, neuromuscular disease including Guillain-Barré Syndrome, pneumonia, hepatitis, and secondary bacterial infections.

Two different HZ vaccines are currently used in Canada: Zostavax II® (Live Zoster Vaccine, LZV), and Shingrix® (Recombinant Zoster Vaccine, RZV, or sub-unit adjuvanted Zoster vaccine, SU-Z). All individuals ≥ 50 years of age without contraindications should receive HZ vaccine, preferably RZV. LZV is contraindicated in those with immunosuppression. In the USA, the CDC recommends that healthy adults 50 years and older get two doses of Shingrix®, 2 to 6 months apart.

WHAT ARE THE RESOURCES FOR IMMUNIZATIONS?

Most guidelines propose tables and immunization calendars for adults that will generally cover vaccines offered in Public Health programs. It is important to refer to your provincial or state health authority for vaccine coverage. The primary objective of provincial immunization programs for adults is to reduce hospitalizations and deaths associated with vaccine-preventable diseases.

Health care providers' goal should be to prevent morbidity and mortality at an individual level.

For vaccines not covered by a Public Health program, a prescription will be required to insure reimbursement for those with insurance coverage or to receive a proper receipt for an income tax deduction related to medical care costs.

Tables 14.1 and 14.2 includes all the vaccines recommended, including those at the expense of the patient.

ANTIBODY LEVELS

Rarely, it will be necessary to do a serology to verify if a patient is protected against vaccine-preventable diseases. Hepatitis B seroprotection is defined as anti-HBs titer of ≥10 IU/L. In adults, the immune response can be affected negatively by immunosuppression, in chronic conditions such as chronic kidney disease, among individuals with diabetes. For immunocompromised individuals, initial annual monitoring of HB antibody levels following HB immunization may be considered.

For yellow fever, for those previously immunized who are at very high risk or for whom a booster dose is recommended, measured neutralizing antibody titer to yellow fever virus can confirm ongoing protection and prevent the need for a booster.

For rabies, in both pre-exposure prophylaxis and post-exposure prophylaxis, a post-vaccination serology 2 to 4 weeks after the last dose should be considered if the person vaccinated is considered immunocompromised.

RESOLUTION OF THE CLINICAL VIGNETTE

Immunization is one of the greatest success stories in medical history. It has improved the lives of every Canadian and American and has saved more lives than any other health intervention. We have seen many diseases such as diphtheria, mumps, measles, and rubella drop by over 99% with the introduction and integration of a vaccine into the immunization program. In older adults, immunization is a powerful tool to protect a vulnerable person from severe infections and their complications.

■ Vaccinations provide efficient protection from infectious diseases.

■ Age-related changes in the immune system may hamper successful vaccination.

■ Vaccines tailored to the needs of the aging immune system will have to be developed.

■ Vaccination schedules will have to be adapted to improve protection in elderly persons.

For this particular couple, each member should have annual influenza vaccination with HD-TIV, and once in their lifetime a pneumococcal vaccine with PC-13 administered 8 weeks prior to PP-23, a shingle vaccination with Shingrix®, and a Boostrix ® vaccine against diphtheria-tetanus-pertussis infections.

Older adults are predisposed to complications from vaccine-preventable diseases due to intrinsic as well as exogenous causes. Aging is associated with a decrease in the efficacity of the immune

Table 14.1 Vaccines for Older Adults

Disease	Vaccines/Administration	Comments
Hepatitis A	Havrix® Vaqta® Avaxim® Combined with hepatitis B: Twinrix Combined with typhoid: Vivaxim Two intramuscular doses: 0 and 6 months	Vaccinate: MSM; users of illicit drugs orally, by inhalation or by injection under unhygienic conditions; inmates in correctional facilities under provincial jurisdiction; people in communities with outbreaks of hepatitis A (e.g., the Hasidic community) or whe hepatitis A is endemic; residential contacts of an adopted chil who has arrived since less than three months and comes from country where hepatitis A is endemic; chronic liver disease; planned travel and stay in endemic areas; some workers.
Hepatitis B:	Engerix®-B (20 µg/ml HBsAg) Recombivax HB® (40 µg/ml HBsAg) Combined with hepatitis A: Twinrix® Three intramuscular doses: 0, 1, and 6 months	Administer 40 µg per dose for vaccination of immunosuppress persons. The dosage of anti-HBs is recommended between 1 and 2 mon after the last dose to check the immune response. The combined vaccine for hepatitis A and Twinrix® hepatitis B (GSK) is not recommended for vaccination of immunosuppre patients. Use monovalent vaccines.
Human Papillomavirus	HPV2: Cervarix® HPV4: Gardasil® HPV9: Gardasil® 9 Three intramuscular doses: 0, 2, and 6 months	HPV vaccines may be administered to women over 45 years o and men 27 years of age and older who are at ongoing risk o exposure to HPV. MSM have a disproportionately high burden of HPV infectior The vaccine can be given even if the person has already had a HPV infection or an HPV infection-related lesion (e.g., condy or abnormal screening test) since the acquired immunity is s (type-specific).
Influenza	Standard dose (SD) trivalent and quadrivalent High-dose trivalent influenza vaccine (HD-TIV) Annually	The quadrivalent live attenuated influenza vaccine (Flumist Quadrivalent) is a live attenuated, reassortant vaccine and is contraindicated in immunosuppressed persons. NACI recommends that high-dose trivalent influenza vaccine (HD-TIV) should be offered over standard-dose TIV to pers years of age and older.
Pneumococcal	PC13: Prevnar 13® (conjugated) PP23: Pneumovax® 23 (polysaccharide) One dose PC13 followed 8 weeks later or more by 1 dose PP23 1 booster dose of PP23 at ≥ 65 (minimum 5 years interval)	Wherever possible, the conjugate vaccine (PC13) should be administered first with a minimum of 8 weeks of polysacch vaccine. If the PP23 was administered first, wait 1 year before adminis the PC13.
Shingles	Recombinant Zoster Vaccine, RZV, or sub-unit vaccine: Shingrix® Live Zoster Vaccine, LZV: Zostavax II® RZV: 2 doses at a recommended interval of 2 months Minimum 4 weeks LZV: 1 dose	RZV: Vaccinate all people aged 50 or over. Preferential use of the RZV over LZV. A person can be vaccinated against shingles regardless of the history of chicken pox, shingles, or varicella vaccination. People with a history of ophthalmic zoster with ocular invol may be vaccinated 12 months or more after the start of the episode if at least 6 months have elapsed since the end of t active treatment. LZV should be used only if RZV is not available or contrain
Tetanus-Diphtheria-Pertussis	Adacel® (dcaT) Boostrix® (dcaT) dT (dT) Booster: 1 dose (dT) every 10 years. Administer at least one dose of vaccine containing the pertussis component in adult life.	People who need a primary vaccination should receive one the Tdap (or Tdap-Polio) vaccine and two doses of the Td Td-Polio) vaccine. In exceptional circumstances (for example, a long stay in a where access to health care is limited), another reminder m given if more than five years have elapsed since the last d Adults should be given a dose of Tdap without adhering usual interval since administering a dose of Td vaccine.

Table 14.2 Vaccines for Travelers

Disease	Vaccines/Administration	Comments
Cholera-ETEC	Dukoral 2 doses orally, 1–6 weeks apart Booster: 1 dose every 3 months (ETEC) or 1 dose every 2 years (cholera)	May be considered for prevention of travelers' diarrhea in persons with chronic illnesses such as chronic renal failure, congestive heart failure, insulin-dependent diabetes mellitus, and inflammatory bowel disease, for whom there is an increased risk of serious consequences from travelers' diarrhea. If more than 5 years have passed since primary immunization or last booster dose, repeat primary series.
Japanese encephalitis	Ixiaro 2 doses	If the risk of exposure persists, give 1 dose after 12 months after a primary vaccination with Ixiaro and a second dose after 10 years.
Meningococcal ACWY	Menactra® Menveo® Nimenrix	Vaccinate those at high risk (asplenia, contact, travel)
Meningococcal B	Bexsero (GSK); Trumenba (Pfizer)	Vaccinate those at high risk (asplenia, contact, travel)
Polio	Imovax-Polio®: 1 booster dose at 0, 1 month	A single polio vaccine booster is indicated for at-risk adults. Routine vaccination of adults (18 years of age or older) is not necessary in Canada.
Rabies	Imovax-Rabies: multiple calendars possible. Refer to guidelines	Pre-exposure immunization with ID is not recommended in immunosuppressed persons.
Typhoid	Injectable, recombinant vaccines: Typhim Vi® or Typherix® Combined, recombinant with Hepatitis A: Vivaxim Oral, live attenuated vaccine: Vivotif®	Booster: a vaccination started with a hepatitis A vaccine or a typhoid vaccine can be continued with the combined vaccine against hepatitis A and typhoid, and vice versa, depending on the schedule and dosage of the vaccine used. Oral, live attenuated vaccine contraindicated in immunosuppressed.
Yellow fever	YF-VAX®: live attenuated vaccine	Since the entry into force of the amendment to the International Health Regulations on 11 July 2016, all international yellow fever vaccination certificates are considered valid for life, including certificates issued more than 10 years ago. Use of a one-time booster dose is recommended for travelers who may have received a primary dose of yellow fever vaccine during a period of reduced immunocompetence. This includes those who were pregnant, taking immunosuppressive medication, received a previous dose which may be inadequate for long-term protection, and individuals diagnosed with an illness associated with an immunocompromised state. Individuals who underwent a hematopoietic stem cell transplant after having received yellow fever vaccine are included in this category (see International Health Regulations, amended for expanded discussion.) A booster dose of yellow fever vaccine every 10 years is recommended for HIV-positive individuals prior to travel to endemic regions.

system to fight infections, called immunosenescence. Therefore it leads to an increase risk of invasive diseases with agents such as pneumococcal infection.

To insure that all your patients keep their immunization status up-to-date, provide them with an immunization booklet and ask them to bring it to every medical consultation.

REFERENCES

1. Protocole d'immunisations du Québec. MSSS. Québec. Mises à jours trimestrielles.
2. http://www.msss.gouv.qc.ca/professionnels/vaccination/protocoled-immunisation-du-quebec-piq/
3. Provincial and Territorial Routine Vaccination Programs for Healthy, Previously Immunized Adults. Public Health Agency of Canada. February 2019. https://www.canada.ca/en/public-health/services/provincial-territorial-immunization-information/routine-vaccination-healthy-previously-immunized-adult.html
4. Sellers SA, Hagan RS, Hayden FG, Fischer WA 2nd. The hidden burden of influenza: A review of the extra-pulmonary complications of influenza infection. *Influenza Other Respir Viruses*. 2017;11(5):372–393. doi:10.1111/irv.12470
5. Hospitalisations et complications attribuables à l'influenza: rapport de surveillance 2017–2018.
6. INSPQ Fevrier 2019. https://www.inspq.qc.ca/publications/2486. https://www.inspq.qc.ca/sites/default/files/publications/2486_hospitalisations_complications_inluenza_2017_2018.pdf
7. Dr. Janet McElhaney. Member, CIHR Institute Advisory Board (IAB) on Indigenous Peoples' Health. http://www.cihr-irsc.gc.ca/e/50234.html
8. Vaccination contre le tétanos: pertinence de doses de rappel chez l'adulte. INSPQ septembre 2018.

15 Management of Older Patients in the Emergency Department

This Man Is Old, But Is It an Emergency?

Cyrille Launay, MD, PhD

CONTENTS

CLINICAL VIGNETTE

An 88-year-old man is brought to the emergency department (ED) by his daughter because he can no longer perform his basic activities of daily living (bathing, dressing, transferring). She also reports that her father was having difficulty preparing his meals and has lost weight. The patient cannot provide details and does not understand why he is at hospital. He has no complaints and states that even if he is "a little bit tired", he wants to go back home. He is coherent but he is not able to say the month or the year. He has a mild cough but has no fever. The chest examination reveals wheezing but no audible crackles. Blood tests available disclose leukocytes 7×10^9/L, CRP 15 mg/L, creatinine 67 umol/L. The physician diagnoses acute bronchitis, proposes discharge home and treatment with an opioid cough suppressant.

WHY ARE OLDER PATIENTS IN THE EMERGENCY DEPARTMENT AT RISK OF MISDIAGNOSIS?

The health status of older patients (i.e., 75 years and older) is highly heterogeneous and is related to the various and cumulative effects of aging, life habits and chronic diseases that are highly prevalent in this age group. Thus, older patients are generally sicker than younger ones and 80% of those aged 75 years and older present with at least 2 chronic diseases that increase the risk of developing acute diseases. Indeed, older patients often experience complex interactions between acute and chronic diseases but also geriatric syndromes (e.g., cognitive impairment) that may induce atypical clinical presentations such as functional decline or increasing disabilities. Thus, they may be admitted to ED with non-specific complaints (feeling "tired" or "weak") that arise due to cognitive impairment and communications problems, functional decline and comorbidities. Geriatric syndromes may not be recognized (misdiagnosed) and not managed (mistreated).

Therefore, 25% of older patients leave ED with no definite diagnosis whereas most of them suffer from an acute disease. Underdiagnosis and underestimation of patients with atypical clinical presentations may lead to adverse outcomes such as higher risk of hospitalization and in-hospital mortality.

How to Deal with Older Patients in the Emergency Department

The adapted care plan of older patients is based on a multidimensional, interdisciplinary diagnostic process to determine the medical, psychological and functional capabilities called the comprehensive geriatric assessment (CGA). CGA is the most validated intervention dedicated to elderly patients and aims at assessing and addressing their needs.

Benefits of CGA have been confirmed through several meta-analyses, which have reported a reduction of admissions and readmissions to hospital, more discharges to home, increased lifetime spent at home, prevention of functional decline and decrease in mortality and in healthcare expenditures.

Despite its benefits, a systematic CGA for every older ED inpatient in daily practice remains impossible to implement because it is a complex and time-consuming process. Furthermore, it requires a multidisciplinary geriatric team that cannot alone support the care of all frail older ED patients due to limited availability.

DOI: 10.1201/9781003344476-17

The usual emergency department's mission is to quickly prioritize patients whose life is in danger; therefore, their triage often fails to detect the complex reasons that lead to the ED visits of older patients.

Thus, a two-step approach seems the best strategy to provide the appropriate care to the right patient at the right time, in order to identify those who are in greatest need of a geriatric intervention.

To implement such an approach, a screening tool is required to identify frail patients or patients at risk of adverse outcomes during hospitalization.

Useful Tools to Identify Vulnerable Patients in ED

Several tools have been developed to identify early frail patients or patients at risk of a prolonged hospital stay, 30-day readmission or mortality. There is currently no consensus on a screening tool for use in ED. The ideal tool would need to be multidimensional. Thus, most of the screening tools in use assess physical function, cognition, malnutrition and disabilities that are the main geriatric conditions.

To date, there is a consensus for the need for a screening tool in ED, but this tool needs to be adapted to the specific conditions of the medical practice in ED. This tool needs to be multidimensional, capable of being quickly performed and easy to use without specific geriatric training. Among those tools, Identification of Senior at Risk (ISAR), Emergency Room Evaluation and Recommendations (ER2) or Prisma 7 are meant to guide the appropriate levels of treatment to provide to older patients. According to their risk stratification, patients considered frail or at risk of prolonged length of hospital stay may require a geriatric intervention (i.e., to be hospitalized in a geriatric unit, or the intervention of a mobile geriatric team).

Key Components of a Comprehensive Geriatric Assessment

Medical Assessment

Problem list
Comorbidities
Medications
Nutritional assessment
Gait and balance assessment

Functional Assessment

Activities of daily living
Instrumental activities of daily living

Psychological Assessment

Cognition
Assessment of mood

Social Assessment

Family support
Home help services

Environmental Assessment

Financial

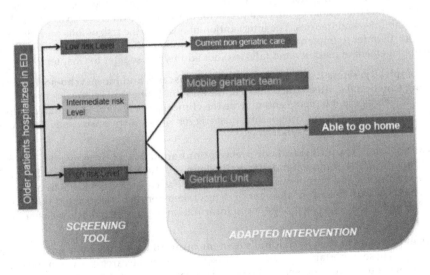

Geriatric assessment and interventions.

If no screening tool is available, an assessment based on the components of the CGA may be performed.

CGA allows a coordinated and integrated plan of treatment, and thus may prevent complicated medical pathways characterized, for instance, by prolonged length of hospital stay. This intervention can be performed in different ways depending on the medical resources and organization of the structure. Most of the time, CGA is delivered on a geriatric ward, or by a mobile geriatric team.

In EDs, mobile geriatric assessment provides an intervention with several objectives. The first one is to diagnose unrecognized geriatric syndromes such as delirium, frailty and gait impairment. Second, the mobile geriatric team may provide guidance on the level of care and recommendations on immediate care, prevention of functional decline or prevention of delirium. Finally, mobile geriatric teams may propose and coordinate a care plan that includes a discharge home or suggest the type of inpatient medical unit that may provide the most adapted care (e.g., a geriatric unit, an internal medicine unit) or institutionalization.

CONTINUATION OF THE VIGNETTE

A mobile geriatric team is asked to assess the patient in order to help with the medical management and to coordinate the discharge.

Their geriatric assessment uncovers several geriatric syndromes. First, cognitive impairment is detected, using the Mini Mental State Examination (MMSE). Second, they gather information that the patient fell many times and always refused a walking aid. Finally, malnutrition is diagnosed considering a weight loss of 7 kg in the last 6 months and a lower than expected weight of 61 kg. The mobile geriatric team provided a plan for immediate care and proposed to transfer the patient to an acute geriatric unit.

How to Deliver a Geriatric Assessment in ED

Several areas must be considered to assess older patients. These areas have been grouped under the acronym of 5 Ms as proposed by the American and Canadian Geriatrics Societies. These 5 Ms stand for:

- **Mind: refers to cognitive impairment and/or delirium and depression:** Delirium is highly prevalent in EDs (up to a quarter of patients) and should not remain unrecognized considering related morbidity and adverse outcomes. The confusion assessment method (CAM) is a simple tool with high predictive performance that may be used to identify delirium. Patients with cognitive impairment are vulnerable and must be managed carefully because of the risk of delirium. Besides, assessing their cognitive status is mandatory to enable a safe return home from ED. For interventions to reduce or manage delirium, please refer to Chapter 8.

- **Mobility: refers to gait impairment and falls:** Half of those aged 80 years and over fall at least once a year. Thus the history of falls is a predictor of future falls and is also associated with greater disabilities and injuries. The intervention may assess the risk of falls and identify their risk factors, in order to implement multidisciplinary interventions to address them. For details on the management of mobility and falls in older adults, please refer to Chapter 9.

- **Multi-complexity: refers to the burden of chronic diseases and bio-psycho-social situations including functional status:** Functional decline and disabilities are relatively common reasons for visits to EDs by older patients and may be the clinical presentation of an underlying disease. That is why such non-specific complaints must trigger an exhaustive assessment of acute and chronic diseases and geriatric syndromes.

- **Medication: refers to optimization of prescriptions and adverse drug events:** Taking 5 different medications or more per day usually defines polypharmacy. Adverse drug effects increase with aging and number of drugs and may be a reason for ED visits in up to 14% of older persons. Furthermore, the number of drugs taken per day is associated with comorbidity burden and diseases' severity. For more information on polypharmacy, please refer to Chapter 34.

- **Matters most: refers to each individual's own meaningful health outcome goals and care preferences:** These important aspects can be discussed with the caregiver when the patient is unable to contribute. Emphasis should be placed on patient-centered care.

RESOLUTION OF THE CLINICAL VIGNETTE

Many geriatric syndromes may be evoked from the beginning of this vignette. The reason for admission is non-specific and the clinical presentation is mainly functional. Such a visit could be considered inappropriate in ED whose aim is intended to treat acute diseases. However, nearly 60% of patients presenting with non-specific complaints to ED suffer from serious medical conditions. Acute functional decline may lead to disabilities. It is mandatory to provide specific interventions that improve the diagnostic process to manage patients adequately and prevent further decline. The main clinical elements suggest acute bronchitis without severity criteria. However an acute disease may expose a vulnerable patient with reduced physiological reserves to dependency.

The patient is described as not able to say the month or the year, suggestive of cognitive impairment. Indeed, temporal disorientation is related to acute and chronic cognitive impairment. Thus this item may help to identify delirium and/or dementia. Consequently, opioid treatment must be used with caution to avoid delirium and is not indicated to treat cough. A brief geriatric assessment that examines cognition is mandatory in this case. Confirmation of a diagnosis of dementia can be completed at a later stage along with a decision on treatment.

Finally, this clinical vignette shows the necessity to go beyond the assessment of acute diseases in ED and to consider geriatric syndromes and chronic diseases. A care plan to prevent functional decline, disabilities and delirium must be elaborated from ED to avoid inappropriate discharge home with its deleterious consequences.

REFERENCES

1. Preston L et al. Southampton (UK): NIHR Journals Library. 2018.
2. Ellis G, Whitehead MA, O'Neill D, Langhorne P, Robinson D. Comprehensive geriatric assessment for older adults admitted to hospital. Cochrane Database Syst Rev. 2011. doi: 10.1002/14651858.
3. Aminzadeh F, Dalziel WB. Older adults in the emergency department: a systematic review of patterns of use, adverse outcomes, and effectiveness of interventions. Ann Emerg Med. 2002;39:238–247.
4. Wachelder JJH, Stassen PM, Hubens LPAM et al. Elderly patients presenting with non -specific complaints: characteristics and outcomes. PlosOne. 2017;12(11): e0188954.
5. Ellis G, Marshall T, Ritchie C. Comprehensive geriatric assessment in the emergency department. Clin Interv Aging. 2014;9:2033–2043.
6. Sternberg SA, Wershof Schwartz A, Karunananthan S, Bergman H, Mark Clarfield A. The identification of frailty: a systematic literature review. J Am Geriatr Soc. 2011 Nov;59(11):2129–2138.

16 Critical Care of the Older Person

Astrid F. Pilgrim, MD, MS and Michael R. Pinsky, MD, CM, Dr hc, FCCP, MCCM, FAPS

CONTENTS

CLINICAL VIGNETTE

An 85-year-old non-smoking Caucasian male widower, previously self-sufficient and living alone, is brought into the Emergency Department by his daughter. She normally spoke to him daily, but the day before when she called him he sounded somewhat confused. On the day of admission she went to his home and found him confused and rambling, but in no acute distress. After calling his primary care physician she brought him into the local hospital Emergency Department. In the Emergency Department he was found to be sleepy but arousable, disoriented, but in no acute distress, with a good nutritional status and no evidence of trauma.

Temperature was 38.2 C, heart rate 85/min and regular, respiration rate 12/min and unlabored, blood pressure 135/60 mmHg. Neurological, cardiac and respiratory examinations were normal. The abdomen was slightly distended with tenderness but no rebound. There were no bowel sounds. Periphery had good pulses without edema. Capillary refill time was 1.5 seconds. Abnormal initial laboratory studies included a serum sodium of 125 mmol/dl, hemoglobin of 10.5 gm/dl, a white blood count of 10,000 with 3% bands and an arterial blood gas on room air of PO2 55 mmHg, PCO2 38 mmHg, pH 7.32. A chest radiography revealed some calcification of the aorta, thoracic vertebral fusion and free air under the diaphragm. An abdominal CT scan revealed free air anteriorly, fluid in the abdominal cavity and thickened descending colon wall.

Based on these findings blood cultures were obtained and the patient placed on broad spectrum antibiotics and resuscitated with 500 ml of 0.9% NaCl. Surgical consultation was obtained and the patient was transferred to the intensive care unit where he was instrumented with a central venous and radial artery catheter. Over the next hour the patient received 1,500 ml of a balanced salt solution, but he progressively became unresponsive. He was electively intubated to protect his airway. Upon intubation, his blood pressure decreased to 95/40 mmHg and his heart rate increased to 95/min. His blood pressure did not respond to 1000 mL bolus infusion of 0.9% NaCl, so norepinephrine was initiated and titrated to achieve a mean arterial pressure greater than 65 mmHg while plans were made for an emergent exploratory laparotomy.

Upon opening the abdomen during laparotomy foul-smelling feculent fluid was observed with fecal soiling; a ruptured descending colonic diverticulum was identified. A diverting colostomy and rectal mucus fistula was created, the abdomen was washed out three times, and then closed. A second look surgery the following day revealed no bowel leak or fluid collections. However, on post-operative day 2 his urine output decreased despite being 5,000 ml positive with a doubling of both BUN and creatinine. He was placed on continuous veno-venous hemofiltration for fluid management, which was weaned off after 5 days. His initial post-operative course was complicated by secondary fungal peritonitis treated with anti-fungal agents. However, his level of consciousness remained depressed despite holding all sedation. He remained ventilator and vasopressor dependent.

At 10 days post intubation, a discussion was had about tracheostomy. A spot cortisol level was drawn and came back 18 mg/dl. He was placed on hydrocortisone 100 mg intravenously every 8 hours. After 36 hours of hydrocortisone, his level of consciousness markedly improved and he was rapidly weaned off the ventilator and 12 hours later off norepinephrine. On his 14th hospital day he was transferred to a regular ward and by day 20 transferred to a skilled nursing facility.

DOI: 10.1201/9781003344476-18

CASE DISCUSSION

This case highlights many of the features of critical illness in the older person. As people age their ability to cope with stress of any kind decreases. First, the typical clinical presentations of pneumonia, sepsis or myocardial infarction are often absent. The most common presentation of older patients with catastrophic illness is confusion and inactivity. This patient presented with confusion and minimal inflammatory changes, like fever and tachycardia, despite severe intra-abdominal sepsis. Some of this blunted response may be due to the immune senescence seen with aging. Also, his initial arterial blood gas revealed hypoxemia with an increased A-a gradient, but no pulmonary infiltrates. Aging causes alveolar dropout or senescent emphysema such that the normal PaO2 of an 85-year-old person is 60 mmHg. With aging, all physiologic systems are impaired and homeostasis becomes "homeostenosis."

Second, when being treated with presumptively correct therapies, he did not rapidly improve. This is also frequent. Critically ill older people do nothing quickly except die. Thus, responses to dialysis, antibiotics and fluids need to be titrated much more closely than in the younger patient. The relative adrenal insufficiency documented on day 10 and treated appropriately would have resulted in a rapid improvement in level of consciousness in a younger patient. Our patient took 36 hours to respond.

Third, the older critically ill patient will recover and, surprisingly, if they had no pre-existing morbidities, carry a similar mortality rate as younger patients. So do not allow age to be a primary factor in determining who to treat for critical illness.

Fourth and finally, the older patient will recover, but their recovery will be protracted so it needs to be viewed within a longer time frame. Our patient did not recover fully for 6 months.

PHYSIOLOGIC CHANGES ASSOCIATED WITH AGING: WHEN HOMEOSTASIS BECOMES "HOMEOSTENOSIS"

After about 25 years of age, further aging is associated with decrements in physiologic reserve of all organ systems although at different interindividual rates (1). These usually do not become noticeable except in elite athletes until the mid-40s and are not physiologically relevant until after age 60. The heart increases in size and weight, atherosclerosis progresses, and pacemaker cells are lost (2). Maximal heart rate and oxygen (O2) delivery are reduced. The lung experiences loss of elastin fibers and collagen as alveoli drop out, causing senescent emphysema, increased closing volumes and arterial to alveolar O2 difference manifested as resting hypoxemia made worse by exercise and prolonged supine positioning (3). Thoracic cage deformity by kyphosis decreases chest wall compliance and increases residual volume in the lungs. The brain loses white matter which usually only manifests itself as confusion during stress. Renal concentrating capacity decreases such that measures of creatinine or BUN underestimate renal dysfunction. The gastrointestinal system displays decreased salivary production, dysphagia, delayed gastric emptying, development of diverticulae and hernias, and impaired vitamin absorption (4). A summary of the measured decrements in physiologic reserve seen with aging is listed in Table 16.1. The functional cumulative result of these decrements in physiologic reserve is fragility leading to the inability to maintain homeostasis in response to an otherwise minimal stressor.

These are important concepts to remember when treating the older patient with critical illness. They often appear well, living independent lives with good mentation and ambulation while handling their activities of daily living (Figure 16.1). Yet with some stressor, which could be as minor as moving to a new environment, they may become confused, belligerent or subdued. Regrettably, these are often the same presenting symptoms as a new infection or organ ischemia. They rarely have high fevers or tachycardia to the level seen in younger patients with the same illnesses. Similarly, they may not appreciate infarction or inflammation as pain. As in our case with fecal peritonitis, there was no rebound tenderness on abdominal examination.

RESUSCITATION OF THE CRITICALLY ILL OLDER PATIENT: SICK OLD PEOPLE DO NOTHING FAST BUT DIE

Due to their markedly reduced physiological reserve, the older critically ill patient needs a more nuanced resuscitation approach that recognizes those differences. Regarding specific therapies for diseases, the same management principles apply to older patients, but with an understanding that too rapid fluid resuscitation, vasopressors and extubation from mechanical ventilation may be as dangerous as delayed resuscitation and prolonged mechanical ventilation.

The fundamental principles of resuscitation of the critically ill patient presenting with cardiorespiratory insufficiency remain unchanged. Regarding ventilation, maintain a pulse oximeter

Table 16.1 Systemic Changes with Aging (2, 4)

System	Physiologic Changes
Neurologic	Decreased number of neurons. Decreased action potential speed. Decreased axon/dendrite branches.
Cardiovascular	Heart increases in size and weight. Progression of atherosclerosis. Loss of pacemaker cells. Increased vascular intimal thickness and stiffness. Increased left ventricular (LV) wall thickness and left atrial (LA) size.
Pulmonary	Loss of elastin fibers and collagen, kyphosis with decreased compliance of chest wall, increased residual volume. Alveoli duct volume increases at the expense of the alveoli resulting in senile emphysema.
Gastrointestinal	Decreased salivary production, dysphagia, diverticulae and hernias, delayed gastric emptying, impaired vitamin absorption.
Genitourinary	Kidney size and weight decreases. The number of functional glomeruli and renal tubules decreases, GFR declines, concentrating ability of kidney declines. The bladder can develop trabeculation and diverticula. There is urethral mucosal atrophy.
Endocrinologic	Increased atrophy of certain glands (pituitary, thyroid, thymus) with resultant changes in hormone levels and function.
Hematologic	Loss of self-renewal capacity of hematopoietic stem cells.
Immunologic	Gradual decline in the acquired immune system ("immunosenescence") including fewer naive and more memory T cells and decreased function of the B cell. Atrophy of the thymus. Increase in innate immune system activation leading to an elevated proinflammatory state marked by increased levels of cytokines and macrophage activation markers.
Musculoskeletal	Decreased bone density. Loss of cartilage thickness in synovial joints resulting in stiffness and less flexibility. Selective loss of type II muscle fibers. Lipofuscin and fat deposited in muscle tissue. Decrease in overall muscle mass.

The Impact of Aging on the Ability to Respond to Stress

Figure 16.1 Schematic diagram of the effect of aging on the ability of the body to adapt to stress effectively.

O2 saturation >90% with supplemental oxygen as needed and defend the airway. If breathing is inadequate to sustain normal gas exchange, an initially non-invasive trial of artificial ventilation could be done, but if not successful, invasive ventilation via endotracheal intubation should be performed.

Regarding cardiovascular support, the priorities are pressure, flow and function. Ensure that mean arterial pressure (MAP) is >65 mmHg or no more than 15 mmHg less than baseline in a previously hypertensive subject in order to sustain cerebral and coronary blood flow. This is usually done by rapid small bolus fluid resuscitation and vasopressor infusions. It is important to note that the recent Lamontagne et al. 65 TRIAL (5) which compared a MAP goal >65 mmHg to >60 mmHg in patients older than 65 with vasodilatory hypotension demonstrated a non-significant trend towards higher mortality with higher MAP goal. While current practice dictates a MAP goal of 65, this may change in the future with more studies.

Once pressure has been corrected, and this should take less than an hour, the focus shifts to maintaining an adequate flow to meet the metabolic demands of the body as assessed by loss of skin mottling, short (<2 sec) capillary refill time, lactate levels falling to <2 mmol/dl and resolution of metabolic acidosis if previously present.

Finally, once global blood flow appears adequate, resuscitating is fine-tuned by adjusting pressure and flow as needed to establish adequate renal blood flow as monitored by urine output, gut blood flow as monitored by bowel mobility and sensorium as monitored by increased level of consciousness and lack of anxiety. Thus, there are no specific issues in management that are different in treatment of the older patients except that complications of those treatments will be more frequent.

A good example of that is the high incidence of confusion and acute psychosis in the elderly in response to sedative therapies. Older adults need time to adjust to treatments and, once treated, to recover. In a landmark study of ICU outcomes of critically ill older adults, Chelluri et al. in 1993 (6) found that in ICU patients aged 65 to 74 as compared to those aged 75 and older there was no significant difference in length of stay, mortality at 1 year, or quality of life at 1, 6 and 12 months. Thus, age alone cannot predict long-term survival or quality of life in older adults admitted to the ICU. The study also suggests that older persons can eventually get back to their baseline function, but it takes more time and requires more involvement. In 2015 Ferrante et al. (7) performed a prospective cohort study on over 700 community-dwelling older adults with three distinct pre and post-ICU functional trajectories—minimal disability, mild to moderate disability and severe disability. They found that while more than half the participants experienced functional decline after critical illness, pre-hospitalization functional status played a more important role than age, with older adults having minimal disability often being able to return to their pre-hospitalization status.

There are certain drugs routinely used during critical care illness (for delirium, stress ulcer prophylaxis, arrhythmias, etc.) which show greater toxicity in the older patient. Every three years the American Geriatric Society (AGS) publishes the Beers criteria: a list of potentially inappropriate medications for older adults (8). Last updated in January 2019, the list includes 30 medications or medication classes to avoid in older adults. Most notable on this list with high quality of evidence and a strong strength of recommendation against use in older adults are tricyclic antidepressants, nifedipine, amiodarone, proton pump inhibitors, and non-selective NSAIDS. Lower on the list, with moderate quality of evidence but a strong strength of recommendation against use in older adults, are anticholinergics, second-generation antipsychotics (except quetiapine, clozapine and pimavanserin), benzodiazepines, non-dihydropyridine calcium channel blockers, and opioids. While the overall management strategies for diseases are the same for geriatric and non-geriatric patients, it's important to recognize the adverse effects that potentially inappropriate drugs can have in the geriatric patient population in case there is an equally efficacious but safer alternative therapy.

END-OF-LIFE CARE IN THE ICU

In an ideal world, end-of-life care is considered in the older person as part of the long-term healthcare discussion and would occur outside of the hospital in a setting where the patient is healthy enough to express their personal values. In reality, many older patients have never discussed end-of-life care and find their last days of life to be in the hospital where they are unable to share their own wishes and personal values and their family/caretakers are overwhelmed and unsure of the patient's personal values. When the place of care is the intensive care unit, this can make dying with dignity a challenge (9). Importantly, end-of-life care is just part of the palliative medicine spectrum of care. Palliative care is often provided within the intensive care environment, and can be done with all the appropriate trappings of dignity and respect for the patient, their wishes and the family's sensitivities. The World Health Organization defines palliative care as "an approach that improves the quality of life of patients and their families facing the problem associated with life-threatening illness" (10). Thus, palliative medicine is complementary to critical care medicine and physicians in general, but intensivists in particular should strive to enhance the patient's quality of life, provide treatment consistent with their personal values, and offer a support system to the patient and family/caretaker. For example, it is reasonable to initiate an aggressive treatment plan for organ failure scenarios in conjunction with palliative care goals. However, if the outcome appears bleak, it is important to realign the treatment plan with the patient's values and if indicated, transition to end-of-life care. This often is associated with withdrawal of life-supporting therapies, like mechanical ventilation and vasopressor therapy. Such a realignment of care goals is a process that will occur multiple times between the medical team and the patient/family over the course of a patient's admission. Overall, with end-of-life intensive care medicine, the prevention and relief of suffering becomes the primary goal.

THE UNEXPECTED CONSEQUENCE OF AGING—COST OF CARE DECREASES

The common belief is that with hospitalization and especially an ICU admission, older adults utilize more resources than their younger cohorts. Surprisingly, older age is actually associated with a lower total hospital cost. This was demonstrated in the 2003 Chelluri et al. (11) study which analyzed the hospital charges of 813 patients requiring mechanical ventilation; after adjusting for severity of illness (APS), ICU type, care insurance, and the Charlson comorbidity score, each decade of life was associated with a measurable decrease in costs. Further analysis showed decreased cost in the elderly occurs early on during the hospital stay and is not due to a limitation in care in the later days of the hospital stay.

RESOLUTION OF THE CLINICAL CASE

The patient remained in the skilled nursing facility for 2 months before being able to return home with daily home care nursing visits. By month 6 he resumed his normal level of activity and independence. His colostomy was taken down at that time without difficulty.

REFERENCES

1. Brummel NE, Ferrante LE. Integrating geriatric principles into critical care medicine: the time is now. Ann ATS 15:518–522, 2017. doi.org/10.1513/AnnalsATS.201710-793IP
2. Strait JB, Lakatta EG. Aging-associated cardiovascular changes and their relationship to heart failure. Heart Fail Clin 8:143–64, 2012. doi:10.1016/j.hfc.2011.08.011
3. Andrews P, Azoulay E, Antonelli M, Brochard L, Brun-Buisson C, De Backer D, Dobb G, Fagon JY, Gerlach H, Groeneveld J, Macrae D, Mancebo J, Metnitz P, Nava S, Pugin J, Pinsky MR, Radermacher P, Richard C. Year in review in Intensive Care Medicine 2006 II. Infections and sepsis, haemodynamics, elderly, invasive and non-invasive mechanical ventilation, weaning, ARDS. Intensive Care Med 33:214–228, 2007. doi:10.1007/s00134-006-0512-z
4. Medina-Walpole A, Pacala JT, Potter JF, eds. Geriatrics Review Syllabus: A Core Curriculum in Geriatric Medicine. 9th ed. New York, NY: American Geriatrics Society; 2016.
5. Lamontagne F et al. Effect of reduced exposure to vasopressors on 90-day mortality in older critically ill patients with vasodilatory hypotension: A randomized clinical trial. JAMA 323:938–949, 2020. doi:10.1001/jama.2020.0930
6. Chelluri L, Pinsky MR, Donahoe MP, Grenvik A. Long-term outcome of critically ill elderly patients requiring intensive care. JAMA 269:3119–3123, 1993.
7. Ferrante LE, Pisani MA, Murphy TE, Gahbauer EA, Leo-Summers LS, Gill TM. Functional trajectories among older persons before and after critical illness. JAMA 175:523–529, 2015. doi:10.1001/jamainternmed.2014.7889
8. 2019 American Geriatrics Society Beers Criteria® Update Expert Panel. American Geriatrics Society 2019 updated AGS Beers Criteria® for potentially inappropriate medication use in older adults. J Am Geriatrics Soc 67:674–694, 2019. doi:10.1111/jgs.15767
9. Cook D, Rocker G. Dying with dignity in the intensive care unit. N Engl J Med 370:2506–2514, 2014.
10. WHO Definition of Palliative Care. World Health Organization, World Health Organization, 28 Jan. 2012. www.who.int/cancer/palliative/definition/en/
11. Chelluri L, Mendelsohn AB, Belle SH, Rotondi AJ, Angus DA, Donahoe MP, Sirio CA, Schulz R, Pinsky MR. Hospital costs in patients receiving prolonged mechanical ventilation. Does age have an impact? Crit Care Med 31:1746–1751, 2003. doi:10.1097/01.CCM.0000063478.91096.7D

17 COVID-19 in Long-Term Care

*Julia Chabot, MDCM, FRCPC, MSc, Philippe Desmarais, MD,
FRCPC, MHSc and Michael Stiffel, MD, FRCPC*

CONTENTS

CLINICAL VIGNETTE

Mrs. C is an 89-year-old woman living in a long-term care (LTC) facility. She is known to suffer from type 2 diabetes and major neurocognitive disorder of moderate intensity (Alzheimer's). Three years ago, she was relocated to an LTC facility closed unit due to behavioural issues: verbal aggressivity and wandering. Her medications include short-acting insulin and quetiapine.

A few days ago, a resident living in the same unit as Mrs. C developed a cough and fever and was isolated. A COVID-19 swab was done on this resident, which turned out to be positive. Ever since, the nursing staff has been closely monitoring Mrs. C. Although she has no fever or cough, the staff has noticed that her appetite has significantly decreased and that she has become more confused than her baseline. She continues to wander on the unit and constantly needs to be reminded to go back into her room.

Physical examination reveals that her blood pressure is 95/60 (her usual is 110/80), her pulse is 105, her respiratory rate is 14 per minute, her oxygen saturation is 95% on room air and her temperature is 36.7 degrees. She appears tired and her mouth is dry. Her cardiac, respiratory and abdominal examinations are unremarkable.

COVID-19 DISCLAIMER

It is important to acknowledge that COVID-19 is a new disease and that our understanding of it is constantly evolving. This text reflects our current understanding of the disease as well as our opinions as geriatricians in accordance with our clinical experience of treating older adults with COVID-19.

VIROLOGY OF SARS-COV-2

COVID-19 is a disease caused by a mutating coronavirus which was discovered in 2019: SARS-CoV-2 (severe acute respiratory syndrome coronavirus 2). This novel coronavirus was first

DOI: 10.1201/9781003344476-19

described in Wuhan, China, in a cluster of individuals suffering from unexplained pneumonia. On March 11th, 2020, the World Health Organization declared COVID-19 a pandemic. At this writing, the ascendant mutation is designated as Omicron.

SARS-CoV-2 is mainly transmitted through droplets and contact. Contact can be direct (direct contact with a contaminated individual) or indirect (contaminated surfaces; fomites). Airborne transmission is also possible in the context of aerosol generating procedures or treatments (endotracheal intubation, for example). To this date, fecal-oral transmission has not been confirmed.

The average incubation period for this virus is 5–6 days. This incubation period may be as great as 14 days, especially in individuals with milder forms of the disease. Typically, symptomatic individuals are contagious for 1 to 3 days prior to onset of symptoms. Asymptomatic individuals can be contagious. It is also known that COVID-19 is more infectious than influenza and carries greater mortality.

EPIDEMIOLOGY OF COVID-19

In the province of Quebec (Canada), although individuals aged 80 years and older represent about 4.7% of total confirmed cases, they represent 71% of the overall mortality. About 50% of deaths happened in long-term care settings (based on INSPQ October 2021). These figures are similar in many states and countries around the world. In the USA for example, this percentage varied from 21% to 81% in different states according to data provided by the Kaiser Family Foundation (May 2020).

Older individuals are at higher risk of morbidity and mortality due to multiple factors, including age (which is a risk factor in itself), as well as multiple comorbidities (diabetes, hypertension, chronic obstructive pulmonary disease, etc.). Individuals living in LTC settings are at a higher risk when compared to the general older population for a variety of reasons; they are vulnerable, frail, and have a higher burden of comorbidities, including dementia. They are also frequently in close proximity to their caregivers and other residents, increasing the risk of transmission.

COVID-19 has been classically described as a respiratory disease with a wide spectrum of clinical presentations (from asymptomatic carriers to critical respiratory failure). Disease severity for COVID-19 is divided into mild, moderate and severe cases. Mild cases represent the most common trajectory of clinical cases where patients present with only minor symptoms such as a low-grade fever, a dry cough or headaches. Moderate cases are defined by the presence of marked, persistent fever and respiratory symptoms such as dyspnea, chest pains and productive cough, which suggest the presence of underlying pneumonia. Finally, severe cases are defined by the presence of respiratory distress (e.g., marked tachypnea, desaturation), respiratory failure and shock. Although no data is available for the LTC population, the Chinese Centre for Disease Control and Prevention reported that mild, moderate and severe cases were reported in 81%, 14% and 5% of the total case load, respectively.

Furthermore, it has been well documented that a clinical syndrome can evolve rapidly in at-risk groups (including older adults and LTC residents).

CLINICAL PRESENTATION

Typical Clinical Manifestations of COVID-19

The classic clinical presentation associated with COVID-19 is that of a viral syndrome, similar in many regards to influenza (influenza is indeed part of the differential diagnosis). This viral syndrome includes fever, chills, myalgia, lethargy, fatigue and an overall reduced general condition. Patients may also present with headaches, joint pains and non-specific chest pains (secondary to pericardial inflammation). In some patients, specifically those in younger and lower-risk groups, the viral syndrome is the only clinical manifestation of COVID-19.

Respiratory Symptoms

Respiratory symptoms usually follow after typical viral syndrome symptoms. These symptoms are variable, and often include a dry cough and dyspnea. Respiratory symptoms are rarely the initial presentation in COVID-19 patients residing in LTC.

Bacterial pneumonia is a possible complication that must be suspected and treated proactively with the appropriate antibiotic options. Additionally, LTC residents are at higher risk for aspiration pneumonia, for a variety of reasons, including underlying neurocognitive disorders and risk of delirium arising from altered mental states. Therefore, bacterial pneumonia should be included in the differential diagnosis of clinical deterioration for COVID-19 patients, especially in LTC facilities.

Non-Respiratory Symptoms

Although COVID-19 typically presents with respiratory and viral symptoms, there are unique and unusual elements which must not be ignored. These particularities are even more significant in older adults, where clinical presentation can be, and often is, atypical and even asymptomatic. Early recognition, supportive care and appropriate treatment options are therefore essential.

Gastrointestinal symptoms are also frequently observed, including loss of appetite, nausea and diarrhea, which can lead to a significant risk of dehydration in certain populations. As we learn more about this new condition, additional symptoms—some of which are less typical in other viral syndromes—have been identified; specifically, the loss or decrease in sense of taste and smell.

Neurological symptoms going beyond the cognitive changes observed in delirium or secondary to the electrolyte imbalances arising from dehydration and hypoxia have also been observed. COVID-19 creates a pro-coagulant state with increased risk of thrombosis at various sites. It is therefore important to consider strokes and TIA in the differential diagnosis of acute neurological symptoms and changes.

The pro-coagulant state associated with COVID-19 is not limited to neurological complications. Thromboembolic events may also occur at various sites and must be taken into account in the clinical evaluation of these patients. Pulmonary embolisms would worsen respiratory symptoms and venous thrombosis could be overlooked in the context of myalgia.

Considerations for the Geriatric Population

It is known that the geriatric population is at high-risk for COVID-19. However, other elements must be taken into account. As previously mentioned, initial symptoms in older adults may present more subtly and atypically (e.g., patients presenting with only loss of appetite), which may in turn delay diagnosis/management. Gastrointestinal symptoms, as well as general fatigue, have been observed in COVID-19 patients, placing LTC residents specifically at higher risk for dehydration. Older patients already have decreased feelings of thirst, and diarrhea combined with any decrease in oral intake will expose them to weight loss and dehydration. Consequently, they may suffer from electrolyte imbalances, renal damage and greater difficulty in controlling certain conditions, such as diabetes with hypoglycemia. It is also important to consider the polypharmacy of patients, as acute illness may affect plasma concentrations of different medications, exposing patients to multiple undesirable and potentially harmful side effects.

CLINICAL APPROACH

General Approach

Screening and Diagnosis

In the context of an increasing number of COVID-19 cases, as may be seen during an epidemic or pandemic, a low suspicion threshold should be set to screen, test and isolate residents in LTC facilities. This is supported by the fact that the virus can spread quickly through asymptomatic carriers, such as facility workers and visiting family members, and that clinical manifestations of the infection in older adults are frequently atypical or subtle. As for the common manifestations of COVID-19—low-grade fever, new onset of weakness, gait impairment or fall, or increased cognitive deficits (e.g., confusion, delirium)—in the absence of a clear etiology, these may be sufficient to warrant the ruling out of COVID-19 if cases have been reported in the LTC facility or if there is community transmission.

Screening of residents for carrier status and suspected COVID-19 diagnoses can be performed by nasopharyngeal swab which must be tested for the presence of SARS-CoV-2 RNA through RT-PCR. False negative results are not uncommon as the test sensitivity is highly dependent on the use of adequate technique to obtain the sample. If the test result is negative but there is a high suspicion of COVID-19, the test should be repeated 24 to 48 hours following the first test.

While the diagnosis of COVID-19 is primarily based on the identification of virus RNA in nasopharyngeal secretions, other investigations may be suggestive of infection. COVID-19 cases frequently present with lymphopenia and thrombocytopenia on CBC, as well as elevated C-reactive protein, d-dimers and fibrinogen, these latter markers having prognostic utility. Pulmonary imaging, such as chest X-rays and CT scans, may show findings suggestive of viral pneumonia (i.e., diffuse interstitial infiltrates and bilateral perihilar peribronchial thickening), as well as findings for bacterial superinfection or acute respiratory distress syndrome (ARDS), both conditions being common complications of COVID-19. Investigations should be performed in keeping with available resources at the LTC facility, according to the resident's personal wishes, goals and objectives (i.e., level of care), and depending on whether results of investigations would alter clinical management.

Strategies for Disease Transmission Prevention and Protection of Workers and Residents

In the context of an epidemic or pandemic episode where a significant proportion of cases occur within one specific region, several strategies should be implemented to prevent an outbreak within LTC facilities. These strategies, which may be recommended or ordered by public health officials, will vary, but usually include:

- Vaccination of personnel and residents.

- Widespread screening of asymptomatic and symptomatic residents and facility workers, especially with regard to new admissions and employees.

- Potential quarantining of residents.

- Reinforcing hand washing, respect of respiratory hygiene/cough etiquette and donning and doffing of face masks for all facility workers, as well as for residents (when they are not alone in their room).

- Limiting visits to asymptomatic primary caregivers of residents wearing appropriate personal protective equipment.

- Limiting personnel movement and deployment on multiple floors and/or units.

- Updating resident level of intervention in personal medical charts.

Additionally, in the case of an outbreak within an LTC residence, the following strategies should be implemented to prevent further transmission within the facility:

- Separate floors and/or units for infected and non-infected residents and adoption of appropriate droplet precautions throughout the facility.

- Workers dedicated to specific floors and/or units (i.e., avoid having workers care for infected and non-infected residents within the same shift).

- Limiting the number and duration of interactions with residents to essential visits, as well as maximizing the number of interventions within a single visit. This can be achieved by:

  - Simplifying the residents' drug regimen by limiting it to essential drugs only, which may reduce the number of daily visits to their room for drug administration. For instance, drugs prescribed for primary prevention indications may be stopped temporarily (e.g., vitamin D, bisphosphonates).

  - Administering drugs to residents during daily mealtime-dedicated visits.

Supportive Care

As is often the case with other viral respiratory infections, there is currently no clinically approved *curative* treatment for COVID-19. Supportive care measures should be provided to infected residents, which include prescribing antipyretic and analgesic drugs for fever and pain, implementing non-pharmacological interventions for persistent and bothersome coughs, ensuring adequate food and liquid intake, and ensuring frequent normal bowel function.

Vaccines

In the United States and Canada, priority in receiving mRNA vaccines was given to the older population and their caregivers. In the first instance, these vaccines were made available to residents of nursing homes and similar long term care facilities. A subsequent "booster" dose is now being recommended.

Some of these vaccines have an efficacy of 94% and over in preventing COVID-19 disease. The messenger RNA instructs the cell to make only part of the SARS-CoV-2 spike protein (so no disease is caused) which in turn activates the immune response, with production of memory T-lymphocytes and B-lymphocytes. Protein subunit vaccines (containing harmless viral proteins) and vector vaccines that carry genetic SARS-CoV-2 material within a different weakened virus are becoming available as well.

Treatment

Treatment approaches currently may include, with appropriate medical care in acute care settings, the administration of anti-SARS-CoV-2 monoclonal antibodies to affected people 65 years of age and above with comorbidities, with the aim of reducing severe disease.

The oral antiviral molnupiravir has emergency FDA approval in the United States. It has a similar mode of action to remdesivir.

Paxlovid is nirmatrelvir, a SARS-CoV-2 protease inhibitor that inhibits the main protease enzyme needed for coronavirus replication, reducing the risk of hospitalization, in conjunction with ritonavir that binds to the protease site, inhibiting the activity of the enzyme. It has an emergency use authorization from the FDA at this writing.

Hospitalized patients with severe disease may have time to recovery shortened by the use of the antiviral remdesivir, which targets viral RNA-dependent RNA polymerase (RdRp), a viral enzyme that is necessary in the synthesis of RNA.

In patients requiring invasive mechanical ventilation, dexamethasone has been shown to decrease mortality to some extent.

Residents with COVID-19 should be closely monitored for commonly seen complications of the infection, such as bacterial superinfection, ARDS, thromboembolic events (e.g., deep vein thrombosis and pulmonary embolisms), delirium, cachexia, dehydration and the emergence of immobility syndrome. Risk of bacterial superinfection can be reduced by ensuring proper oral hygiene and appropriate diet (to avoid aspiration in the context of dysphagia). If a bacterial superinfection is suspected, antibiotics should be promptly initiated, such as azithromycin with ceftriaxone. Although not part of common LTC clinical practices, residents suffering from a clinically moderate to severe case of the disease should be prescribed anti-thrombotic prophylaxis, as thromboembolic events are particularly frequent and lethal.

Palliative Care

Since older adults residing in LTC facilities usually present with multiple comorbidities and are frail, mortality due to COVID-19 is unsurprisingly high, especially considering that the disease can evolve quickly toward respiratory distress and death. Despite the extraordinary precautions and strategies necessary to reduce the risk of contamination, appropriate palliative care can be achieved within an LTC facility and every medical team has the capacity to provide adequate end-of-life care. In cases where palliative care is chosen, interventions should be implemented to actively ensure the resident's physical and mental well-being.

All unnecessary IV accesses, tubes and cannulae may be discontinued, but a subcutaneous access should be kept for easy administration of medication. Respiratory distress protocol to alleviate terminal symptoms should be prescribed the moment that end-of-life care is chosen by the resident and his or her family, as respiratory distress may occur dramatically quickly with the disease. Given their potent analgesic properties, opioids should be prescribed to treat tachypnea, aiming for a breathing rate below 24/min. Antipsychotics and benzodiazepines may be prescribed for agitation and anxiety. Nausea and vomiting may be addressed with diphenhydramine or ondansetron. Haloperidol may also be used for nausea, as well as agitation. Constipation should be aggressively treated with laxatives in order to avoid abdominal discomfort.

If possible, families should be allowed to visit for humanitarian reasons. It is important for the team to accompany these families, both to provide support but also to ensure the correct use of appropriate personal protective equipment.

When to Transfer to an Acute Care Facility

According to the resident's level of care and the disease's evolution, residents presenting with clinically moderate to severe cases of the disease may have to be transferred to an acute care facility in order to receive interventions which cannot be performed within an LTC facility. Examples include respiratory and circulatory failure requiring invasive respiratory support and fluid resuscitation, as well as scenarios where appropriate palliative care cannot be provided locally.

Specific Interventions for Older Adults

Loss of Appetite, Dehydration and Poor Oral Intake

COVID-19 is notably associated with anosmia and dysgeusia, which may cause loss of appetite, cachexia and dehydration in older adults. Additionally, the infection and its associated hyperinflammatory state increase catabolism, which accelerates cachexia and dehydration. To reduce the risk of acute undernutrition and its complications, restricted diets (e.g., low carbohydrates, low salt and low fat) should be avoided. Nutrition consultants and speech specialists, when available, should be quickly involved as they can design and implement specific interventions which may improve the residents' nutritional state.

Residents should be stimulated and, if needed, assisted when eating and drinking at every meal. Sufficient time should be allotted to meal intake. Dietary supplements may be used (after a meal and not to replace a meal) in order to increase caloric intake. Water pitchers should be provided to residents and hydration should be encouraged at every room visit. While IV fluids are generally to be avoided in LTC facilities, they may be utilized in specific cases.

Immobility Syndrome and Falls

Immobility syndrome is particularly frequent in older adults with COVID-19, partly as a side effect of confinement and respiratory isolation measures. Cachexia, sarcopenia, respiratory symptoms (i.e., dyspnea) and hypoactive delirium may also contribute to immobility and falls. IV tubes, oxygen cannulae and Foley catheters may promote immobility and precipitate falls as well. Mobile residents should be encouraged to move about their room as much as possible, to use their walking aid appropriately, and to carry out daily living activities in whatever capacity they can. The use of catheters and tubes should be discontinued if feasible in order to reduce the risk of falls and to promote ambulation. When available, physiotherapists should be involved as they can design personalised exercise programmes. If residents become confined to their bed (i.e., bedridden), adequate therapeutic surfaces should be utilized to reduce the risk of pressure ulcers and residents should be moved in their bed as frequently as possible.

Delirium and Behavioural Issues

Fever, dehydration and hypoxemia, as well as confinement and isolation, may precipitate delirium in LTC residents. Delirium may also be secondary to another underlying medical problem and should therefore be investigated and treated appropriately. Behavioural issues in the context of delirium or dementia (i.e., Behavioural and Psychological Symptoms of Dementia: BPSD) represent a significant challenge in the context of precautions and strategies seeking to reduce the risk of transmission and contamination. Residents presenting behavioural issues may break droplet precaution and confinement orders. Non-pharmacological interventions (i.e., behavioural approaches) should be favoured, at first, to manage behavioural issues. These include:

- Reminding the resident at every visit of the importance of staying in their room.

- Providing them with cognitive or physical activities to do in their room.

- Putting a "stop" sign on their door or other visual stimuli to keep them in their room.

- Asking a family member or volunteer to talk to them on the phone frequently.

Another avenue to consider is having a volunteer, in appropriate personal protective equipment, stay near the door of the resident's room, to remind them to stay inside. If these behavioural approaches fail and droplet precaution rules are repetitively broken by an infected resident, the possibility of locking the resident's door, using physical restraints (e.g., an abdominal belt while sitting in a chair), or prescribing pharmacological interventions (e.g., low dose antipsychotics) may be considered, but only as a last resort and after having carefully weighed the risks and benefits of such measures. The resident's family should be informed of these issues and be involved in the decision-making process regarding the measures which should be implemented. The least limiting measure should be selected, its indication and success should be reviewed frequently, and it should be discontinued whenever feasible and appropriate.

CASE SUMMARY

Mrs. C lives in an LTC facility, on a closed unit. Recently, a resident from her unit was diagnosed with COVID-19 and was isolated in his room. Mrs. C is known to suffer from major neurocognitive disorder of moderate intensity (Alzheimer's) and presents with a clear change from her baseline behaviour and general state; her increased confusion suggests that she is suffering from delirium. It is also important to recognize that delirium can be both hyperactive and hypoactive. Therefore, patients can become either more agitated or lethargic.

She does not present with any viral syndrome or respiratory symptoms but does suffer from a decrease in appetite. Although she is afebrile and saturating well without signs of respiratory distress, she is already showing signs of dehydration (tachycardia and decreased blood pressure).

Considering that a resident on her unit has tested positive for COVID-19, all the residents from this unit, including Mrs. C, should be tested and isolated to prevent the propagation of the virus. It is important to frequently reassess the clinical status of Mrs. C as COVID-19 is a disease which can evolve rapidly. Furthermore, the person in charge of making medical decisions for Mrs. C should be frequently informed of her clinical status and the objectives for her care should be discussed. The vaccination status of Mrs. C should be reviewed. If she is not vaccinated, this should be offered either as soon as she has passed the isolation period (this delay would be longer should she receive monoclonal antibodies). Other preventative measures, as described previously, should be implemented:

- Nutrition and hydration: Mrs. C should be encouraged to eat and drink. She may also benefit from dietary supplements to increase her caloric intake. Considering her tachycardia, IV fluids could be considered.

- Mobility: She should be encouraged to move to prevent deconditioning while respecting current isolation measures. (Mrs. C should ambulate in her room.).

- Diabetes: Mrs. C is known to suffer from insulin-dependent diabetes. In the context of her decreased oral intake, her dose of insulin should be adjusted to avoid hypoglycemia.

- Wandering behaviour: As described, non-pharmacological interventions (i.e., behavioural approaches) should be favoured. Pharmacological measures may be needed, but these should only be undertaken as a last resort.

- Delirium: Mrs. C's cognitive status should be frequently re-evaluated. Her oral intake, sleep, mobility, skin care and elimination should be optimized. If she were to become lethargic, her dose of quetiapine should be decreased.

- Monitoring of respiratory status: As mentioned previously, LTC residents are at high risk of aspiration pneumonia. There is also a risk of bacterial superinfection (pneumonia) with COVID-19. The need for antibiotics should be frequently reassessed.

REFERENCES

1. D'Adamo, H., Yoshikawa, T., & Ouslander, J. G. (2020). Coronavirus disease 2019 in geriatrics and long-term care: the ABCDs of COVID-19. *Journal of the American Geriatrics Society, 68*(5), 912–917.
2. https://www.inspq.qc.ca/covid-19/donnees
3. Wu, Z., & McGoogan, J. M. (2020). Characteristics of and important lessons from the coronavirus disease 2019 (COVID-19) outbreak in China: summary of a report of 72,314 cases from the Chinese Centre for Disease Control and Prevention. *Jama, 323*(13), 1239–1242.
4. https://www.cdc.gov/coronavirus/2019-ncov/vaccines/different-vaccines.html
5. https://www.canada.ca/en/public-health/services/immunization/national-advisory-committee-on-immunization-naci/guidance-prioritization-initial-doses-covid-19-vaccines.html
6. https://www.fda.gov/news-events/press-announcements/coronavirus-covid-19-updatefda-authorizes-monoclonal-antibodies-treatment-covid-19
7. https://www.nejm.org/doi/full/10.1056/NEJMoa2007764
8. https://www.biospace.com/article/releases/government-of-canada-signs-new-agreement-for-a-covid-19-antibody-therapy/#:~:text=Today%2C%20the%20Honourable%20Anita%20Anand,monoclonal%20antibody%20therapy%20Bamlanivimab%20(LY%2D
9. https://www.canada.ca/en/health-canada/services/drugs-health-products/covid19-industry/drugs-vaccines-treatments/remdesivir-update.html
10. https://www.merck.com/news/merck-and-ridgebacks-investigational-oral-antiviral-molnupiravir-reduced-the-risk-of-hospitalization-or-death-by-approximately-50-percent-compared-to-placebo-for-patients-with-mild-or-moderat/
11. https://www.drugs.com/history/paxlovid.html
12. https://go.drugbank.com/drugs/DB00503
13. https://www.nature.com/articles/d41573-021-00202-8?utm_source=Nature+Briefing&utm_campaign=747c808df9-briefing-dy-20211207&utm_medium=email&utm_term=0_c9dfd39373-747c808df9-42544483
14. https://www.fda.gov/news-events/press-announcements/coronavirus-covid-19-update-fda-authorizes-first-oral-antiviral-treatment-covid-19

PART III
CARING

18 Arthritis in the Older Person

Linda Yue, MD, Kevin Yip, MD, and Joseph A. Markenson, MD

CONTENTS

PATIENT SCENARIO

Rosie is 79-year-old woman who presents to your office complaining of long-term hand pains for over a decade bilaterally. She notes this has been getting worse, complains of an achy feeling in her fingers with stiffness and a cramping sensation. Sometimes they feel swollen and tender at the end of the day, particularly after she spends the afternoon gardening and potting plants. In the last few years she has thought her fingers have started to look more "crooked" than before and developed hard lumps at the creases of her finger joints. Rosie remembers her mother had similar looking hands towards the end of her life and that she would often complain of discomfort in her hands too.

Her other medical conditions include obesity—BMI 32 kg/m²—hypertension and mild asthma. The patient's medication list includes amlodipine 5 mg daily and albuterol inhalers PRN. Her PCP told her she may have a type of arthritis in her hands and she wants to understand what that means and if anything can be done to help.

What Is Osteoarthritis (OA)?

Osteoarthritis is also known as "wear and tear" arthritis and is the most common cause of joint problems worldwide. As we age, the cartilage that cushions joints will break down and this can lead to damage of the bones and joints themselves. Eventually, it can lead to deformities of the structures of the joint leading to stiffness, pain and loss of function and mobility. Although it can affect any joint, it most commonly affects the fingers, hands, knees, hips and spine.

Risk factors of osteoarthritis include:

- Older age.

- Overuse (for example jobs or sports that stress the same joint repeatedly).

- Past trauma or injury to a joint.

- Obesity (due to increased weight on areas that bear load).

DOI: 10.1201/9781003344476-21

- Female gender.

- Family history (those with family members with OA are more likely to develop it).

- Other musculoskeletal issues (can lead to misalignment of body mechanics and predispose other joints to arthritis).

Epidemiology of Arthritis

Arthritis affects a significant proportion of the population with estimates that 22.7% of adults (52.5 million) in America have some form of joint problem and 9.8% (22.7 million) have some limitation in their activities due to their arthritis [1]. This figure increases in adults over the age of 65 years old with arthritis; 45.4% reported that their arthritis limited their activity [2].

The Impact of Arthritis

Osteoarthritis is one of the five main causes of disability for non-hospitalized adults [3] and disproportionally affects older persons. Evidence suggests that patients with arthritis were more likely to have less physical activity, be smokers and have poorer physical and mental health than those without arthritis [4]. This is particularly relevant in older adults where it has been found that worse arthritis pain is associated with higher levels of depressive symptoms [5]. It was estimated in 2003 that arthritis is a substantial economic burden in the USA, leading to $128 billion in medical costs and lost wages [6].

Inflammatory Arthritis

In patients who have at least one swollen joint, the presence of an inflammatory arthritis could be considered rather than osteoarthritis in the right clinical setting. Inflammatory arthritis is a group of conditions rather than a single entity, and is estimated to affect up to 2% of the population [7]. Examples of such conditions that can be seen in the elderly population are discussed in following sections. These types of arthritis affect not only the synovial lining of joints but also the surrounding cartilage, ligaments and insertion points of tendons [7]. Patients will often complain of significant warmth and swelling at joints, especially smaller joints of the hands, wrists and feet. Another common symptom will be joint stiffness that is worse in the morning lasting more than an hour, which tends to improve with continued movement and exercise throughout the day. These symptoms will occur periodically even without provoking actions, and last for days unless targeted medication is used.

Although osteoarthritis can also be characterized by inflammation and swelling as described in the previous section, the underlying mechanism that generates the inflammatory response is different from that seen in the inflammatory arthritis group. In these latter conditions, synovial inflammation leads to progressive and irreversible damage [8]. There are several different pathways that result in this inflammatory response, including activation of macrophages, osteoclasts and T-cells [7, 8]. In several forms of inflammatory arthritis that are closely associated with autoantibody formation, such antibodies drive the formation of immune complexes that serve to mediate further inflammatory response at the joint [7]. While there is no cure for inflammatory arthritis, many treatments now exist that target steps in the inflammatory pathway to halt activity [8]. The specific choice of treatment depends on the form of inflammatory arthritis, but in general will consist of symptomatic and targeted medications.

In addition to improving quality of life, it is also essential to identify and treat inflammatory arthritis as these conditions increase the risk of comorbidities. In older persons many of these may already be present and can thus be exacerbated by an untreated inflammatory condition. Of particular note, the severity of rheumatoid arthritis is significantly associated with cardiovascular disease as well as lymphoma [9].

COMMON RHEUMATOLOGIC CONDITIONS THAT ARE SEEN IN OLDER PERSONS
Rheumatoid Arthritis (RA)

RA is a chronic autoimmune disorder in which the body's immune system attacks the joints as well as other organ systems. In particular the immune system affects the synovium of joints, resulting in joint pain, swelling, and stiffness, and if untreated can result in permanent damage and deformity. RA is one type of inflammatory arthritis that is associated with antibodies, namely anti-cyclic citrullinated peptide antibodies (ACPA) and rheumatoid factor (RF) [7]. These antibodies are directly involved in the generation of joint inflammation in RA. Affected patients complain of symptoms at joints of the wrists, hands at knuckles, ankles and feet. Classically joints on both sides of the body are involved. The inflammatory process of RA can also affect the skin, blood vessels, eyes, and lungs, leading to vasculitis, uveitis and interstitial lung disease. These disease manifestations outside of the joints has been shown to have correlation with the specific antibodies found in RA [10].

Gout

This type of inflammatory arthritis is very common in older patients. It is characterized commonly by sudden, severe and recurrent attacks of joint pain with swelling that is hot to the touch. The involved joint will often be very red as well, and incredibly tender such that even the lightest touch may be exquisitely painful. Gout can involve one or more joints at once, with the classic location involving the big toe [11]. Attacks are caused by a buildup of uric acid crystals in the body that then deposit at joints. The body's immune system reacts to these deposits, causing the intense inflammation that is associated with this arthritis [11]. However, it should be noted that a high level of uric acid in the body alone may not lead to the patient having gout [12]. Treatment should thus be based on a combination of factors, involving the frequency of symptoms and any existing sign of damage from inflammation. A commonly used treatment is colchicine, which stops inflammatory cell types from responding to deposition of uric acid crystals and generating the typical hot swollen joint of gout attacks [13]. It is important to note that colchicine should be dosed appropriately in elderly patients who may have reduced renal function as a result of chronic disease.

Pseudogout

Similar to gout, pseudogout is an inflammatory arthritis common in older persons that is caused by deposits of crystals at joints. Instead of uric acid crystals, however, the crystals involved are calcium pyrophosphate [11]. This leads to the alternate name for pseudogout, which is calcium pyrophosphate deposition disease (CPPD). Pseudogout is also characterized by attacks of joint pain, redness and warmth when it presents in the acute form. It may also exist in a chronic form that coexists with osteoarthritis. Pseudogout tends to affect larger joints on one side of the body, such as the shoulder or hip.

Polymyalgia Rheumatica

Rather than a type of arthritis, polymyalgia rheumatica is an inflammatory condition that predominantly affects older persons. Most people who develop this condition are over the age of 60, and rarely under the age of 50. This disorder causes muscle aching and stiffness, especially at the shoulders and hips. The symptoms generally present suddenly, are worse in the morning, and affect both sides of the body. Constitutional symptoms may be associated, including low grade fever, a general feeling of fatigue or malaise, and unintentional weight loss. The first line treatment is steroids when the condition is suspected, and should be started even if the evaluation is not yet completed. Referral to a rheumatologist should be prompt given the association of polymyalgia rheumatica with a type of vasculitis known as temporal arteritis [14]. Vasculitis is discussed in additional detail under the section "Other Rheumatologic Conditions".

Reactive Arthritis

The hallmark of this arthritis is its association with infection, typically following a gastrointestinal or genitourinary infection [15]. Oftentimes a few medium or large joints on one side of the body become tender and swollen. In addition to joint symptoms there is a classic association with eye inflammation, back pain, ongoing urinary symptoms and inflammation of tendons and tendon insertion points (known as enthesitis). The Achilles' tendon is one example of one of these insertion points.

Septic Arthritis

This is a form of severe arthritis in which bacteria introduced into the bloodstream by an injury then travels to a joint and results in a joint infection [16]. Older adults can be especially susceptible to developing a septic arthritis given their weakened immune systems. The classic symptom is involvement of a single large joint such as the knee, hip or shoulder that is hot and incredibly painful to the point of limited movement. Treatment needs to be prompt with drainage of fluid and often surgery to clean the joint, followed by antibiotics.

Psoriatic Arthritis (PsA)

This form of arthritis is characterized by inflammatory joint symptoms (pain, swelling, and stiffness) in patients who also have psoriasis [17]. The type and pattern of joints affected are often different from that seen in RA. Patients with PsA often have symptoms at the spine, pelvis and tips of fingers with predominantly one side of the body affected.

OTHER RHEUMATOLOGIC CONDITIONS

Myositis

Myositis is an autoimmune inflammatory condition characterized by an immune system attack on muscle groups throughout the body. In the older patient this commonly presents as specific weakness when completing certain activities, such as keeping the arms lifted or standing up from a sitting position. This can be mild at first, and as the extent of muscle damage continues, the weakness gradually worsens. There is an increased incidence of a subtype of myositis, inclusion body myositis, seen in the over age 50 population that instead presents as insidious onset distal weakness [18]. Certain other types of myositis known as dermatomyositis can also be associated with a red-violet rash around the eyes, over the shoulders and back, or over the knuckles and knees. Other types of myositis are known to be associated with medications, including statin cholesterol-lowering medications or certain types of cancer immunotherapy treatments.

Vasculitis

Also known as inflammation of blood vessels, vasculitis can affect patients of all ages. In the older age group over 50, the most common type of vasculitis is known as giant cell arteritis, or temporal arteritis [14]. This is defined as inflammation of the lining of arteries at the temples, hence leading to the alternate condition name. Characteristic symptoms are new onset headaches, tenderness of the scalp and especially over the temporal arteries, jaw heaviness with continued movement such as chewing, and vision blurring or loss. This type of vasculitis is important to be aware of as it can lead to permanent vision loss if it is left untreated. There is also an association with a separate inflammatory condition discussed earlier, polymyalgia rheumatica; a proportion of patients with polymyalgia rheumatica may have coexisting temporal arteritis as well [14]. When either polymyalgia rheumatica or temporal arteritis is suspected, urgent rheumatology referral at minimum is necessary. Treatment is with prompt initiation of steroids, which should result in rapid relief of symptoms [14].

Systemic Lupus Erythematosus (SLE)

SLE, or lupus, commonly affects women especially in young or middle age. Though rare, lupus may present in older individuals over the age of 50–65 [16]. It can affect almost all body systems and lead to many symptoms that can be seen in other conditions, making diagnosis difficult in some cases. Common symptoms include joint pain with stiffness and swelling, unexplained fever, persistent fatigue, rash (especially a characteristic "butterfly rash" over the bridge of the nose). Chest pain, difficulty breathing, headaches and confusion can also be symptoms caused by lupus.

What Specialists Are Involved with Arthritis Care?

Arthritis treatment should take a team-based approach and generally is divided into invasive or noninvasive management, although specialists should be involved in both. Physical therapy has been found to be an important part in arthritis care. It has been shown that aerobic activity and muscle strengthening exercises can improve quality of life, function and reduce disability in arthritis [19]. Physical and occupational therapists are experts in guiding stretching and teaching exercises in a graded and safe manner for the patient.

Orthotics are often used to help brace joints, ligaments or tendons in a manner to help offload stress in arthritic joints [20, 21]. It is important to get these carefully fitted to a person's body shape and biomechanics for comfort and efficacy.

A rheumatologist specializes in the evaluation and treatment of types of arthritis and many other autoimmune conditions. Rheumatologists are able to perform a specific and detailed history and physical exam to differentiate between types of arthritis. A diagnostic evaluation of inflammatory arthritis will typically involve a survey of number and size of joints involved, as well as the pattern of symptoms [22]. Based on the information a rheumatologist gathers, additional labs and imaging studies may be ordered. If there is high suspicion for an inflammatory arthritis, labs can be used to confirm the presence of inflammation, autoantibodies, and to exclude other diagnoses [22]. X-rays may be ordered by a rheumatologist to detect cartilage loss and bone damage. Because x-rays may not be able to detect early signs of damage, other imaging tests including MRI can provide more detailed images of the joint and surrounding cartilage, tendons and ligaments [22]. Ultrasound imaging can also be useful, especially when looking for fluid in joints and to assist with localization when removing fluid from or injecting medication into joints [22].

Pain management specialists can guide the type of medications used to control the chronic pain that is often seen in arthritis. Interventionists may also perform procedures that can include joint injections or nerve blocks that can help reduce discomfort if appropriate.

Orthopedic surgeons are often involved, particularly in end stage disease, for evaluation of potential surgery which can involve repairing ligaments, bones or even joint replacements. However surgeries are not without risk and due to the limited lifespan and efficacy of prostheses, these interventions may not be suited for everyone. Increasingly focus has moved to preventative and pharmacologic approaches which are particularly important for elderly patients who are often frail and have comorbidities that can make surgery dangerous [23, 24].

How Do We Treat Arthritis Medically?

Although surgical interventions can be a definitive approach to arthritis, the majority of cases are managed with physical therapy and with different types of medications that can control pain and therefore restore some level of function. There currently is no widely accepted medicine that can reverse damage from osteoarthritis.

Lifestyle modifications are an often-overlooked treatment option with minimal risk and good improvement of function and pain. Regular exercise and reduction of weight in obese patients are effective in improvement of osteoarthritis as well as general health [25, 26]. Studies have shown that physical therapy can improve function and pain in hip osteoarthritis even without surgery [27, 28].

Drugs such as acetaminophen (Tylenol), non-steroidal anti-inflammatory drugs (NSAIDs), duloxetine and opiates are the common analgesic treatment options for osteoarthritis; however controversies exist in the use of opioids for this purpose [29, 30]. Here we will discuss the common approaches to these medicines and how they affect the older person in particular.

Acetaminophen is a very commonly used analgesic around the world and is often available over the counter. It is believed that acetaminophen acts via various pathways including COX inhibition, the cannabinoid system and TRPV1 [36]. Generally it is a safe drug with few side effects and for this reason is often one of the first-line therapies tried for pain [37]. Caution should be used in patients with liver problems or those with a significant alcohol intake. In these cases a lowered total daily dose can be considered, or the medication avoided altogether.

Non-steroidal anti-inflammatory drugs (NSAIDs) are one of the mainstays of arthritic treatment as they not only work as painkillers but also reduce local inflammation around the joint (for example associated tendinitis) [38]. NSAIDs not only relieve pain but increase mobility and function for approximately 60% of patients with osteoarthritis [39]. Many medical bodies are now suggesting them as first-line treatment or second-line treatment [32, 34, 35].

It should be noted that NSAIDs do have drawbacks and consideration must be given when prescribing, particularly to older persons or over a longer timeframe. Evidence suggests that around

Summary of Pharmacologic Treatment Guidelines for OA from Various Professional Societies

Group	Site(s)	NSAIDs	Tramadol	Other Opioids	Ref.
AAOS[a]	Knee	(+)	(+)	(~)	[31]
ACR[b]	Hand/Hip/Knee	(+/+/+)	(+/+/+)	(–/~/~)	[32]
ACSQHC[c]	Knee	(+)	unspecified	(+) ("limited role")	[33]
DoD[d]	Hip/Knee	(+)	(+)	(+) (second line)	[34]
OARSI[e]	Knee	(+)	(~)	(~) 'uncertain'	[20]
NICE[f]	Unspecified	(+)	unspecified	(+) (second line)	[35]

Note: a: American Academy of Orthopedic Surgeons, b: American College of Rheumatology, c: Australian Commission on Safety and Quality in Health Care, d: United States Department of Defense, e: Osteoarthritis Research Society International, f: National Institute for Health and Care Excellence

1–2% of NSAID users will have some form of gastrointestinal bleeding, resulting in over 10,000 deaths annually [40]. In addition, NSAIDs should not be used in those with kidney disease or cardiovascular history as it can induce renal dysfunction and increase the risk of heart problems. These are problems particularly common in the elderly and lowered/shortened courses of NSAIDs are recommended with close monitoring. NSAIDs are also available as topical gel or cream formulations, which can avoid the adverse side effects of the oral route and may be preferable. Other topical ointments and creams contain active ingredients such as menthol that can interfere with pain signaling and should also be considered in combination with other treatments.

Duloxetine has become increasingly popular for osteoarthritis. Originally used as a type of antidepressant, it has been shown to be useful in osteoarthritis of the back and knees as well as fibromyalgia and neuropathic pains [41, 42]. It belongs to a class of medicines known as serotonin-norepinephrine reuptake inhibitors and is believed to have an effect on central pain pathways. Unlike acetaminophen and NSAIDs, it generally takes a longer timeframe to start working and is slowly up-titrated over weeks. It is generally well tolerated; however, it may interact with other antidepressant medications. Some patients may complain of gastrointestinal upset, headache and drowsiness [43]. Older persons with the syndrome of inappropriate antidiuretic hormone secretion (SIADH) or low sodium levels should avoid duloxetine in particular.

Opiates (codeine, oxycodone, tramadol, morphine, fentanyl) continue to be a widespread treatment for chronic musculoskeletal pain despite a lack of convincing evidence [44] of superior efficacy. Although sometimes used for acute pain, it is generally discouraged to prescribe opiates over a prolonged period. The SPACE trial evaluated adults with back, hip and knee osteoarthritis in primary care clinics and found that pain-related function, as well as intensity of pain, improved for those who were prescribed opiates and non-opiate therapies with no significant difference between them [45]. Chang et al. examined the use of opiates in the context of acute extremity pain in the emergency department and found that there was no clinically significant difference in pain reduction between opioids and non-opioids (ibuprofen + acetaminophen) [46]. Others have found that those receiving opiates for musculoskeletal pain showed increased risk of all-cause mortality cardiovascular death [47].

One should exercise particular caution in older persons as opiates can commonly lead to constipation, dizziness, drowsiness and delirium. Over long timeframes dependence and tolerance can develop, leading to higher doses, which can lead to dangerous side effects such as respiratory depression.

Corticosteroids remain a mainstay of arthritis treatment due to their capacity to reduce inflammation. They can be administered as oral tablets, intramuscular injections or direct injections into the joint. As with NSAIDs and opiates, these should also be used cautiously given a number of important side effects in older persons. When used there should monitoring for exacerbation of conditions already commonly seen in this population, such as glaucoma, osteoporosis, skin thinning and bruising, and steroid-associated delirium.

Several alternative therapies are on the horizon promising efficacy and safety although there still exists significant contention in use, efficacy and safety profile and they are not routinely offered by most providers. PRP (platelet-rich plasma) therapy has been used over the last 10 years and preliminarily shows a unique way to improve function and pain, although there is significant debate about its efficacy [48, 49]. Hyaluronic acid has also been injected into joints in a similar fashion and sadly also lacks robust evidence demonstrating a difference over placebo in clinical studies [50]. Stem cell therapy has also shown potential in limited animal and human trials for cartilage repair and improvement of discomfort but is still in its infancy as a form of therapy [51, 52]. Genicular nerve blocks may also be utilized in some patients with chronic pain, although the technique is not widely practiced [53, 54].

Disease Modifying Antirheumatic Drugs (DMARDs)

DMARDs are used to slow the progression of damage from joint inflammation. They can be divided into two large categories, conventional and biologic drugs. These differ primarily in their mechanism of action and drug targets. Side effects, including lowering of blood counts or kidney and liver toxicity, are specific to each drug group, but all increase the risk of infections. As a result, the use of DMARDs in the older population can present challenges due to potential comorbidities in this patient group. It is thus important to ensure that the older patient has a thorough general health assessment, consistent primary care to address underlying comorbid medical conditions, and that older persons are up to date with their vaccination series in order to protect against the elevated risk of systemic infections with the use of biologic DMARDs [55].

WHEN TO REFER?

Situations that necessitate referral to rheumatology or orthopedic specialties will generally be those in which there is any suspicion for one of the clinical entities discussed earlier. When there is a characteristic pattern of joint swelling that raises concern for an inflammatory arthritis, such as the typical bilateral small joint involvement of RA, or a constellation of joint pain with other constitutional symptoms that are otherwise unexplained, a more detailed examination by a rheumatologist is beneficial. Depending on their evaluation, further tests or treatment may be indicated.

Another commonly encountered situation is that of unexpected positive lab tests, especially autoimmune antibodies. These should be interpreted with caution as their presence alone does not indicate the presence of an autoimmune condition. The antinuclear antibody (ANA) in particular has been reported to be quite prevalent in general healthy populations without corresponding disease [56]. It should be especially noted that the incidence of autoimmune antibodies increases with age as well [56]. Ordering these antibody tests should thus be undertaken with caution, and is often best decided after an evaluation by a rheumatologist.

Other important reasons to refer an older patient with joint pain are suspected infection or trauma. If a patient presents with an inflamed joint and systemic sign of infection, it is important to consider the possibility of an infected joint given the emergent nature of this presentation as noted earlier [57]. When there is a history of recent fall or injury and presence of a fracture on imaging, a surgical specialist should be involved in the management [58]. In both of these cases, evaluation by an orthopedic specialist is warranted. Finally, malignancy should be kept in mind when caring for this patient group given its increased incidence with age. Alarming features of presentation include insidious and worsening long bone or back pain, especially at night, as well as fractures with no, or insufficient, trauma history or fractures with minor trauma [58]. In these cases, further workup for an undetected malignancy should be completed. Care should be taken to ensure that patients have up-to-date routine cancer screenings.

REVISITING THE SCENARIO

After seeing Rosie in your office, you are better able to tease out the pattern and timing of her symptoms. As she described to you, the sensation of aching pain and swelling in both her hands is worse at the end of her day. Her pain is also worse with the more activity she does, rather than alleviating her pain or stiffness. While she feels the need to "stretch her hands a little" in the morning to "get going", you clarify with her that this feeling goes away quickly and well within 30 minutes. On your exam you note the following features:

- Degenerative changes at the fingertips (distal interphalangeal joints), including the presence of Heberden's nodes.

- Enlargement of the proximal knuckles (metacarpophalangeal joint) that are cool to the touch. There is no redness overlying them.

- There is elicitable pain with palpation at the base of both thumbs (carpometacarpal joint). This area appears somewhat enlarged and "square" in shape.

- You do not feel any appreciable swelling at the wrist or fingers.

Based on your history and exam, you discuss with Rosie that she has "wear and tear" arthritis in her hands. This has developed with use over time, and resulted in her pain and stiffness. You did not identify any signs of an inflammatory type arthritis in either her story or exam, and she is happy to hear this news as she was concerned about having "rheumatism". You reassure her that there are several options available to manage her arthritis now.

Rosie reports she has only been using trolamine salicylate (Bengay) on her hands. You advise her to start using prescription topical diclofenac gel at the base of her hands and finger creases where her pain occurs. If there is no improvement, or her pain begins to last all day, you will talk with her about starting acetaminophen (Tylenol). Because she has some difficulty grasping objects tightly or opening jar lids, you also recommend working with an occupational therapist to help her perform daily activities important to her.

TAKE HOME POINTS

- There are two major forms of arthritis, degenerative (or mechanical) and inflammatory. Although both can result in joint pain, damage and signs of local inflammation, the underlying mechanism leading to the manifestations is different.

- Inflammatory arthritis presents with important features that differentiate it from degenerative arthritis. The associated morning joint stiffness and pattern of joint involvement are two such characteristics.

- If there is either suspicion for an inflammatory condition, or uncertainty regarding whether one should be considered, early referral to a rheumatologist for specialty evaluation is warranted.

- In cases of mechanical joint disorders or injuries, evaluation and management together with an orthopedic or sports medicine specialist is beneficial.

- The management of both degenerative and inflammatory arthritis should consist of a multidisciplinary approach. Treatment should involve a combination of pharmacologic therapy, physical and/or occupational therapy, and rheumatology or orthopedic specialty co-management.

REFERENCES

[1] J. M. Hootman, C. G. Helmick, K. E. Barbour, K. A. Theis, and M. A. Boring, "Updated projected prevalence of self-reported doctor-diagnosed arthritis and arthritis-attributable activity limitation among US adults, 2015–2040," (in eng), *Arthritis & Rheumatology (Hoboken, N.J.)*, vol. 68, no. 7, pp. 1582–1587, Jul 2016.

[2] J. M. Hootman, C. G. Helmick, and S. M. Schappert, "Magnitude and characteristics of arthritis and other rheumatic conditions on ambulatory medical care visits, United States, 1997," (in eng), *Arthritis and Rheumatism*, vol. 47, no. 6, pp. 571–81, Dec 15 2002.

[3] "Prevalence and Most Common Causes of Disability Among Adults—United States, 2005," *Morbidity and Mortality Weekly Report (MMWR)*, Accessed on: May 1 [Online]. Available: https://www.cdc.gov/mmwr/preview/mmwrhtml/mm5816a2.htm

[4] J. M. Hootman and W. Y. Cheng, "Psychological distress and fair/poor health among adults with arthritis: state-specific prevalence and correlates of general health status, United States, 2007," (in eng), *International Journal of Public Health*, vol. 54 Suppl 1, pp. 75–83, Jun 2009.

[5] J. E. Lee, E. Kahana, B. Kahana, and K. Barnes, "Positive affect, depressive symptoms, and arthritis pain of elderly people over time," (in eng), *Healthy Aging Research*, vol. 4, 2015.

[6] "National and state medical expenditures and lost earnings attributable to arthritis and other rheumatic conditions—United States, 2003," (in eng), *MMWR. Morbidity and Mortality Weekly Report*, vol. 56, no. 1, pp. 4–7, Jan 12 2007.

[7] M. H. Chang and P. A. Nigrovic, "Antibody-dependent and -independent mechanisms of inflammatory arthritis," (in eng), *JCI Insight*, vol. 4, no. 5, Mar 7 2019.

[8] C. Deng *et al.*, "Targeted apoptosis of macrophages and osteoclasts in arthritic joints is effective against advanced inflammatory arthritis," (in eng), *Nature Communications*, vol. 12, no. 1, p. 2174, Apr 12 2021.

[9] C. Turesson, "Comorbidity in rheumatoid arthritis," (in eng), *Swiss Medical Weekly*, vol. 146, p. w14290, 2016.

[10] M. L. Westedt *et al.*, "Rheumatoid factors in rheumatoid arthritis and vasculitis," (in eng), *Rheumatology International*, vol. 5, no. 5, pp. 209–214, 1985.

[11] A. Sidari and E. Hill, "Diagnosis and treatment of gout and pseudogout for everyday practice," (in eng), *Primary Care*, vol. 45, no. 2, pp. 213–236, Jun 2018.

[12] K. Yip, R. E. Cohen, and M. H. Pillinger, "Asymptomatic hyperuricemia: is it really asymptomatic?," (in eng), *Current Opinion in Rheumatology*, vol. 32, no. 1, pp. 71–79, Jan 2020.

[13] A. Slobodnick, B. Shah, S. Krasnokutsky, and M. H. Pillinger, "Update on colchicine, 2017," (in eng), *Rheumatology (Oxford, England)*, vol. 57, no. suppl_1, pp. i4–i11, Jan 1 2018.

[14] R. Dammacco *et al.*, "Giant cell arteritis: the experience of two collaborative referral centers and an overview of disease pathogenesis and therapeutic advancements," (in eng), *Clinical ophthalmology (Auckland, N.Z.)*, vol. 14, pp. 775–793, 2020.

[15] A. García-Kutzbach, J. Chacón-Súchite, H. García-Ferrer, and I. Iraheta, "Reactive arthritis: update 2018," (in eng), *Clinical Rheumatology*, vol. 37, no. 4, pp. 869–874, Apr 2018.

[16] D. Lazaro, "Elderly-onset systemic lupus erythematosus: prevalence, clinical course and treatment," (in eng), *Drugs & Aging*, vol. 24, no. 9, pp. 701–715, 2007.

[17] A. Ogdie, L. C. Coates, and D. D. Gladman, "Treatment guidelines in psoriatic arthritis," (in eng), *Rheumatology (Oxford, England)*, vol. 59, no. Suppl 1, pp. i37–i46, Mar 1 2020.

[18] A. Balakrishnan, R. Aggarwal, V. Agarwal, and L. Gupta, "Inclusion body myositis in the rheumatology clinic," (in eng), *International Journal of Rheumatic Diseases*, vol. 23, no. 9, pp. 1126–1135, Aug 2020.

[19] G. A. Kelley, K. S. Kelley, J. M. Hootman, and D. L. Jones, "Effects of community-deliverable exercise on pain and physical function in adults with arthritis and other rheumatic diseases: a meta-analysis," (in eng), *Arthritis Care & Research*, vol. 63, no. 1, pp. 79–93, Jan 2011.

[20] T. E. McAlindon *et al.*, "OARSI guidelines for the non-surgical management of knee osteoarthritis," *Osteoarthritis and Cartilage*, vol. 22, no. 3, pp. 363–388, 2014.

[21] K. D. Gross and H. J. Hillstrom, "Noninvasive devices targeting the mechanics of osteoarthritis," *Rheumatic Diseases Clinics of North America*, vol. 34, no. 3, pp. 755–776, 2008.

[22] S. A. Paget, A. Gibofsky, and J. F. Beary, *Hospital for Special Surgery Manual of Rheumatology and Outpatient Orthopedic Disorders: Diagnosis and Therapy*. Philadelphia: Wolters Kluwer Health, 2005.

[23] R. Pivec, A. J. Johnson, S. C. Mears, and M. A. Mont, "Hip arthroplasty," *The Lancet*, vol. 380, no. 9855, pp. 1768–1777, 2012/11/17/ 2012.

[24] A. J. Carr *et al.*, "Knee replacement," *The Lancet*, vol. 379, no. 9823, pp. 1331–1340, 2012/04/07/ 2012.

[25] R. Christensen, E. M. Bartels, A. Astrup, and H. Bliddal, "Effect of weight reduction in obese patients diagnosed with knee osteoarthritis: a systematic review and meta-analysis," *Annals of the Rheumatic Diseases*, vol. 66, no. 4, pp. 433–439, 2006.

[26] E. W. Gregg *et al.*, "Association of the magnitude of weight loss and changes in physical fitness with long-term cardiovascular disease outcomes in overweight or obese people with type 2 diabetes: a post-hoc analysis of the Look AHEAD randomised clinical trial," *The Lancet Diabetes & Endocrinology*, vol. 4, no. 11, pp. 913–921, 2016.

[27] K. E. Heiberg, V. Bruun-Olsen, A. Ekeland, and A. M. Mengshoel, "Effect of a walking skill training program in patients who have undergone total hip arthroplasty: followup one year after surgery," (in eng), *Arthritis Care Res (Hoboken)*, vol. 64, no. 3, pp. 415–23, Mar 2012.

[28] H. P. French *et al.*, "Exercise and manual physiotherapy arthritis research trial (EMPART) for osteoarthritis of the hip: a multicenter randomized controlled trial," (in eng), *Archives of Physical Medicine and Rehabilitation*, vol. 94, no. 2, pp. 302–14, Feb 2013.

[29] A. Spitz, A. A. Moore, M. Papaleontiou, E. Granieri, B. J. Turner, and M. C. Reid, "Primary care providers' perspective on prescribing opioids to older adults with chronic non-cancer pain: a qualitative study," *BMC Geriatrics*, vol. 11, no. 1, p. 35, 2011.

[30] K. Yip and J. Oettinger, "Why are we still using opioids for osteoarthritis?," (in eng), *International Journal of Clinical Practice*, vol. 74, no. 1, p. e13416, Jan 2020.

[31] J. C. Richmond *et al.*, "American Academy of Orthopaedic Surgeons clinical practice guideline on the treatment of osteoarthritis (OA) of the knee," *Journal of Bone and Joint Surgery, American Volume*, vol. 92, no. 4, pp. 990–993, 2010.

[32] M. C. Hochberg *et al.*, "American college of rheumatology 2012 recommendations for the use of nonpharmacologic and pharmacologic therapies in osteoarthritis of the hand, hip, and knee," *Arthritis Care and Research*, vol. 64, no. 4, pp. 465–474, 2012.

[33] *Osteoarthritis of the Knee Clinical Care Standard*. Sydney: ACSQHC: Australian Commission on Safety and Quality in Health Care, 2017.

[34] "VA/DoD Clinical Practice Guideline For The Non-Surgical Management Of Hip & Knee Osteoarthritis," US Department of Defense, 2014.

[35] "Osteoarthritis: care and management," *NICE*. Accessed on: February [Online]. Available: https://www.nice.org.uk/guidance/cg177/chapter/1-Recommendations#pharmacological-management

[36] M. Jóźwiak-Bebenista and J. Z. Nowak, "Paracetamol: mechanism of action, applications and safety concern," (in eng), *Acta Poloniae Pharmaceutica*, vol. 71, no. 1, pp. 11–23, Jan-Feb 2014.

[37] T. E. Towheed, L. Maxwell, M. G. Judd, M. Catton, M. C. Hochberg, and G. Wells, "Acetaminophen for osteoarthritis," (in eng), *The Cochrane Database of Systematic Reviews*, vol. 2006, no. 1, p. Cd004257, Jan 25 2006.

[38] V.-K. Bournia, G. Kitas, A. D. Protogerou, and P. P. Sfikakis, "Impact of non-steroidal anti-inflammatory drugs on cardiovascular risk: is it the same in osteoarthritis and rheumatoid arthritis?," *Modern Rheumatology*, vol. 27, no. 4, pp. 559–569, 2017/07/04 2017.

[39] J. R. Vane and R. M. Botting, "Mechanism of action of aspirin-like drugs," *Seminars in Arthritis and Rheumatism*, vol. 26, pp. 2–10, 1997/06/01/ 1997.

[40] B. Cryer, "NSAID-associated deaths: the rise and fall of NSAID-associated GI mortality," *The American Journal of Gastroenterology*, vol. 100, no. 8, pp. 1694–1695, 2005.

[41] Z. Y. Wang *et al.*, "Efficacy and safety of duloxetine on osteoarthritis knee pain: a meta-analysis of randomized controlled trials," (in eng), *Pain Medicine (Malden, Mass.)*, vol. 16, no. 7, pp. 1373–85, Jul 2015.

[42] C. Weng, J. Xu, Q. Wang, W. Lu, and Z. Liu, "Efficacy and safety of duloxetine in osteoarthritis or chronic low back pain: a Systematic review and meta-analysis," (in eng), *Osteoarthritis and Cartilage*, vol. 28, no. 6, pp. 721–734, Jun 2020.

[43] S. H. Gao, J. B. Huo, Q. M. Pan, X. W. Li, H. Y. Chen, and J. H. Huang, "The short-term effect and safety of duloxetine in osteoarthritis: a systematic review and meta-analysis," (in eng), *Medicine*, vol. 98, no. 44, p. e17541, Nov 2019.

[44] D. B. Reuben *et al.*, "National institutes of health pathways to prevention workshop: the role of opioids in the treatment of chronic pain," *Annals of Internal Medicine*, vol. 162, no. 4, pp. 295–300, 2015.

[45] E. E. Krebs *et al.*, "Effect of opioid vs nonopioid medications on pain-related function in patients with chronic back pain or hip or knee osteoarthritis pain: the SPACE randomized clinical trial," (in eng), *Jama*, vol. 319, no. 9, pp. 872–882, Mar 6 2018.

[46] A. K. Chang, P. E. Bijur, D. Esses, D. P. Barnaby, and J. Baer, "Effect of a single dose of oral opioid and nonopioid analgesics on acute extremity pain in the emergency department: a randomized clinical," *Jama*, vol. 318, no. 17, pp. 1661–1667, 2017.

[47] W. A. Ray, C. P. Chung, K. T. Murray, K. Hall, and C. M. Stein, "Prescription of long-acting opioids and mortality in patients with chronic noncancer pain," (in eng), *Jama*, vol. 315, no. 22, pp. 2415–23, Jun 14 2016.

[48] M. S. Dhillon, S. Patel, and R. John, "PRP in OA knee—update, current confusions and future options," (in eng), *SICOT J*, vol. 3, pp. 27–27, 2017.

[49] M. Ranade, H. Pandit, and K. Kothari, "Does intraarticular PRP injection improve function, pain and quality of life in patients with OA of knee? Case control study of 50 patients," *Journal of Arthroscopy and Joint Surgery*, vol. 5, no. 3, pp. 171–174, 2018/09/01/ 2018.

[50] D. Jevsevar, P. Donnelly, G. A. Brown, and D. S. Cummins, "Viscosupplementation for osteoarthritis of the knee: a systematic review of the evidence," (in eng), *The Journal of Bone and Joint Surgery. American Volume*, vol. 97, no. 24, pp. 2047–60, Dec 16 2015.

[51] F. Davatchi, B. Sadeghi Abdollahi, M. Mohyeddin, and B. Nikbin, "Mesenchymal stem cell therapy for knee osteoarthritis: 5 years follow-up of three patients," *International Journal of Rheumatic Diseases*, vol. 19, no. 3, pp. 219–225, 2016.

[52] A. Mobasheri, G. Kalamegam, G. Musumeci, and M. E. Batt, "Chondrocyte and mesenchymal stem cell-based therapies for cartilage repair in osteoarthritis and related orthopaedic conditions," *Maturitas*, vol. 78, no. 3, pp. 188–198, 2014/07/01/ 2014.

[53] Z. L. McCormick *et al.*, "Cooled radiofrequency ablation of the genicular nerves for chronic pain due to knee osteoarthritis: six-month outcomes," *Pain Medicine*, vol. 18, no. 9, pp. 1631–1641, 2017.

[54] D.-H. Kim *et al.*, "Ultrasound-guided genicular nerve block for knee osteoarthritis: a double-blind, randomized controlled trial of local anesthetic alone or in combination with corticosteroid," *Pain Physician*, vol. 21, no. 1, pp. 41–52, 2018.

[55] C. Lahaye, Z. Tatar, J. J. Dubost, A. Tournadre, and M. Soubrier, "Management of inflammatory rheumatic conditions in the elderly," (in eng), *Rheumatology (Oxford, England)*, vol. 58, no. 5, pp. 748–764, May 1 2019.

[56] X. Li *et al.*, "Epidemiological survey of antinuclear antibodies in healthy population and analysis of clinical characteristics of positive population," (in eng), *Journal of Clinical Laboratory Analysis*, vol. 33, no. 8, p. e22965, Oct 2019.

[57] A. S. Hassan, A. Rao, A. M. Manadan, and J. A. Block, "Peripheral bacterial septic arthritis: review of diagnosis and management," (in eng), *Journal of Clinical Rheumatology: Practical Reports on Rheumatic & Musculoskeletal Diseases*, vol. 23, no. 8, pp. 435–442, Dec 2017.

[58] A. Y. L. Wong, J. Karppinen, and D. Samartzis, "Low back pain in older adults: risk factors, management options and future directions," (in eng), *Scoliosis and Spinal Disorders*, vol. 12, p. 14, 2017.

19 Stroke Prevention in the Elderly

Liam Durcan, MD, FRCPC

CONTENTS

A 74-year-old right-handed woman who had been previously healthy is seen in clinic following her presentation to the emergency department. She relates a history of suddenly losing the ability to speak for 15 minutes on the previous day. She was able to understand all that was said to her during the event. She denied having had any headache or other neurological symptoms. By the time she presented to the emergency department her symptoms had resolved and her neurological exam was normal. Her blood pressure was 160/95.

Brain imaging (a non-contrast CT scan) showed no acute stroke nor hemorrhage. The only abnormality on a carotid doppler done the same day was an 80% stenosis of the right internal carotid artery. ECG revealed normal sinus rhythm.

Her fasting glucose was 6 mmol/l and her LDL was 3.8 mmol/l. She is a non-smoker.

The diagnosis of isolated expressive aphasia, due to a transient ischemic attack, was made.

PREAMBLE

Stroke is a leading cause of death and disability. Risk of stroke is age-related and age is the most important non-modifiable risk factor. Modifiable risk factors for recurrent stroke include hypertension, diabetes, dyslipidemic states, smoking, symptomatic carotid stenosis and atrial fibrillation.

The incidence of stroke increases with age, doubling for each decade after age 55. Among adults ages 35 to 44, the incidence of stroke is 30 to 120 of 100,000 per year, and for those ages 65 to 74, the incidence is 670 to 970 of 100,000 per year.

Stroke risk is further heightened after TIA and minor stroke-observational and risk-stratification studies have shown between 2% and 17% within the first 90 days. In patients who have had a transient ischemic attack, one in five will have a subsequent stroke, heart attack or die within one year, with stroke being the most common outcome.

One of the challenges in stroke prevention in the elderly is the application of evidence-based treatment or investigational recommendations in an age group who have often been excluded from randomized trials on which those recommendations are based. Unlike in younger adults where the evidence for secondary stroke prevention is well established and supported by randomized clinical trial data, evidence is often less clear in older adults.

What Is the Risk to This Patient?

A recent TIA is associated with a significant increase of subsequent stroke. Tools such as the ABCD2 score can give some insight to the degree of that heightened risk as well as risk-stratify patients according to their demographics, vascular risks and clinical presentation. (Tables 19.1 and 19.2) This patient's ABCD2 score is 4—her risk of event recurrence, using this data, is moderate.

What Are Her Risk Factors Associated with This Presentation?

Age, hypertension and hyperlipidemia.

106

DOI: 10.1201/9781003344476-22

Table 19.1 ABCD2 Score

ABCD2 Score	Points
Age > 60 years	1
BP > 140/90 at presentation	1
Clinical features of the TIA	1
Speech disturbance without weakness or unilateral weakness	2
Duration of symptoms	1
10–59 minutes	2
> 60 minutes	
Diabetes in patient's history	1

Table 19.2 Risk of Stroke Following Various ABCD2 Scores

Total Risk	Scores	2 days	7 days	90 days
Low	0–3	1.0	1.2	3.1
Moderate	4–5	4.1	5.9	9.8
High	6–7	8.1	12.0	18.0

HYPERTENSION

Following a stroke or transient ischemic attack, blood pressure lowering treatment is recommended to achieve a target of lower than 140/90 mm Hg. For patients who have had a small subcortical stroke, blood pressure lowering treatment is recommended to achieve a systolic target lower than 130 mm Hg. In patients with diabetes, blood pressure lowering treatment is recommended for the prevention of first or recurrent stroke to attain systolic blood pressure targets consistently lower than 130 mm Hg and diastolic blood pressure targets consistently lower than 80 mm Hg.

Reducing blood pressure is more important than the agent used.

Hypertension in the Very Elderly Trial confirmed the benefit of treating hypertension in patients over the age of 80. Patients were randomized to indapamide or placebo with a target BP of 150/90. No significant differences in adverse events—primarily syncopal episodes and falls of any kind—were noted between the treatment and placebo group. The number-needed-to treat (or NNT) at 2 years was 94 for stroke and 40 for mortality. (The NNT is an epidemiological measure of the effectiveness of an intervention. It is the average number of people who need to be treated to prevent one additional bad outcome compared to the control group. The lower the number the more effective the treatment.)

Carotid stenosis is an important and potentially treatable risk factor for recurrent stroke, with the most important determinants of risk being the degree of stenosis and whether the stenosis is symptomatic. The most important initial decision-point is whether the stenosis is symptomatic: an asymptomatic carotid stenosis of greater than 70% carries a per year risk of 1–3% and current guidelines recommend maximal medical therapy over endarterectomy. This relatively low risk is contrasted with a 28.3% 3-year risk of symptomatic carotid stenoses of the same degree.

It is also important to note that risk of recurrent ipsilateral stroke in symptomatic stenosis greater than 70% is markedly increased in the period immediately following the TIA or minor stroke—with ipsilateral recurrence risk ranging from 11.5% to 25% at 14 days. Pooled data from the North American Symptomatic Carotid Endarterectomy Trial and the European Carotid Stenosis Trial showed performing carotid endarterectomy within two weeks gave optimum results.

Atrial fibrillation is a cardiac arrhythmia associated with an increased risk of ischemic stroke and peripheral embolization. The arrhythmia is associated with a gradual increase in left atrial volume and can be associated with presence of a thrombus in the left atrial appendage. Patients may have a number of symptoms with atrial fibrillation, but it must be remembered that many patients may experience subclinical atrial fibrillation and that symptoms of palpitations are neither sensitive nor specific for atrial fibrillation.

Non-valvular atrial fibrillation increases stroke risk by a factor of 5 and valvular atrial fibrillation by a factor of 17. Atrial fibrillation becomes more clinically relevant with age: the attributable risk of stroke from AF is estimated to be 1.5% for those aged 50–59 years, and it approaches 30% for those aged 80–89 years. Women are at a higher risk of stroke due to AF than men. Strokes attributed to atrial fibrillation are more severe and TIAs attributed tend to last longer than those attributed to other etiologies.

The diagnosis of atrial fibrillation is most often made from the electrocardiogram—whether it is a single ECG exam, the 24- or 48-hour evaluation of a Holter monitor or more prolonged cardiac monitoring. The Embrace Study compared 30-day ambulatory monitoring with a 24-hour Holter monitor to detect atrial fibrillation in cryptogenic (unknown cause) stroke. The 30-day monitoring arm detected atrial fibrillation in 16.1% compared to 3.2% in the group investigated with 24-hour Holter.

Clinical scores—such as the CHADS2 score and CHA2DS2-VASc score—have been developed to help predict the risk of stroke and systemic embolism in patients with AF, in order to determine whether that risk is sufficient to warrant the bleeding risks associated with anticoagulant therapy. In a patient who presents with stroke or TIA and is found to be in atrial fibrillation, the ischemic event alone carries enough value in these scoring systems to warrant anticoagulation.

Hyperlipidemia—many observational studies have described the relationship between lipid abnormalities and elevated stroke risk, implicated in both intracranial and extracranial atherosclerosis. The pivotal study showing benefit of lipid-lowering regimes in stroke prevention was the SPACL study, which randomized patients to atorvastatin 80 mg or placebo. The treatment group had an absolute risk reduction of 2.2% for a number needed to treat of 45 to prevent one stroke at 5 years.

DIABETES

Through mechanisms such as accelerated atherosclerosis and endothelial dysfunction, diabetes increases not only the risk for stroke, but is also associated with increased post-stroke mortality and poorer clinical outcomes for survivors. Most recently, GLP-1 agonists have shown to have a modest benefit in prevention of stroke in Type II diabetics. (Absolute risk reduction of 0.81% or NNT of 125.)

SMOKING

Cigarette smoking is associated with an approximate doubling of stroke risk. A recent study has also shown a dose–response relationship for the risk, with an odds ratio ranging from 1.46 for those smoking < 11 cigarettes per day to 5.66 for those smoking 40+ cigarettes per day, indicating that while cessation is the ultimate goal, reduction of amount smoked can confer an important risk reduction.

What Would Be an Appropriate Initial Intervention and Further Investigations?

As the patient has presented more than a day after her event and has no residual deficits, *she is not a candidate for acute revascularization therapies* (intravenous tPA or endovascular thrombectomy).

Tempo of Assessment and Intervention—The EXPRESS Study prospectively looked at 90-day recurrent stroke rates in patients seen in clinic before and after an expedited assessment program was put into place. The establishment of expedited assessment (with a reduction of median time to evaluation of 3 days to 1 day) resulted in an absolute risk reduction of recurrent stroke at 90 days of 8.2%.

The combination of low-dose aspirin and clopidogrel (Plavix) has been found to reduce the risk of recurrent stroke and disability compared with aspirin alone when started as soon as possible after a high-risk transient ischemic attack (TIA) or minor ischemic stroke without persistent disabling neurologic deficit and continued for 10 to 21 days.

Three randomized controlled trials comparing dual antiplatelet therapy with aspirin monotherapy in more than 10,000 patients provided evidence that dual therapy decreased nonfatal recurrent strokes (number needed to treat [NNT] = 53). Dual antiplatelet therapy had no effect on all-cause mortality or the incidence of myocardial infarction or recurrent TIA, and had some associated harms of minor (number needed to harm [NNH] = 143) and moderate to major (NNH = 500) extracranial bleeding.

As the patient is hypertensive and is neurologically stable, *antihypertensive medication* can be started. The choice of agent may be influenced by a number of other health variables or patient preferences.

A more conservative approach is often indicated in patients with an acute and persistent neurological deficit as they may be depending on elevated blood pressure to maintain cerebral perfusion to potentially endangered brain tissue. Often, antihypertensives may be held for 48 to 72 hours following a stroke, assuming the elevated BP is not causing end-organ damage elsewhere.

Cholesterol-lowering agents—Statins are started after stroke, with many stroke specialists using dosages in higher range (Atorvastatin 40–80 mg daily) to achieve a reduction of LDL below 2 mmol/l.

INVESTIGATIONS

TTE

Transthoracic echocardiographic evaluation is recommended for most stroke patients, primarily to investigate the conditions associated with atrial fibrillation and to assess valvular structures, which may influence the type of antithrombotic agent used.

Holter

Paroxysmal AF may not be detected on serial ECGs or short-term cardiac monitoring. In cases of acute cerebral ischemia where the diagnosis of atrial fibrillation is not already made, a 24- or 48-hour Holter monitor is indicated. If these investigations are negative but atrial fibrillation is still clinically suspected (cryptogenic stroke, no evidence of large vessel atherosclerosis, increased left atrial volume on TTE, excessive number of premature atrial beats (e.g. > 500 per 24 hrs of monitoring) ambulatory cardiac monitoring for 30 days is suggested.

Education

All patients are counseled on lifestyle changes that have positive effects on reducing stroke recurrence. As well, a key part of any initial assessment is ensuring the patient understands the symptoms of stroke, to be better able to present immediately should they experience recurrent symptoms.

RESOLUTION OF THE CLINICAL VIGNETTE

The patient remained asymptomatic. At 21 days post-event, clopidogrel (Plavix) was stopped and low-dose (81 mg daily) enteric-coated acetylsalicylic acid (aspirin) was continued. The patient was started on atorvastatin 40 mg daily and perindopril 4 mg/indapamide 1.25 mg daily. Her hemoglobin A1c was not elevated.

In this case, the carotid stenosis, although greater than 60%, is in the right internal carotid artery and the patient's stroke is localized to an area supplied by the left carotid artery. The right carotid stenosis is an *asymptomatic stenosis* and best managed medically. Endarterectomy is not indicated.

The patient had a trans-thoracic echocardiogram that showed slightly increased left atrial volume without structural abnormality of the valves. A 48-hour Holter monitor did not detect atrial fibrillation but did show greater than 1500 premature atrial beats per 24 hours. A 30-day implanted device revealed prolonged episodes of atrial fibrillation. The patient was started on Apixaban 5 mg BID. Aspirin was stopped.

REFERENCES

1. Dual antiplatelet therapy for high-risk TIA and minor stroke: BMJ rapid recommendation. *BMJ*. December 2018;363:k5130.
2. Gladstone D et al. Atrial fibrillation in cryptogenic stroke. N Engl J Med 2014;370:2467–2477.
3. Johnston SC et al. Validation and refinement of scores to predict very early stroke risk after transient ischaemic attack. Lancet. 2007 27;369(9558):283–292.
4. Rothwell et al. Effect of urgent treatment of transient ischaemic attack and minor stroke on early recurrent stroke (EXPRESS study): a prospective population-based sequential comparison. Lancet. October 2007;370(9596) 20–26, 1432–1442.
5. Markidan J et al. Smoking and risk of ischemic stroke in young men. Stroke. 2018;49:1276–1278.

20 Advances in Cardiac Care for Older Persons

P. David Myerowitz, MD, FACS, FACC

CONTENTS

ADVANCES IN CARDIAC CARE FOR OLDER PERSONS

Many of the advances in cardiac care in the last two decades have focused on minimally invasive procedures especially aimed at the elderly and vulnerable. This chapter will attempt to chronicle these treatments, mainly surgical and invasive cardiological, but also some new drug therapies that have proven especially advantageous to the older cardiology patient. For the purpose of this chapter I will use age 65–84 as elderly and over 85 as very elderly. Since new procedures, devices and drugs are continuously added to the clinician's armamentarium, this chapter is not meant to be comprehensive. Nor is it written for cardiac care physicians. Rather it is a plain language description of the latest advances in cardiac care available to older patients designed to improve both length and quality of life.

Since the concept of frailty was discussed in an earlier chapter, I will not repeat the discussion. Although there are objective measures, such as the Charlson Comorbidity Index, for most of my career as a cardiac surgeon, the concept of frailty was more a subjective assessment (i.e. you'll know it when you see it). That said, my first heart transplant in 1984 was in a man over 50 years old which at that time was pushing the age limit (he survived over ten years to see multiple grandchildren born). I also remember a blind, formerly active 90-year-old man confined to his bed with severe aortic stenosis whom I was pushed to operate on in the 1980s and whose family sent me a picture ten years later of him celebrating his 100th birthday. In my opinion, age alone should not definitively rule out most if not all available options for cardiac care.

In fact, there is a quarterly journal, *Journal of Geriatric Cardiology*, devoted to the care of the older patient with cardiovascular disease.

HEART FAILURE (DECREASED OR PRESERVED EJECTION FRACTION) AND HYPERTENSION

Definitions and Medical Therapy

Heart failure occurs when the heart is unable to pump enough blood to keep up with the oxygen demands of the body. Some of the typical symptoms include shortness of breath, fatigue, peripheral edema (swelling of the legs), persistent cough, rapid weight gain and confusion. The common measurement used to define this condition and which is easily obtained by a noninvasive test called an echocardiogram is the ejection fraction, the percentage of the volume of blood in the left ventricle (the heart's main pumping chamber) that is ejected with each heartbeat. Normally this is greater than 50%. A value below 40% is consistent with heart failure and is labeled heart failure with reduced ejection fraction (HFrEF).

DOI: 10.1201/9781003344476-23

The New York Heart Association, for the classification of heart failure, describes four categories based on severity of symptoms: Class I is no symptoms with no limitation of activity; Class II is symptoms on normal activity with slight limitation of activity; Class III is marked limitation of activity with symptoms on less than normal activity; and Class IV is symptoms on any activity with inability to perform any activity. Roughly one third of patients are in Class I, a third in Class II and a third in Class III and IV.

Studies show that 1–5% of the population have chronic heart failure and 50% of these heart failure patients are over 75 years of age. Eighty-five percent of first-time hospitalizations for heart failure are patients over 65 and 60% are over 75 years old with one-third of these patients dying within 6 months of diagnosis.

Fifty percent of patients, and increasing in frequency, comprise a second group of patients with heart failure with preserved ejection fraction (HFpEF). These patients have characteristic symptoms of heart failure but a normal ejection fraction. This diagnosis can also be made by echocardiogram and most likely results from stiffness of the muscle of the left ventricle. I will first discuss heart failure with reduced ejection fraction.

The mainstay of treatment for HFrEF is drug therapy and perhaps the most commonly used categories of drugs are the angiotensin-converting enzyme inhibitors (ACE inhibitors) and angiotensin receptor blockers (ARBs) that block the release of substances that cause narrowing of blood vessels. There are many affordable brand-name and generic versions of these drugs available. By dilating peripheral blood vessels the workload of the heart is reduced, much like opening a nozzle on the end of a hose reduces the workload on a water pump. Unfortunately, multicenter studies show that these drugs are vastly underutilized, especially in the older population, and when used are given in much lower doses than recommended.

High blood pressure and hypertension commonly accompany heart failure in the elderly. The target for systolic blood pressure (upper number), however, has been a moving target for those heart councils recommending treatment. While 120/80 (mmHg) is the classic normal blood pressure, treatment for decades was recommended for blood pressures over 130 systolic and 90 diastolic, with numbers in between these two levels termed pre-hypertension. Recently the recommendation for target systolic pressure was lowered to 120; however, management in the elderly remains controversial. While the diastolic pressure (lower number) target remains the same, in the elderly a systolic of 130 seems realistic with a level of 150 in those over 80 to avoid the complications of sudden drops in blood pressure leading to syncope and falls.

A newer combination drug, an angiotensin receptor blocker–neprilysin inhibitor (brand name Entresto in the United States) has been shown to be even more effective in the treatment of HFrEF and should be used in patients who have a suboptimal response to the aforementioned drugs. Though somewhat more complicated in its action, the neprilysin inhibitor increases the activity of substances that block the retention of sodium, a common problem in heart failure patients.

Another commonly used category of drugs used in heart failure are diuretics which prevent fluid retention, presenting as fluid in the lungs as well as peripheral edema or swelling of the legs. Leg edema in the elderly may also be caused by venous insufficiency, poor nutrition with low protein levels in the blood and adverse drug effects (e.g. use of calcium channel blockers), resulting in frequent misdiagnosis especially in the very elderly. A recent blood test, B-type natriuretic peptide, is significantly elevated in heart failure and may be useful to confirm or rule out the diagnosis. Hydrochlorothiazide and spironolactone are commonly used affordable diuretics that are also effective in treating hypertension and HFrEF. With refractory or acute fluid retention, furosemide (brand name Lasix) is extremely effective in eliminating fluid retention demonstrated by sudden weight gain, but frequently causes a potentially dangerous lowering of potassium in the blood which can lead to heart rhythm disturbances.

Low-dose beta blockers such as carvedilol and metoprolol are also commonly used to treat both heart failure and hypertension. If tolerated, a heart rate target of less than 70 should be achieved.

Side effects may occur with any of these drugs and include elevated blood potassium causing heart rhythm abnormalities and kidney dysfunction with ACE inhibitors, spironolactone and ARBs; vertigo, asthma-like bronchial constriction, depression and cognitive impairment with beta blockers; and low blood sodium with kidney failure and delirium for diuretics. These drugs must be monitored carefully as new drugs are added or their doses increased to prevent hypotension (low blood pressure). Orthostatic hypotension—a drop in blood pressure when one stands from sitting or lying down—is common, but may be transient and respond to temporary cessation of a drug followed by a more gradual increase in dose to allow accommodation. Bradycardia or a slow heart rate is a common side effect of all beta blockers. Heart rates of 60 to 70 are usually well tolerated.

Ancillary office personnel should do regular checks inquiring as to shortness of breath, dizziness or falls and patients should be instructed on regular two- or three-times-a-day home monitoring of blood pressure using an automated device and daily weight. Most automated blood pressure cuffs (many cuffs are accurate and easy to use) also provide heart rate and store measurements for later review by caregivers. Patients should be instructed to report a rapid change up or down in weight, blood pressure or heart rate, especially if accompanied by dizziness.

In very elderly patients and all older patients with frailty demonstrated by muscle wasting, poor appetite, depression, lack of exercise and comorbidities such as diabetes and renal insufficiency, all of these drugs must be used with extra caution. Drug levels tend to be higher in this population at the same doses as younger patients.

Multicenter studies have shown that these drugs, though highly effective, are not prescribed for many heart failure patients, especially the elderly, and, even if ordered, are not given in recommended dosages. With careful monitoring, these drugs can and should be prescribed for the older patient with symptomatic heart failure with reduced ejection fraction and/or hypertension.

The incidence of heart failure with preserved ejection fraction is increasing in the elderly and now represents half of all patients with heart failure. Nonetheless, this group of heart failure patients is less well understood and has no effective therapy. Echocardiographic studies frequently demonstrate diastolic dysfunction or stiffening of the left ventricle.

Treatment of associated conditions such as coronary artery disease and hypertension should be addressed. However, despite treatment regimens similar to heart failure with reduced ejection fraction, few gains have been achieved in reducing mortality, the need for re-hospitalization or improving symptoms and quality of life as has been accomplished with HFrEF. Nonetheless, the same drugs discussed earlier should be tried in these patients in hopes of achieving some improvement.

No discussion of the treatment of heart failure in the older person would be complete without a discussion of end-of-life care. Hospitalizations are frequent, and at some point, options for additional therapy run out. Since most adults with heart failure die in a hospital, palliative care at home may be appropriate treatment for this cohort in an attempt to improve quality of life and reduce costs associated with repeat hospitalizations.

CARDIAC RESYNCHRONIZATION THERAPY (CRT)/INTRACARDIAC DEFIBRILLATOR (ICD)

Nearly a century ago, researchers found that heart rhythm abnormalities led to impaired heart function. Eighty years later, in the 1990s, heart failure patients with electrical conduction abnormalities on their electrocardiogram (ECG), specifically a left bundle branch block (LBBB) producing delayed contraction between the right and left ventricles, showed significant improvement in ejection fraction when a pacemaker was used to correct this abnormality. Not all patients show improvement, with a third not responding at all.

The technique involves the transvenous insertion of electrodes into the right atrium, right ventricle and a third electrode through the coronary sinus into a vein on the back of the left ventricle. Initiation of contraction begins with sensing of an electrical impulse in the right atrium followed by simultaneous firing of the right ventricle and left ventricle electrodes so their contractions occur simultaneously. This provides optimal filling of the left ventricle and, in two-thirds of patients, reduction in symptoms and improvement in heart function. The addition of defibrillator function to the device also reduces the incidence of sudden death.

All heart failure patients in Class III or IV heart failure with the likelihood of significant survival who demonstrate a left bundle branch block on ECG should be considered for a CRT pacemaker insertion.

HEART TRANSPLANTATION AND MECHANICAL PUMPS

As I mentioned in my introduction, in its early years, heart transplantation was restricted to the young—under age 50—with no other organ dysfunction. The number of donors per year has struggled to keep up with an expanding pool of recipients including the elderly, resulting in longer waiting lists and the search for alternative solutions. Comparing 2008 to 2018, the percent of adult heart transplant recipients over the age of 65 increased from 13.9% to 22.2% in the United States. In absolute numbers, 660 heart transplants were performed in 2018 in people over the age of 65. The push for this expansion came as multiple single center studies showed similar survival rates in the elderly as in younger than 65 recipients. At the same time, the percent of adults receiving a heart transplant for coronary artery disease decreased while the percent performed for cardiomyopathy increased, most likely the result of improved treatment of coronary artery disease as well as the increase in end-stage heart failure patients.

Part of the explanation is the expanded donor pool during this time which until 2010 had been stagnant at about 2500 a year. But in the second half of the last decade, numbers jumped to 3500, perhaps partly as a result of expanding acceptable criteria for donors and older population growth. These new criteria included increasing donor age to 65; accepting Hepatitis C positive donors and then treating the hepatitis with a newly discovered, expensive but very effective treatment in the recipient; and accepting marginal hearts requiring corrective procedures (such as coronary bypass or valve repair) or a period of mechanical support for recovery of function. Many of these marginal donor organs were used in older recipients with good results.

The technique of heart transplantation has basically not changed since first performed in the late 1960s. The results, however, have greatly improved with current one-, three-, and five-year survival at 90%, 85% and 80% respectively.

Much of the improved survival is a result of safer and more effective immunosuppressive drugs such as cyclosporine and more recently tacrolimus and mycophenolate mofetil/mycophenolic acid. These drugs have reduced the frequency and severity of acute rejections and possibly chronic rejection as demonstrated by diffuse coronary artery vasculopathy, a common cause of late mortality. They have also allowed the more aggressive and early tapering of corticosteroids, another immunosuppressive mainstay which has severe side effects. These newer drugs are especially important in the older recipient in whom the side effects of corticosteroid therapy such as hypertension and diabetes are more frequent.

Other factors leading to improved survival, with heart transplants performed since 2000 experiencing a median survival of 12 years, include better preservation of donor hearts and mechanical devices used pretransplant to stabilize and improve multi-organ dysfunction in severely ill recipients. These pumps have developed along two distinct pathways, ventricular assist devices (VADs) and total artificial hearts (TAHs). A VAD is attached to the patient's existing heart while a TAH replaces the heart. Most patients can be managed with a single left-sided VAD since the predominant problem is left ventricular dysfunction, and a single VAD connected to the apex of the left ventricle with outflow to the ascending aorta is able to pump the entire cardiac output to the systemic circulation. If there is additional right ventricular dysfunction, either an additional right sided VAD may be implanted or, if available, a TAH can be implanted. Currently available TAHs are more complicated to insert and, of course, eliminate any chance for native heart recovery and removal.

Mechanical pumps have been effectively used as a bridge to transplantation for almost 40 years. Unlike earlier pulsatile pumps, more recent models are continuous flow (the patients do not have a pulse), use floating blades to propel the blood and require less anticoagulation than earlier models. Patients on transplant waiting lists who are failing medical therapy can be supported for months or years while multi-organ failure is reversed and they are stabilized prior to transplantation. They can be discharged to home with much improved quality of life awaiting a suitable donor. The poster child for an older person with this therapy is former Vice President Dick Cheney. He underwent implantation of a VAD at age 69, appeared in a television interview while on the device and subsequently, at age 71, underwent a successful heart transplant in 2012.

The next stage of development of particular importance to those heart failure patients over 65 is the use of VADs or total heart replacement with a mechanical pump as destination therapy, rather than as a bridge to transplant. Most patients only require support of the left ventricle which can be accomplished with a VAD. For those with damage to both the right and left ventricles, a total artificial heart may be necessary. In fact, I wrongly predicted shortly after I started our heart transplant and mechanical pump/artificial heart program at The Ohio State University in 1986 that heart transplantation would be obsolete in ten years, replaced by mechanical pumps. With vast improvements in technology, we are finally getting closer. Recent studies show two-year survival in these critically ill terminal heart failure patients receiving destination therapy with a VAD of 50–80%, making this option viable. Over 10,000 patients worldwide have undergone implantation of a HeartMate II VAD.

Unfortunately, it is estimated that 300,000 patients would benefit from implantation of a VAD for end-stage heart failure. Obviously, the cost, estimated at $200,000 to $300,000 an implant, would be prohibitive. How this technology will be applied to the thousands of terminal heart failure patients over 65 remains in question.

CORONARY ARTERY DISEASE

Heart attacks and angina (crushing chest pain usually described as a weight on the chest rather than sharp pain and frequently confused with indigestion) occur when one or more of the three major arteries or their branches on the surface of the heart (coronary arteries) suffer restricted flow or blockage. The average age at presentation with acute coronary syndrome, a constellation of symptoms occurring during a heart attack (ACS), is 65 for males and 72 for females, the delay in the latter being perhaps due to the protective effects of estrogen in earlier life. Two-thirds of myocardial infarctions, heart attacks, occur in those over 65 years of age and 85% of the mortality in ACS is in the Medicare population.

Age impacts not only the risk of cardiovascular events (heart attacks, strokes and peripheral vascular disease), but also the selection of treatment and the outcomes and complications of therapy. Older patients tend to have more complex disease of the arteries as well as more comorbidities including hypertension, heart failure, heart rhythm abnormalities, anemia and kidney failure which contribute to the risk of the use of blood thinners or the recommendation for invasive therapy.

ACS presents differently in the elderly than it does in those under 65 years of age. Chest pain, the hallmark of heart attack, occurs in less than half of those over 85 compared with over three-quarters of those under 65 years of age. Older patients more frequently exhibit shortness of breath, profuse sweating, nausea and vomiting and syncope. Because of muscle stiffness and frequent diffuse disease of all three major coronary arteries, the older patient frequently is diagnosed with heart failure which delays appropriate interventions designed to limit heart muscle damage from a heart attack.

Once a diagnosis of ACS is made, two treatment options exist if the event is less than 12 hours old: clot busting drugs given intravenously or an invasive procedure. Most often for the last decade the invasive procedure in this acute setting is percutaneous coronary intervention (PCI) which is done in the catheterization laboratory by a cardiologist. Under sedation, a tube is threaded from the groin or arm into the artery or arteries exhibiting blockage, a balloon inflated to open the narrowing and a metal cage or stent placed to keep the artery from closing again. The options of types of stents (bare metal, drug eluting and absorbable) and manufacturers is beyond the scope of this chapter and each design has its specific application; however, drug eluting stents seem to have the best results and widest application at the time of this writing. Occasionally the anatomy is unfavorable and the only option is coronary artery bypass surgery (CABG) where veins from the leg or an artery from the chest wall or both are used to bypass the blockage by providing a new route for oxygen-rich blood to flow beyond the obstruction.

These same two options apply to patients with angina or episodic heart failure but who do not present with an impending heart attack. The debate over which procedure is superior in this elective setting, percutaneous coronary intervention vs. coronary artery bypass graft surgery, is neverending and constantly evolving and to some extent depends on the aggressiveness of the catheterization laboratory cardiologist. PCI is now used for virtually all categories of coronary artery disease including left main coronary artery disease—obstruction of the main artery supplying most of the left ventricle—a subcategory of anatomy that used to be reserved for surgery. Recent studies suggest that diabetics, including elderly diabetics, have better outcomes with CABG than PCI. Indeed, older patients with complex multivessel disease may be better served with surgery than with a difficult PCI.

As with all invasive procedures in the elderly, careful consideration of comorbid conditions such as kidney failure, previous stroke, dementia, frailty and biological as well as chronological age should be considered when deciding which or if invasive therapy is indicated.

After either invasive therapy, a cardiac rehabilitation program with monitored increasing exercise should be recommended. This is especially important in the elderly where in addition to improved cardiovascular performance, the patient may benefit from improved physical fitness, balance, muscle strength and instruction in fall prevention.

In addition, medical therapy if not already in place should be instituted to reduce the likelihood of recurrent disease. All patients should be treated with high dose cholesterol-lowering or statin drug therapy. If the blood pressure is elevated or not already treated, the drugs already discussed for the treatment of hypertension should be instituted. Low dose beta blocker as well as aspirin if no bleeding contraindication should also be instituted. However, doses should be adjusted for kidney function and begun judiciously with increases based on tolerance. Frequent visits or calls as drugs are adjusted are required and a cardiac rehab facility is another venue that can oversee these changes. The risk of side effects from drugs increases from around 10% with two medications to nearly 40% with four and over 80% with seven or more.

VALVE DISEASE

Aortic Valve Disease

As with coronary disease in the 1970s, the treatment of valve disease has undergone a revolution in the last decade due to development of new minimally invasive technology. The aortic valve controls the unidirectional flow of blood from the left ventricle to the aorta (major artery taking oxygen-rich blood to the body). Calcific aortic stenosis, a degenerative disease of this valve mainly in older patients, affects around 5% of people over 65 and is moderate to severe in half of those. Up to half of these patients are asymptomatic, yet once they develop symptoms, expected survival is less than three years. Because many of these asymptomatic patients have other comorbid conditions or a high frailty index, in the past up to half of them received no further evaluation and were not referred for surgery. There is no effective medical therapy option for aortic stenosis as it is a fixed blockage preventing blood from leaving the left ventricle. With the advent of Transcatheter Aortic Valve Replacement (TAVR), this has all changed.

TAVR was first performed in 2002 in France. Originally designated for use only in older patients deemed inoperable by the usual open surgical technique, the FDA (Food and Drug Administration) approved them for use in 2011. Currently they are FDA approved for use in all patients and offered routinely to older patients instead of the open surgical procedure.

The procedure is performed under awake sedation and local anesthesia usually through an artery in the groin, where a 5–6 mm catheter or tube containing the collapsed valve is threaded up and through the aortic valve. The metal cage or stent containing the valve is released and expanded, opening the native valve and allowing the artificial valve leaflets attached to the stent to expand and function. The stents are metal and the leaflets are composed of preserved pericardium (the sack that surrounds the heart) from cows or pigs. Once expanded the new valve provides instantaneous relief of the obstruction. This improved opening allows improved blood flow to the body, reduced strain and workload on the left ventricle of the heart and improvement in symptoms.

Two manufacturers (Edwards and Medtronic) supply most of the valves currently used. They produce different versions of their valves and of its insertion technology, both aspects of which continue to be refined. Smaller catheters make insertion easier and less risky for vascular complications. At first Edwards relied on balloon expansion of the stent containing the three semilunar valve leaflets fashioned from preserved bovine pericardium and Medtronic, a self-expanding stent. Currently, Edwards has both technologies available in different models.

Surgical valve replacement under direct vision offers some advantages over this much less invasive technique including thorough removal of calcium deposits on the valve which crumble much like dried dirt, assurance that the openings of both coronary arteries aren't obstructed, avoidance of the heart's electrical conducting system and assurance that there are no leaks around the valve. Coronary obstruction is a rare complication with a properly seated TAVR and newer models can be repositioned if this occurs. There continue to be issues post-procedure with paravalvular leaks (leaks occurring between the stented valve and the heart tissue) and heart block requiring a pacemaker. These are troubling problems which may limit the extension of the TAVR valve to a population that would also be amenable with low risk for surgical replacement.

The lack of the ability to debride calcium deposits from the valve tissue resulting in embolization (breaking off and causing strokes or damage to other organs) seems to have been at least partially resolved by new technology. Many centers now insert a second catheter with nets that deploy in the arteries to the brain or in the aorta above the valve to protect the entire body. Embolized chunks of calcium are captured in the nets and retrieved when the nets are closed and the catheter is withdrawn. This new technology seems to be effective.

Another long-term issue which may limit the use of these valves in younger patients (those under 65) and perhaps even the elderly is the durability of the valve tissue. Although surgically implanted pericardial valves have been used for decades with good long-term results, the different stresses on the pericardial tissue within a metal stent may have an impact. At five-year follow-up in one trial comparing the two different TAVR technologies, there were no significant differences between the balloon expandable and self-expanding valves in one thousand patients; half of these high risk patients were dead and half of those deaths were of cardiovascular causes. Deterioration of the valve tissue was more common in the balloon expandable valves and must be watched closely for further acceleration which would frustrate, in my opinion, those who optimistically assert that TAVR will be the procedure of choice in the future. There have been recent studies comparing surgical valve replacement with TAVR that have shown comparable or superior results with TAVR, but I remain somewhat skeptical. In older patients with limited life expectancy,

TAVR is the procedure of choice. Even in those who are likely to survive for more than ten years, if structural valve deterioration occurs, a second TAVR can be placed inside the original one (valve-in-valve procedure) expanding the indications for this procedure.

Mitral Valve Disease

The mitral valve is the one-way valve between the upper left heart chamber or left atrium (LA) which receives oxygen-rich blood from the lungs and the lower left heart muscular pumping chamber or left ventricle (LV) which pumps the oxygen-rich blood to the body. The valve has two leaflets and a number of fibrous chords (chordae tendineae) which attach the free edge of the leaflets to the papillary muscles in the wall of the left ventricle. When the valve is closed it resembles a flat parachute. When functioning properly, this valve opens to allow blood to fill the left ventricle from the atrium and then closes when the left ventricle squeezes, preventing blood from leaking back into the left atrium and the lungs. Diseases affecting the mitral valve produce stenosis (blockage, MS), regurgitation (leakage, MR) or both. For simplicity I will deal with the pure forms of stenosis and regurgitation.

Mitral stenosis is at this time a surgical disease with no approved catheter-based treatment yet available. One cause, rheumatic heart disease, is rare in developed countries due to the rapid diagnosis and treatment of streptococcal infections which, when left untreated, lead to rheumatic disease and valve calcification. As discussed in the aortic valve section, stenosis may also be caused by calcific degeneration. In either case the valve is treated by open or, in select centers, robotic/minimally invasive procedures. If the valve is pliable, a commissurotomy may be performed using a scalpel to divide the fused leaflets and supporting structures of the valve. In most instances the valve is too heavily diseased and is replaced by a mechanical valve in younger patients or a biological valve in the elderly.

It is likely in the near future that transcatheter mitral valve replacement will become more accepted. Major stumbling blocks are the difficulty in gaining access to the mitral valve and past problems with rapid degeneration of biological valves in the mitral position. Exposure can only be obtained by either punching a hole in the atrial septum (the tissue dividing the right and left sided upper chambers of the heart) or by surgically exposing the apex of the left ventricle and opening a hole in that location. That said, several companies are working on this technology which will enter mainstream therapy, especially in the elderly, soon.

Mitral regurgitation (MR) may be primary or secondary. Primary mitral regurgitation may be caused by non-calcific degeneration of the valve tissue, stretching of the opening to which the leaflets attach (annulus) and lengthening or tearing of the supporting cords (which attach the leaflets to the heart muscle in the left ventricle and keep the valve from prolapsing into the left atrium). The degeneration of the valve tissue is termed myxomatous degeneration. The physiological abnormality is mitral valve prolapse where the leaflets upon closure do not adjust to the annulus or coapt, but travel into the left atrium allowing blood to leak backwards. This results in greater work for the left ventricle muscle and may produce high pressure over time in the lungs. If left untreated, the result is heart failure with a dilated left atrium and left ventricle. This process may take years to decades. Earlier intervention regardless of symptoms may prevent these changes. If surgery is delayed due to age and lack of symptoms, careful follow-up is required to allow consideration of intervention (especially with newer catheter-based techniques to be described) before irreversible damage has occurred.

Surgical intervention with valve repair has been the gold standard for three decades. Removing redundant parts of leaflets, placing Gore-Tex sutures to replace torn cords and placing a cloth-covered ring to cinch up the annulus (the fibrous ring to which the leaflets are attached) are performed in various combinations to accomplish a competent valve in most patients. Some centers now do these repairs using minimally (small incisions) invasive or robotic techniques. All require cardiopulmonary bypass. If repair is not possible, valve replacement is performed.

Secondary (or functional) mitral regurgitation occurs when the valve leaks secondary to dilatation of the left ventricle and atrium but the valve tissue itself is normal. The dilatation stretches the annulus so the leaflets, though normal in size, fail to coapt. Once a patient has severe symptoms, valve repair or replacement fails to improve survival and, in some cases, may make symptoms worse by placing a greater workload on the left ventricle. A new device, the Mitra Clip, is approved for both primary and secondary MR. The cloth-covered metal clip is inserted through a catheter which punctures the inter-atrial septum. The clip grasps and approximates the middle section of the two leaflets of the mitral valve, thus decreasing the amount of leakage. For primary MR the need for reoperation within a year for 20% or more of patients is too high compared to surgical repair for younger patients. However, in high-risk older patients it would seem to be worth a try. For secondary MR, the advantage of Mitra Clip over medical therapy alone is controversial. Two studies with a mean patient age of 70 recently showed improved survival and reduced hospitalization for heart failure in one and not the other. A third study including both primary and secondary MR patients with a mean age of 80 compared valve repair to Mitra Clip with significantly better results with surgery.

This technology will continue to improve (there is already a newer version of the Mitra Clip). Other devices, including annular rings that can be implanted through a catheter, and further improvements in the technique and devices for transcatheter mitral valve replacement will also occur. While all catheter-based technologies hold the promise of quicker recovery, less pain and lower risk in high-risk patients, surgical techniques of mitral valve repair have proven themselves effective and long lasting in all age groups for 30 years. In the end, the patient, regardless of age, should be presented all options. A healthy 70-year-old might not want to risk a repeat operation at age 80 when a surgical valve repair has a proven long-term excellent result.

Tricuspid Valve Disease

The tricuspid valve is the right heart equivalent of the mitral valve on the left, a one-way valve separating the right ventricle (lower pumping chamber) from the right atrium that receives the blood returning to the heart from all the veins in the body. Although tricuspid regurgitation (TR) is estimated to afflict 1.6 million people in the United States, corrective surgery is performed less than 500 times a year. The leakage is almost always secondary to left-sided muscle or valve disease resulting in heart failure. With heart failure the pressure in the left ventricle is elevated and this pressure elevation backs up into the left atrium. The elevated pressure in the left atrium is transmitted back into the vessels in the lungs (pulmonary hypertension) and the right atrium with secondary dilatation of the right ventricle and tricuspid annulus.

Despite the few surgeries currently performed, I believe, because of the ease of access to the tricuspid valve and annulus through a major neck or groin vein, that this technology will be used more often in the future. There are at least two other leaflet coaptation devices like the Mitra Clip in development as well as seven or more transcatheter annuloplasty rings. Once proven on the right side with easier access, I believe many of the annuloplasty devices designed to cinch the annulus tighter and reduce leakage will be reconfigured for use on the left side or mitral annulus. As of this writing there is not enough information to warrant a positive recommendation for routine use of any of these devices with perhaps the exception of the Mitra Clip on the tricuspid valve.

ARRHYTHMIA—ATRIAL FIBRILLATION

It is estimated that 75% of patients exhibiting this rhythm are between the ages of 65 and 85 years. Up to 10% of those over 80 years of age will exhibit atrial fibrillation with a four to five times greater risk of stroke.

With newer home monitoring devices being advertised daily (Kardia, Apple watch) that can detect this abnormal rhythm, and because of the serious and debilitating complication of stroke which frequently accompanies it, there is increased awareness of treatment to eliminate atrial fibrillation.

The normal heart rhythm is called sinus rhythm where the electrical stimuli that trigger contraction of the heart (right and left atria followed by right and left ventricle) progresses in an orderly fashion. The stimulus begins in the SA node, an area of specialized tissue in the right atrium with spontaneous automaticity (firing off an electrical stimulus at a rate of 60–80 beats per minute) that is also influenced to increase or decrease that rate by both the nervous system (sympathetic and parasympathetic) and hormonal influences. Examples of these effects are the increase in heart rate when frightened or during exercise. The subsequent contraction of the right and left atria tops off the preceding passive filling of the left and right ventricles by adding up to an additional 20% to the volume of blood in these chambers. The stimulus then travels to the AV node at the top of the interventricular septum, the muscle separating the left and right ventricles, from which it spreads to both ventricles to initiate an orderly contraction of these two pumping chambers.

In atrial fibrillation, the right atrium is bombarded with fast recurrent stimuli originating spontaneously from the areas where the pulmonary veins enter the left atria. Instead of an orderly contraction, the atria quiver, sending a barrage of stimuli to the AV node, only some of which are conducted through this area to stimulate contraction of the ventricles. In addition to not fulfilling their role of topping off the ventricles, the sluggish flow of blood in the atria allows clots to form in finger-like outpouchings (atrial appendages) off of the main body of the atria which can then break loose and in the case of the left atrium go to the brain causing a stroke. Physiologically this rhythm can reduce the cardiac output (the amount of blood the heart pumps) by 20%. The heart rate at which the ventricles pump is frequently quite rapid (100–175 beats per minute at rest) which can result in a drop in blood pressure, light headedness and syncope. Patients may exhibit symptoms of their heart pounding rapidly (palpitations), shortness of breath, fatigue and chest pain.

Medical Therapy and Cardioversion

When first diagnosed, patients with non-valvular atrial fibrillation of recent onset frequently present with severe symptoms of low cardiac output and low blood pressure due to the drop in filling of the left ventricle and the rapid heart rate. Depending on severity of symptoms, chemical cardioversion with medications may be tried over hours to a few days, or, if severely symptomatic, electrical cardioversion in the ER is feasible. Commonly, a dose or two of a calcium channel blocker drug (e.g. cardizem) will frequently convert to sinus rhythm. If successful, maintenance drug therapy with any number of drugs may be used. If not, electrical cardioversion should be attempted after performing a trans-esophageal echocardiogram (TEE) to rule out a clot in the left atrium or appendage. If present, cardioversion is delayed and full anticoagulation is started. Awake sedation is used since the procedure is painful.

After successful cardioversion, maintenance drug therapy, depending on which drug is tolerated, and anticoagulation with a non-warfarin drug (NOAC—novel oral anticoagulant) in the elderly is recommended, although in practice up to 50% of elderly patients are not placed on anticoagulation due to the fear of falls resulting in bleeding into the brain (intracerebral hemorrhage). NOACs have been shown to be as effective as warfarin (the previously used anticoagulant) with a lower bleeding risk.

One alternative to cardioversion is to leave the patient in the abnormal rhythm and use drugs to control the heart rate. A target heart rate of less than 80 at rest and less than 110 with moderate exercise should be set. Although a number of drugs singly or in combination have been used, beta blockers are the first line drug. An intravenous form of the drug can be started in symptomatic patients who are not candidates for cardioversion and subsequent oral doses should be gradually increased until therapeutic. Other drugs can be added or substituted if needed, including calcium channel blockers such as cardizem. Digoxin may also be used although some have cautioned that it may increase mortality. The evidence for this is unclear especially in light of its use for over a century.

Ablation—Pulmonary Vein Isolation

The aim of pulmonary vein isolation is to return the patient to sinus rhythm. This is accomplished by interrupting the pathways from the openings of the pulmonary veins from which signals are transmitted to the atria by creating physical barriers of scar tissue by either balloon cryoablation (cold) or radiofrequency (heat). In addition to isolating the pulmonary vein openings, additional sites of origin within the left atrium may require ablation. The success rate regardless of age appears to be 70–80%. The main complications are perforation due to full-thickness penetration into the pericardium with tamponade, pulmonary vein narrowing due to excessive scarring and stroke. The frequency of these complications does not seem to be age related and varies in different series from 0–10%.

Post-procedure anticoagulation is required for at least 3 to 6 months at which time, if the patient has maintained sinus rhythm, therapy may be discontinued. As with cardioversion, with the increased risk of warfarin anticoagulation in the elderly the newer drugs (NOACs) with a better safety profile are preferred.

In patients undergoing open heart surgery for coronary or valvular heart disease and who are in atrial fibrillation or have been in and out of this rhythm, pulmonary vein isolation combined with left atrial appendage exclusion may be added expeditiously with little increased risk.

Ablation—AV Node Ablation and Pacemaker

Another alternative for rate control, though less desirable, is AV node ablation with the mandatory insertion of a permanent pacemaker. AV node ablation produces complete heart block by completely interfering with any electrical conduction from the atria to the ventricles. This makes the patients 100% dependent on a pacemaker while leaving the atria in most cases in fibrillation. The incidence of heart failure is more than double that with pulmonary vein isolation and afflicts more than half the patients treated with this strategy. In addition, over time right ventricular pacing may further compromise cardiac function although these effects may be improved with the use of biventricular pacing (synchronizing the contraction of the right and left ventricles with wires in each ventricle) or atrial sensing in the third of patients who convert to sinus rhythm (a wire in the right atrium senses a stimulus and then fires a stimulus to the ventricle, much like a normal heart beat).

In order of desirability, in the setting of acute onset atrial fibrillation an attempt at medical or electrical cardioversion should be attempted. If unsuccessful or if atrial fibrillation recurs more than once or twice (except in the very frail elderly or those with limited survival potential) pulmonary vein isolation should be attempted once or twice. If that is unsuccessful, rate control first with medical therapy and as a last resort with AV node ablation and pacemaker should be used. NOACs unless absolutely contraindicated should be used for anticoagulation in those in whom a rate control strategy is adopted and at least for 3–6 months in those undergoing pulmonary vein isolation.

Watchman Device for Stroke Prevention in Atrial Fibrillation

Surgical closure of the left atrial appendage either from the outside by over-sewing or applying a clip to the base of this thumb-like outpouching off the left atrium or by use of a purse string suture excluding its opening from inside the left atrium during mitral valve surgery has been used by some for 70 years. Unfortunately, there is no good data to prove the effectiveness of this additional procedure. I routinely excluded the left atrial appendage from inside in all mitral valve surgeries in patients with a history of atrial fibrillation since it made sense (the left atrial appendage is the site of stroke causing emboli in up to two-thirds of patients in atrial fibrillation) and added less than five minutes to the procedure. There is currently a large randomized multicenter study to answer the question. However, especially in atrial fibrillation patients with a contraindication to anticoagulation, one would assume this simple procedure would be of benefit.

A catheter-based technique has been introduced recently to simulate internal closure of the appendage. The Watchman device is an umbrella-shaped metal expandable stent with a fabric covering that is deployed inside the opening of the left atrial appendage, excluding it from the circulation. Studies have shown that this device reduces the risk of stroke to the same level that oral anticoagulation does. However, there are significant, frequent complications with this technique including dislodgement, leakage of blood into the pericardium (the sac surrounding the heart) and stroke. Therefore, although I believe that surgical closure will prove to be a useful adjunct in open heart surgery, further experience with the Watchman with further reduction in complications will be necessary before it can be a first-line therapy.

PALLIATIVE CARDIAC CARE

While palliative or hospice care has been well defined for cancer patients, such treatment for end-stage heart failure or valvular heart disease has only recently been recognized especially for the elderly. Not only do these patients suffer the common symptoms of heart disease including shortness of breath, fatigue and fluid accumulation in the periphery (edema) and abdomen (ascites), but they also exhibit pain, nausea, anxiety and depression. While heart transplant and/or permanent ventricular assist devices may be applicable to some, many patients may either not be a candidate for such therapy or may not be willing to subject themselves to the demands of such therapy. The topic of palliative care is rarely included in cardiology journals or national meetings and is not routinely part of cardiology training programs.

Prognosis in end-stage cardiac disease is more variable than with cancer, with many patients' survival extending for months to over a year with exacerbations and remissions. Medicare approval for some home therapies such as inotropes (intravenous infusions of drugs to improve heart function) frequently are not approved and hospice-level care at home and in extended care facilities may require repeat certification. Functional status may decline for prolonged periods of time, requiring long periods of support for patients and caregivers. Prolonged psychosocial support both inpatient and at home is required.

Many of the medical and catheter-based therapies discussed in this chapter may also be applied in the palliative setting. Only after a thorough discussion with the patient and caregivers outlining all reasonable options based on both the patient's age and functional status should a course of action be undertaken. As with all palliative care, quality of life is important and, I believe, especially in the uncertain prognostic arena of end-stage heart failure, should take precedence over quantity.

SUGGESTED ADDITIONAL READING

Abdel-Wahab, M, Neumann, FJ, et al. 5-year Outcomes After TAVR With Balloon-Expandable Versus Self-Expanding Valves: Results From the CHOICE Randomized Clinical Trial. JACC Cardiovasc Interv 2020; 13(9):1071–1082.

Daneshvar, DA, Czer, LSC, et al. Heart Transplantation in the Elderly: Why Cardiac Transplantation Does Not Need to be Limited to Younger Patients But Can Be Safely Performed in Patients Above 65 Years of Age. Ann Transplant 2010; 15(4):110–119.

Holmes, DR Jr., Kar, S et al. Prospective Randomized Evaluation of the Watchman Left Atrial Appendage Closure Device in Patients with Atrial Fibrillation Versus Long-Term Warfarin Therapy: The PREVAIL Trial. J Am Coll Cardiol 2014; 64(1): 1–12.

Jankowska, EA, Vitale, C, et al. Drug therapy in elderly heart failure patients. Eur Heart J Suppl 2019; Dec 21(Suppl L):L8–L11.

Kapa, SK, Bala, R. Ablation of Atrial Fibrillation in the Elderly: Current Evidence and Evolving Trends. J Atr Fibrillation 2011; 4(2): 341–353.

Leyva, F, Nisam, S, et al. 20 Years of Cardiac Resynchronization Therapy. J AmColl Cardiol 2014; 64:1047–1058.

Stehlik, J, Kobashigawa, J, et al. Honoring 50 Years of Clinical Heart Transplantation in Circulation In-depth State-of-the-Art Review. Circulation 2018; 137:71–87.

Shah, M, Jorde, UP. Percutaneous Mitral Valve Interventions (Repair): Current Indications and Future Perspectives. Front Cardiovasc Med 2019; 6: 88–123.

Sepheri, A, Beggs, T, et al. The Impact of Frailty on Outcomes after Cardiac Surgery: A Systematic Review. J Thorac Cardiovasc Surg 2014; 148(31): 3110–3117.

Teuteberg, JJ, Teuteberg WG. Palliative Care for Patients with Heart Failure. www.acc.org/latest-in-cardiology/articles/2016/02/11/08/02/palliative-care-for-patients-with-heart-failure

21 Could My Patient Be at Risk of Orthostatic Hypotension?

Eric T. Hedge, MSc and Carmelo Mastrandrea, MD, PhD

CONTENTS

CLINICAL VIGNETTE

A 78-year-old man presents to his family physician with an increasing frequency of dizziness on standing over the past few months that is especially pronounced in the early afternoon. He states that he occasionally suffered from similar episodes in the past, but managed to cope by taking his time when he stood up. There is no history of weakness, loss of consciousness or falls, and he otherwise remains well. He admits that he has become more sedentary recently following the COVID-19 lockdown, and rarely performs any physical activity. For the last few years he has been taking Losartan 50 mg OD and Clorathalidone 25 mg OD for hypertension (which is well controlled), and Metformin 500 mg OD for diabetes (recent Hb A1c 5.2%). He was recently diagnosed with benign prostatic hypertrophy, managed well with Doxazosin 4 mg OD, up-titrated from 2 mg four months ago.

Given this history, there is a need to assess for possible orthostatic hypotension and falls risk, and propose a plan for management of his symptoms.

WHY IS ORTHOSTATIC HYPOTENSION AN IMPORTANT CLINICAL PROBLEM?

Orthostatic hypotension (OH) is very common in older adults. A 2020 systematic review of OH in around 23,000 people 60 years of age or older identified a prevalence of one-in-five for community-living individuals, increasing to almost one-in-four for those living in long-term care (1). However, postural symptoms often remain unreported, with many people modifying their lifestyles to manage mild orthostatic symptomatology at home without ever presenting to a medical professional. Furthermore, OH may remain completely symptomless, with unexplained falls occurring without preceding warning. Indeed, many individuals do not experience any symptoms during formal tilt-table testing despite significant and sometimes sudden reductions in blood pressure and cerebral blood flow, which lead to an often-imminent loss of consciousness and collapse. When reported, symptoms include, but are not limited to, dizziness or lightheadedness on standing, blurred vision, weakness, confusion, nausea, hot flushes, sweating, syncope and falls. Unfortunately, formal testing and diagnosis of OH by clinicians typically requires prompting by the patient or relatives, and often occurs after episodes of discrete symptomatic events. Therefore, and rather regrettably, it is not unexpected for OH-induced falls to lead to emergency admissions with associated head trauma and long-bone fractures as the first presentation without prior clinical diagnosis and/or management of OH. Additionally, OH is an independent risk factor for multiple cardiovascular conditions, including myocardial infarction and heart failure, atrial fibrillation, and stroke. It may also indicate otherwise undiagnosed autonomic and neurodegenerative conditions. Given the certainty that OH remains vastly undiagnosed in the community, it represents a source of great morbidity and even mortality, especially in older populations.

Orthostatic hypotension is the inability of the body to maintain adequate blood pressure during movement to an upright position because of gravity. However, there are other notable causes for reductions in blood pressure and/or cardiac output, which can be provoked by postural challenge, that are in fact due to structural or electrophysiological abnormalities that prevent normal homeostatic blood pressure regulation. For example, arrhythmias, aortic stenosis and cardiomyopathies may severely and sometimes suddenly limit cardiac output, leading to symptoms of dizziness and potential loss of consciousness. In people with these conditions, the additional stress on the heart inherent

DOI: 10.1201/9781003344476-24

in postural changes may provoke events that are otherwise manageable at rest. Other, non-cardiac causes of OH-related symptoms include atypical seizures, hypoglycemia and other metabolic disturbances. They are significant disease states that require independent investigation and management. Clinical assessments of patients who experience postural symptoms should not ignore these potential causes.

WHAT ARE THE RISK FACTORS FOR ORTHOSTATIC HYPOTENSION?

On standing, immediate venous pooling in the legs and splanchnic vasculature leads to a reduction in cardiac filling, which limits pressure generation as described by the Frank-Starling relationship (stroke volume of the left ventricle increases as the left ventricular volume increases). Subsequent reductions in pressure within the arterial system reduce stimulation of the carotid baroreceptors, leading to reflex elevations in sympathetic tone and subsequent positive chronotropic (increasing heart rate), dromotropic (increasing rate of conduction through AV node), inotropic (increasing contractility) and lusitropic (increasing relaxation of myocardium during diastole) effects. Simultaneous activation of the arterial and cardiopulmonary baroreflexes increases arterial smooth muscle tone, which elevates total peripheral resistance (TPR). These control mechanisms maintain arterial pressure and represent normal cardiovascular responses to an orthostatic challenge.

Orthostatic hypotension stems from the cardiovascular system's inability to maintain physiologically adequate blood pressure during postural challenge and represents a breakdown of the previously described mechanisms. Subsequently, this leads to hypoperfusion of cerebral tissues and consequent symptomology. Therefore, one must consider any factors that impair the cardiovascular system's ability to generate consistent and adequate perfusion pressures. The Canadian Geriatrics Society provides the 4D-AID framework for assessing and prioritizing contributing factors for OH, which includes Deconditioning, Dysfunctional heart, Dehydration and Drugs (4Ds; causes with intact compensatory tachycardia) and Autonomic dysfunction, Idiopathic and Drugs (AID; causes without compensatory tachycardia) (2). Here, we propose a slightly different categorization using the following groups in order to help explain the physiological mechanisms leading to OH risk factors: 1) alterations to intrinsic cardiac function, 2) alterations to normal cardiovascular control and 3) reductions in cardiac filling.

1. *Alterations to intrinsic cardiac function.* Any circumstances that alter the rhythmical contractile properties of the heart may predispose an individual to OH. Possibilities include reductions in cardiac contractility (e.g., following previous myocardial infarction and subsequent heart failure), aortic stenosis, and medications.

   Areas of reduced cardiac muscle contractility curtail the inotropic response to postural challenges, which subsequently increases the risk of OH via reduced force of contraction and an inability to mount sufficient increases in blood pressure. Heart failure is a significant risk factor for the presence of OH, depending on the severity (NYHA class) and presence of acute decompensation; Gorelik and colleagues' 2016 review identified that up to 83% of elderly hospitalized patients with heart failure also experience OH (3).

   Medications can alter the contractile capabilities of cardiac myocytes, or suppress heart rate responses. For example, beta-blockers reduce the inotropy and chronotropy of the heart, which can impair the cardiac response that is needed to maintain blood pressure and stroke volume during orthostatic challenge. Calcium channel blockers are an example that reduce both the force and speed of cardiac contractions. Any medication that interferes with normal cardiac physiology may increase the risk of orthostatic intolerance.

2. *Alterations to normal cardiovascular control.* Effective cardiovascular responses to blood pressure changes during postural transitions require rapid and appropriate magnitude autonomic reflexes. Age, and its related vascular stiffening, reduces arterial baroreceptor sensitivity and limits accurate blood pressure sensation, thereby blunting cardiovascular responses. Increasing age alone is an independent risk factor for the presence of orthostatic hypotension (4). Primary neurological impairment leading to autonomic dysfunction, such as Parkinson's disease, primary autonomic failure and Lewy body disease, will blunt cardiovascular responses to orthostatic challenge. Secondary neurological impairment, such as spinal cord lesions interrupting normal neuronal pathways, or peripheral neuropathies that develop with diseases, such as diabetes mellitus, all prevent normal autonomic control of postural responses and may predispose individuals to OH.

Heat stress, including fever from infectious disease, alters the cardiovascular response to standing and increases the risk of orthostatic intolerance. When a patient is hot, cutaneous vascular conductance increases and results in a reduction in TPR. When low TPR is combined with the orthostatic stress of standing up, cardiac output may fall to levels that fail to adequately maintain systemic blood pressure and cerebral perfusion. Heat-induced reductions to TPR can be further compounded by secondary effects of fluid status, as dehydration can also reduce circulating volume and cardiac filling.

Any medications that interfere with control of vascular tone may alter normal physiological responses to orthostatic challenges. Antihypertensive medications, such as calcium channel blockers, promote smooth muscle relaxation, limiting the elevations in TPR required to maintain blood pressure while standing. Another example includes alpha adrenoceptor blockers, which are commonly used to treat benign prostatic hypertrophy, that also inhibit the magnitude of vascular smooth muscle contraction and prevent normal elevations in TPR. Any medication known to interfere with normal autonomic control of the vascular system and baroreflex mechanisms must be part of a risk-factor list for OH.

3. *Reductions to cardiac filling.* Any reduction in total circulating blood volume will limit venous return to the heart and predispose an individual to increased risk of OH. Total body blood volume losses that may occur with dehydration from any cause, blood loss or even volume depletion due to periods of immobility or prolonged bed-rest, can severely exacerbate OH. Among causes of dehydration in older adults, one has to consider changes in thirst perception with reduced fluid intake, inaccessibility to fluids due to mobility impairment, and increased fluid losses with vomiting, diarrhea or bleeding. However, reduced venous return may also occur without changes to total blood volume. For example, hyperemia of the splanchnic circulation and increased mesenteric vessel blood flow following a meal results in pooling of blood in these tissues and a temporary reduction in venous return to the heart; it may well be that those suffering with OH find that their symptoms are much worse following a large meal. Another common condition of OH without changes in total blood volume in older adults that may be overlooked by clinicians is venous insufficiency from incompetent veins in the lower extremities and their valves. The venous blood pooling in the legs causes OH by the mechanism described previously. Finally, medications can reduce circulating volume leading to reductions in cardiac filling. Diuretics lower circulating volume via their effects on normal kidney function; however, other medications to consider include laxatives, antacids and ACE inhibitors (via their effects on aldosterone production and inhibition of sodium retention).

How Is the Diagnosis of Orthostatic Hypotension Made?

On history taking, any symptoms related to postural changes, such as unexplained falls or episodes of lightheadedness, dizziness, changes in vision or blurring of vision, sweating, feeling of warmth, nausea, headaches, confusion, palpitations or other abnormal symptoms described by patient, could be indicative of orthostatic hypotension. These symptoms may be common early in the morning, following long periods of immobility, and/or following a meal. Medication review is paramount.

On physical examination, any evidence of bruising or unexplained injuries may be indicative of falls and should prompt questioning regarding their etiology. A quick assessment can provide evidence for the presence of orthostatic hypotension if there is a sustained reduction in systolic blood pressure of at least 20 mmHg, or diastolic blood pressure of at least 10 mmHg within 3 minutes of standing (5). A simple testing algorithm would include the following (Table 21.1):

1. Have the patient lie down for 5 minutes.

2. Measure blood pressure and heart rate.

3. Have the patient stand up.

4. Repeat blood pressure and heart rate measurements after standing for 1 and 3 minutes.

Tilt-table testing provides formal assessment of an individual's cardiovascular response during a passive postural challenge. Venous pooling in the lower limbs reaches a level far greater than that during normal standing, as the test eliminates the need for normal postural muscle contractions in the legs and abdomen that are usually required to maintain balance. The cardiovascular system is therefore stressed to a greater degree, especially during the early stages of the postural transition,

Table 21.1 Testing for Orthostatic Hypotension

Position	Time Point	Measures	Symptoms
Lying	5 minutes	BP ____/____ HR_____	
Standing	1 minute	BP ____/____ HR_____	
Standing	3 minutes	BP ____/____ HR_____	

and eliminates any active or reflex lower limb muscle contraction that may temporarily raise venous return, stroke volume and blood pressure. Close monitoring of the patient's vital signs (continual ECG/EKG and blood pressure monitoring) will allow for a more in-depth assessment of autonomic cardiovascular control, and diagnosis of orthostatic hypotension. There is significant concern for patients with evidence of severe sinus bradycardia, sinus standstill or atrioventricular block during this test. Closer follow-up and cardiovascular consultation is warranted before submitting these persons to a tilt-table test.

WHAT ARE THE INTERVENTIONS TO REDUCE ORTHOSTATIC HYPOTENSION?

The ideal intervention for orthostatic hypotension is one that maintains a patient's standing blood pressure without causing hypertension while lying down, reduces orthostatic symptomatology and improves the patient's ability to perform daily tasks. In practice, this is very difficult as many patients who experience OH already have concomitant supine hypertension. No single intervention is perfect, but a combination of different treatment strategies can be effective at improving patients' quality of life. Interventions are grouped into non-pharmacological and pharmacological.

Appropriate assessment for orthostatic hypotension (and more generally falls) in older adults is an important and somewhat overlooked aspect in many community medical assessments. Formal falls assessments of older adults should be routine, especially for those who are frail or live relatively isolated lives. Assessment on admission to nursing homes and residential retirement facilities would reduce incidence of falls in high-risk populations. Given that patient education remains an important part of the management of OH, routine assessment as part of an overall risk-aversion strategy for falls should be encouraged.

Non-Pharmacological Interventions

Patient education and trigger avoidance will help individuals understand their diagnosis, and may prevent future symptoms and falls. Ensuring that the patient comprehends that they are at risk when standing suddenly, especially at night if they need the toilet, could prevent a fall. Encourage slow postural changes with pauses. For example, ask the patient to allow for a minute or two of sitting rest between lying to standing transitions, allowing more time for physiological adaptation to upright posture. Physical maneuvers during standing, such as leg muscle contraction, forward bending of the torso, leg crossing and squatting, may also aid in maintaining blood pressure in those suffering from OH. Respiratory techniques such as sniffing and breathing in through pursed lips may also be beneficial. Volume support and increasing salt intake can increase circulating volume; however, such measures should be considered carefully in those with hypertension and/or heart failure. In some cases, raising the head of the bed or using more pillows to decrease hydrostatic pressure on the kidneys and reduce glomerular filtration can contribute to decreased nocturia/fluid loss. Further explanations of the aforementioned techniques are summarized well in Wieling et al.'s review on the topic (6). For patients who experience OH after eating a meal, a simple and low-cost treatment strategy is to limit the size of meals, and compensate by increasing meal frequency. Eating smaller meals with lower levels of carbohydrates more often throughout the day instead of a few high-carbohydrate meals will help reduce the magnitude of post-prandial splanchnic hyperemia, leading to fewer and less severe symptoms.

Controlled exercise and physical activity, such as swimming, aerobics and walking, can be a useful part of an OH management plan. Mild exercise can help to reduce venous pooling and increase plasma volume, while potentially also helping to combat other comorbidities. Isometric exercise or exercise where the patient may strain and hold their breath is not advisable, as this may result in reductions in venous return, leading to orthostatic intolerance. In cases where upright exercise is too risky due to the orthostatic drop in blood pressure, recumbent cycling is a safe alternative.

Reviewing medications in individuals with OH, especially in those that are symptomatic, is an important aspect of their management plan. Typically, this requires risk management, especially in older adult populations with comorbidities, by a multidisciplinary medical team, with a poly-pharmaceutical management plan. Depending on the particular circumstances, ceasing medications or dose reduction should be considered for drugs that offer minimal benefit, or when the risk of falls exceeds other benefits. Discussions with the patient and family are paramount to ensure everyone understands why certain treatments may have been attenuated or stopped.

Another non-pharmaceutical modality is the use of compression garments that can reduce the amount of venous pooling that occurs while standing, and include leg stockings up to the thighs and abdominal binders. Some older patients will require assistance from homecare services to wear these garments. Finally, offering a medical alert button may also provide a level of security for concerned patients and family.

Pharmacological Interventions

Medications are available to assist in the management of symptomatic OH in conjunction with non-pharmaceutical measures, or in the eventuality that all non-pharmaceutical measures have been instituted without success. The addition of the mineralocorticoid fludrocortisone will increase circulating volume and support greater cardiac filling volumes. It is generally recommended to start at a daily dose of 0.05 mg and if OH is not controlled in two weeks one should consider increasing the dose to a maximum of 0.1 mg OD. The effect on blood pressure may take up to two weeks until the circulating volume is expanded. Patients should be informed of the possibility of developing peripheral ankle edema. Due to effects in the handling of sodium/potassium (Na^+/K^+) by the kidneys, it is recommended to check K^+ within one month due to the risk of developing hypokalemia, and to treat accordingly. The combination of domperidone, a peripheral acting dopaminergic antagonist, at 10 mg TID has been shown to be helpful, especially in patients suffering from Parkinson's disease. Vasopressors, such as midodrine, raise TPR, and can be helpful in the management of OH. Usual doses start at 5 mg BID which can be titrated up to 10 mg TID. Another more recent drug is droxidopa, a pro-drug that is converted to norepinephrine by the enzyme aromatic L-amino acid decarboxylase in the body providing α and β agonist effects with increases in blood pressure. Although droxidopa is stated to treat neurogenic OH associated with conditions such as Parkinson's disease and primary autonomic failure, its use has been tried in non-neurogenic cases with some success. The initial dose of droxidopa is 100 mg TID and it can be titrated up to 600 mg TID, in accordance with blood pressure response and tolerance.

A frequent problem encountered in patients with OH is recumbent hypertension. Overcoming this problem could involve elevating the head with pillows to about 30° and providing low-dose antihypertensive medication such as enalapril 2.5 mg in the evening before going to bed.

RESOLUTION OF THE CLINICAL VIGNETTE

The lack of any neurological history or other malaise would lead us to deduce that this gentleman is likely suffering from a gradual worsening of a longstanding tendency towards postural hypotension. It can be deduced from the history that his symptoms started to get worse and more frequent soon after the increase in the dose of the alpha-adrenergic blocker (Doxazosin) for his benign prostatic hypertrophy. It is likely that the combination of this drug, along with his long-standing angiotensin receptor blocker and diuretic, are causing the problem. The history of diabetes may alert us to possible autonomic neuropathy, but the limited medication required to control his glycemia and the normal Hb A1c would make it unlikely that he has neuronal involvement. His recent immobility will also increase his risk of postural symptoms.

After full examination to rule out any underlying condition, including checking the state of the venous system of his lower extremities, the clinician can perform postural blood pressure testing as described previously. It should be noted that this may still not show OH, but his strong history should still elicit some form of medical management of his symptoms. It is likely that he has periods of hypotension during the day.

This gentleman should be encouraged to increase his activities during the day, not only to ameliorate his orthostatic hypotension, but also to improve his general health. Education concerning the likely cause of his OH and techniques to reduce the likelihood and severity of episodes should be provided to him. Ambulatory blood pressure monitoring or home blood pressure recordings throughout the day can provide the clinician with an idea of any periods of recurrent hypotension.

In certain cases the timings of medications can be altered to try to eliminate cumulative hypotensive effects occurring in the early afternoon following receiving all antihypertensive medication at once in the morning, with the goal of achieving better 24-hour blood pressure control. This patient's diuretic should be stopped, especially if the 4 mg of Doxazosin is needed to maintain symptomatic control of his BPH. Finally, this gentleman should be followed up after initiation of the medical plan, to reassess his symptoms and review his blood pressure. If the OH persists, in subsequent visits, adding 1 g of salt with each meal and prescribing venous stockings may be necessary before considering pharmacological treatment of his OH.

REFERENCES

1. Saedon NI, Pin Tan M, Frith J. The prevalence of orthostatic hypotension: a systematic review and meta-analysis. *J Gerontol A Biol Sci Med Sci* 75: 117–122, 2020. doi: 10.1093/gerona/gly188
2. Molnar F, Frank CC. Determining the causes of postural hypotension. *Canadian Family Physician* 64: 40, 2018.
3. Gorelik O, Feldman L, Cohen N. Heart failure and orthostatic hypotension. *Heart Fail Rev* 21: 529–538, 2016. doi: 10.1007/s10741-016-9541-z
4. Monahan KD. Effect of aging on baroreflex function in humans. *Am J Physiol Regul Integr Comp Physiol* 293: R3–R12, 2007. doi: 10.1152/ajpregu.00031.2007
5. Freeman R, Wieling W, Axelrod FB, Benditt DG, Benarroch E, Biaggioni I, Cheshire WP, Chelimsky T, Cortelli P, Gibbons CH, Goldstein DS, Hainsworth R, Hilz MJ, Jacob G, Kaufmann H, Jordan J, Lipsitz LA, Levine BD, Low PA, Mathias C, Raj SR, Robertson D, Sandroni P, Schatz I, Schondorff R, Stewart JM, van Dijk JG. Consensus statement on the definition of orthostatic hypotension, neurally mediated syncope and the postural tachycardia syndrome. *Clin Auton Res* 21: 69–72, 2011. doi: 10.1007/s10286-011-0119-5
6. Wieling W, van Dijk N, Thijs RD, de Lange FJ, Krediet CTP, Halliwill JR. Physical countermeasures to increase orthostatic tolerance. *J Intern Med* 277: 69–82, 2015. doi: 10.1111/joim.12249

22 The Care of Chronic Obstructive Pulmonary Disease in Older Adults

Bryan Ross, MD, MSC, FRCPC and Jean Bourbeau, MD, MSC, FRCPC, FCAHS

CONTENTS

CLINICAL VIGNETTE

A 79-year-old man with chronic obstructive pulmonary disease (COPD) presents to clinic for his routine follow-up. He has severe COPD and had previously experienced on average 1–2 acute respiratory attacks (acute exacerbations of COPD) per year which required outpatient treatment with short-acting inhalers, oral antibiotics, and corticosteroids but not with emergency department visitation or hospitalization. Since the time of his last clinic visit, however, he had been admitted to hospital for a severe acute exacerbation of COPD and was subsequently discharged home. Short-acting beta-agonists and anti-muscarinic antagonists were used sparingly during his hospitalization due to perceived concerns of a co-morbid cardiac history and due to perceived concerns of the use of anti-cholinergics in the elderly. In addition to a past medical history of COPD, he also has a history of paroxysmal atrial fibrillation, osteoarthritis with knee and small digit (hand) involvement, and he also wonders if his hearing is starting to decline. His COPD controller medications include an inhaled long-acting muscarinic antagonist (LAMA), an inhaled long-acting beta-2 agonist (LABA) and an inhaled corticosteroid (ICS) in three separate inhaler device types. He lives at home alone in a 2-storey house. He suffered his first fall 6 months ago, which he attributes to shortness of breath after walking up the flight of stairs to his second floor too quickly. He discontinued smoking more than 10 years ago. His anti-pneumococcal vaccines are up to date, he receives his annual flu vaccination, and his COVID vaccination status is in keeping with the latest recommendations. He knows very little about COPD, and he wishes to learn more about the early signs of an exacerbation and what to do about them when they occur. He has never previously participated in a Pulmonary Rehabilitation (PR) program, but after his recent hospitalization for an acute exacerbation of COPD and his fall earlier this year, he is interested to learn more about whether he is a candidate.

WHAT IS CHRONIC OBSTRUCTIVE PULMONARY DISEASE (COPD)?

Chronic obstructive pulmonary disease (COPD), an umbrella term encompassing both emphysema and chronic bronchitis, is a very common, often preventable, and treatable disease that affects many older adults. In fact, it is the third leading cause of global morbidity and has become the third leading cause of death worldwide. With population aging, COPD prevalence has increased by roughly 44% from 1990 to 2015 in Canada, and this same pattern is observed around the world. Globally, the most recently reported prevalence of COPD is approximately 10–13%, although this is underestimated considering that approximately 70% of COPD worldwide may be underdiagnosed. There are particular concerns of underdiagnosis in the elderly due to a small but sizeable proportion who cannot perform acceptable/reproducible spirometry manoeuvres to confirm the diagnosis.

COPD can develop from a variety of separate causes and conditions, each of which lead to airflow obstruction which is not fully reversible. Airflow obstruction is detected by testing lung function using post-bronchodilator spirometry. The forced vital capacity (FVC—the maximum volume of air during a full, forced exhalation manoeuvre following a full inhalation) of an individual is compared with the forced expiratory volume in 1 second (FEV_1—the expiratory volume in the first second of a forced vital capacity manoeuvre). A low FEV_1 to FVC ratio (an FEV_1/FVC ratio of less than 0.7, or a ratio less than the predicted lower limit of normal (LLN) value) which is not completely reversible supports a diagnosis of COPD. The magnitude of FEV_1 impairment indicates

DOI: 10.1201/9781003344476-25

Table 22.1 Classification of Airflow Limitation Severity in COPD

CLASSIFICATION OF AIRFLOW LIMITATION SEVERITY IN COPD (BASED ON POST-BRONCHODILATOR FEV_1)		
In patients with FEV1/FVC < 0.70:		
GOLD 1:	Mild	$FEV_1 \geq 80\%$ predicted
GOLD 2:	Moderate	$50\% \leq FEV_1 < 80\%$ predicted
GOLD 3:	Severe	$30\% \leq FEV_1 < 50\%$ predicted
GOLD 4:	Very Severe	$FEV_1 < 30\%$ predicted

Source: Retrieved from https://goldcopd.org/gold-teaching-slide-set/ (obtained with permission)

the spirometric 'severity' of airflow obstruction and is classified as *Global Strategy for Prevention, Diagnosis and Management of COPD* ('GOLD') 1 to 4 (presented in Table 22.1).

The natural history of COPD entails a progressive decline in lung function over time and is also characterized by discrete episodes or 'acute lung attacks' known as acute exacerbations of COPD or AECOPD. These AECOPD episodes carry a large burden to the older adult living with COPD and can lead to subsequent lung function decline. The severity and frequency of AECOPDs are an important risk factor for COPD mortality, and hospitalization for AECOPD is a leading budgetary cost of most developed healthcare systems around the world. It is not uncommon for patients to experience ≥2 moderate to severe exacerbations per year. It is imperative to identify individuals at risk for frequent exacerbations and to employ optimal strategies to minimize the risk of these events. The modern approach that includes pharmacologic and non-pharmacologic treatment offers great promise in the ability to individualize care and improve outcomes for patients with COPD (controlling symptoms, preventing AECOPDs), particularly for older patients in whom it is critical to maintain a high quality of life and maximize independence.

WHAT ARE THE RISK FACTORS FOR COPD?

COPD can develop in individuals following the chronic inhalation of noxious inhaled gases and particles. The most widely studied association is cigarette smoking, and therefore the cumulative smoking history (commonly measured in 'pack-years') is an important risk factor for developing COPD, as is passive (second-hand) smoke exposure and, possibly, regular marijuana use. Around the world, the persistent inhalation of toxic particles at work (occupational exposures), indoor cooking/heating fuels (biomass exposure), and outdoor ambient air pollution are other important exposures and risk factors. A past medical history compatible with asthma and/or severe childhood respiratory disease are also known risk factors for COPD. Further knowledge on the natural history and risk factors for the older patient with COPD is being researched by cohorts such as the *Canadian Cohort Obstructive Lung Disease* (CanCOLD—www.cancold.ca), which has an average age of greater than 65 years in COPD participants and is the first population-based long-term COPD cohort study in Canada that aims to address such challenging and important research questions.

In normal individuals without COPD, pulmonary function (as measured by FEV_1) improves from childhood into early adulthood, peaks around age 20, and then gradually declines thereafter over the typical lifespan. Given that COPD is a disease associated with exposure to noxious inhaled stimuli over many years, advanced age (a reflection of cumulative years of noxious exposure) can also be considered a risk factor in itself, not only for the development of COPD but moreover for the severity of disease.

The complicating factors particularly relevant to the older adult living with COPD are nicely summarized in Figure 22.1 from the excellent review article by RA Incalzi et al. (2014), which demonstrates the complicated interplay between relevant factors in the elderly such as malnutrition, co-morbidities (including osteoporosis, depression, and anxiety), and social isolation with COPD-relevant factors such as symptoms of dyspnea and AECOPD events.

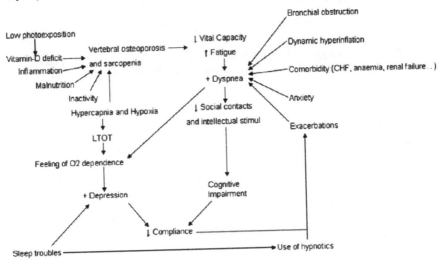

Figure 22.1 The complicating factors relevant to the older adult living with COPD (obtained with permission)

WHAT ARE THE PHARMACOLOGIC TREATMENTS FOR OLDER ADULTS LIVING WITH COPD?

An important pearl in the management of older patients with COPD is that age and disease severity should *not* be perceived as acceptable reasons to withhold evidence-based therapies. The most recent updates on the pharmacologic management of COPD were published by the Canadian Thoracic Society in 2019 (*Canadian Thoracic Society Clinical Practice Guideline on Pharmacotherapy in Patients with COPD—2019 Update of Evidence*) and by the American Thoracic Society in 2020 (*Pharmacologic Management of Chronic Obstructive Pulmonary Disease: An Official American Thoracic Society Clinical Practice Guideline*). They provide a comprehensive approach to improving both symptoms and activity limitations as well as reducing the risk of future AECOPDs.

Every adult chronic disease (both respiratory and non-respiratory) is unique in regard to the natural history, progression, and disease-specific end-of-life care strategies. These disease-specific particularities may inform the removal of treatments felt to be of little additional benefit or even harmful in older adults (for example, the regularly updated recommendations of the *Beers Criteria® for Potentially Inappropriate Medication Use in the Elderly*). The disease trajectory of COPD is that of a slow progressive decline which takes place over many years. Even in very advanced disease in elderly patients, palliative symptoms of dyspnea can and should be aggressively treated. Dyspnea is one of the most distressing symptoms and its significance is often under-appreciated. Clinical tools such as the *modified Medical Research Council (mMRC) Dyspnea Scale* (presented in Table 22.2) can be used to record the severity of dyspnea. The older patient living with COPD must not be deprived of treatments which can provide the most effective disease control possible, as doing so deprives the potential for better symptom control and a better quality of life throughout the entire span of the natural history of the disease.

Because most pharmacologic COPD treatments have not reliably demonstrated mortality benefits, the latest national and international COPD guidelines such as the 2019 Canadian Thoracic Society Guideline and the 2022 *Global Strategy for Prevention, Diagnosis and Management of COPD* place a particular emphasis on targeting the two most relevant aspects of disease when tailoring chronic therapies: reducing/managing shortness of breath (dyspnea) and reducing/minimizing the risk of future AECOPD events. Inhaled therapies are the cornerstone of the *pharmacologic* treatment of COPD and should be used before the consideration and/or addition of oral therapies. A general helpful rule is that *dyspnea* should be aggressively treated with long-acting bronchodilators (LAMAs, LABAs, or both), while *future AECOPD risk* should be treated with add-on ICS (particularly in those with prior hospitalization for AECOPD, with multiple outpatient AECOPDs, with elevated blood eosinophil counts and/or with co-morbid asthma).

Table 22.2 The Modified Medical Research Council (mMRC) Dyspnea Scale

> **MODIFIED MRC DYSPNEA SCALE[a]**

PLEASE TICK IN THE BOX THAT APPLIES TO YOU | ONE BOX ONLY | Grades 0 - 4

mMRC Grade 0.	I only get breathless with strenuous exercise.	☐
mMRC Grade 1.	I get short of breath when hurrying on the level or walking up a slight hill.	☐
mMRC Grade 2.	I walk slower than people of the same age on the level because of breathlessness, or I have to stop for breath when walking on my own pace on the level.	☐
mMRC Grade 3.	I stop for breath after walking about 100 meters or after a few minutes on the level.	☐
mMRC Grade 4.	I am too breathless to leave the house or I am breathless when dressing or undressing.	☐

[a] Fletcher CM. BMJ 1960; 2: 1662.
TABLE 2.5

Source: Retrieved from https://goldcopd.org/gold-teaching-slide-set/ (obtained with permission)

The main COPD therapies are administered through inhaled devices. Unfortunately, misuse is common, and factors associated with inhaler misuse independent of device type are older age, lower education level, and lack of instruction from a healthcare professional. Particularly in the older adult with COPD, there are many challenges with the use of inhalation therapy. Many of these challenges are nicely summarized in Figure 2 of the review article by Usmani (2019). These include patient-specific factors including cognitive, neuromuscular, and musculoskeletal function; the patient's ability to use the device; and their own personal preferences. This underscores the importance of appropriate and individualized device selection.

Time should be spent on tailoring the inhaler device type based on co-morbid medical conditions, hand dexterity, and hand-mouth coordination capacity, and the inspiratory flow capable of being generated by the patient. When using metered-dose inhalers (MDI), a spacer device (also known as a valved holding chamber) will facilitate effective medication delivery to the lungs. It is important to ensure that proper technique is reviewed considering that poor inhaler technique is associated with worse outcomes. Given the reality of polypharmacy in older adults, strategies to simplify inhaler therapy regimens (such as 2-in-1 or 3-in-1 inhaler devices when 2 or 3 separate drug classes are medically appropriate) should also be pursued whenever feasible. Patients who use multiple devices with similar inhalation technique have better clinical outcomes than those using devices that require a variety of inhalation techniques. If medication cost is suspected to be limiting device purchase or adherence in an older patient on a limited budget or pension, local exception codes for elderly patients should be sought and used and involvement of social worker services may help to navigate the most appropriate prescription strategies. An excellent English and French video resource demonstrating proper inhaler technique for a variety of puffer types was created by the Canadian Thoracic Society and is openly available at https://cts-sct.ca/covid-19/how-to-properly-use-an-inhaler/.

Notable oral controller therapies include theophylline, azithromycin, phosphodiesterase-4 (PDE-4) inhibitors (such as roflumilast), and opioids such as morphine. Theophylline has a narrow therapeutic window and can also have important drug-drug interactions and as such should largely be avoided in older patients with COPD. Azithromycin can effectively reduce future AECOPDs in selected patients and is largely well tolerated by older adults; however the benefit must be weighed against the risks of potential microbial resistance, hearing impairment, and QT-prolonging drug interactions. Baseline and routine audiology screening may be prudent in older patients at risk, as well as a baseline electrocardiogram (ECG). PDE-4 inhibitors are particularly useful for patients with COPD with a chronic bronchitis phenotype with excessive sputum production and a prior history of AECOPDs; however because of well-known gastrointestinal side effects (including diarrhea, nausea, reduced appetite, and weight loss) it should be used cautiously or avoided in older patients with malnutrition or who are underweight. Opioids such as morphine have been used for years in very advanced COPD in those patients with intractable breathlessness. Immediate-release morphine reduces dyspnea intensity and extends exercise endurance time in over half of patients with advanced COPD. The approach of using morphine for symptom control has to be conceptually differentiated from the management of terminal patients close to death. A measured approach, including the sage prescriber adage to 'start low and go slow' (and importantly, to *remain* low such that the benefits of dyspnea control continue to outweigh the risks), can reassure the clinician and patient alike. Concerns of side effects in the elderly are generally valid and close monitoring is advised; however, notably, this should not be a deterrent to the effective and well-established symptom burden treatment with oral opioids or other therapies.

THE ACUTE MANAGEMENT OF AECOPDS IN OLDER ADULTS

The acute management of an AECOPD includes effective bronchodilation (including additional short-acting bronchodilator therapy), anti-infective and anti-inflammatory treatments (antibiotics and systemic corticosteroids), oxygen, and even non-invasive ventilatory strategies when warranted, and general supportive care. AECOPDs are important and potentially life-threatening events and should be treated aggressively regardless of the age of the patient. An all-too-common scenario is the withholding of effective therapies such as short-acting beta-agonists (SABAs) in older patients with co-morbid cardiac conditions such as arrhythmias, or withholding short-acting anti-muscarinic antagonists (SAMAs) in older patients due to concerns of causing delirium or other anti-cholinergic sequelae such as urinary retention. The deprivation of much-needed timely AECOPD treatments risks worsening the severity and duration of the AECOPD as well as the prolongation of the subsequent recovery period. Therefore, much like the philosophy of aggressively managing chronic symptoms of COPD in older adults with effective controller therapies, the acute management of AECOPDs must also be aggressive and comprehensive. To quote the common slogan of a large number of national lung association organizations, "When you can't breathe, nothing else matters".

WHAT ARE THE NON-PHARMACOLOGIC TREATMENTS FOR OLDER ADULTS LIVING WITH COPD?

Non-pharmacological treatments should include but are not limited to smoking cessation and adherence to age- and disease-appropriate vaccination schedules. Two crucially important non-pharmacological interventions for any COPD patient including the older adult living with this condition include pulmonary rehabilitation and self-management education. Patients suffering from COPD have reported inadequate education regarding their disease, its treatment options, strategies for self-management, and exacerbation prevention strategies. Decisions are made on essentially a daily basis by the patient as to whether medical treatments and/or a healthy lifestyle will be started or continued. For self-management intervention to be effective requires an iterative process of interaction between participant and healthcare provider, and ideally also includes the establishment of personal goals and the provision of longitudinal feedback. The precise content of the self-management intervention will depend upon the individual patient's disease severity (and complications such as recurrent exacerbations), the presence of co-morbid conditions, and the patient's own capacity to manage their disease (cognition, self-efficacy, literacy, and numeracy).

However, a self-management intervention is not an alternative to Pulmonary Rehabilitation. Society guidelines define Pulmonary Rehabilitation as

> a comprehensive intervention based on a thorough patient assessment followed by patient-tailored therapies, which include, but are not limited to, exercise training, education, and behaviour change, designed to improve the physical and psychological condition of people with chronic respiratory disease and to promote the long-term adherence of health-enhancing behaviors.

Pulmonary Rehabilitation is based on a robust evidence base and improves dyspnea, exercise capacity, and quality of life. Recent evidence further supports the longstanding notion that Pulmonary Rehabilitation participation in the immediate post-AECOPD hospitalization period additionally confers a mortality benefit. Pulmonary Rehabilitation is an effective multidisciplinary non-pharmacological intervention that represents the standard of care in COPD management, comprising exercise training, education, and self-management behaviour modification as fundamental elements. Programs are individually tailored to the participant. Since rehabilitation goals and exercise prescriptions are highly personalized, by extension in the older patient with COPD, *age, frailty, or COPD severity* are *not* exclusion criteria for participation. Pulmonary Rehabilitation can benefit almost every patient with COPD irrespective of disease severity, sex, ethnicity, or age. In fact, Pulmonary Rehabilitation participation can effectively target frailty, lower extremity weakness, and sarcopenia (age-related loss of muscle mass and strength) through a combination of longitudinal endurance and resistance exercises. Some programs additionally offer balance-specific exercises in selected participants with the aim to reduce the risk of future falls. The use of adjuncts and exercise equipment can support the older patient with COPD during and after the program. For example, particularly in older adults with advanced COPD who may be at risk of falls or may require supplemental oxygen as an outpatient, the use of a rollator can help recruit accessory respiratory muscles on exertion, can support balance, can provide a means to sit and rest during bouts of exertion, and can also help transport heavy oxygen tanks and supplemental equipment during ambulation.

The Pulmonary Rehabilitation participants themselves must actively engage in the program in order to be equipped with the tools to subsequently manage their own disease on a day-to-day basis. Education on self-management is an important component of Pulmonary Rehabilitation which promotes behaviour change and the adoption of healthy habits at any age and allows for the many benefits to persist well after program completion. Lastly, in addition to the social aspect of meeting and fraternizing with peers who are also living with a chronic respiratory disease, many COPD and Pulmonary Rehabilitation clinical programs connect the participant to a dedicated Case Manager who becomes their 'coach' and represents their link to the clinical program. Case Managers provide valuable guidance, education, and patient empowerment through motivational interviewing methods. Older adults with COPD, particularly those who may be socially or geographically isolated, can greatly benefit from longitudinal Case Manager care as part of an effective multidisciplinary approach.

A fantastic bilingual resource available to any healthcare provider and to any patient following a simple account sign-up is the Living Well with COPD (LWWCOPD) platform (www.livingwellwithcopd.com). LWWCOPD equips patients and healthcare providers alike with the tools to effectively manage COPD.

RESOLUTION OF THE CLINICAL VIGNETTE

This older adult living at home independently with advanced COPD has had a recent severe AECOPD hospitalization and a fall at home attributed to a dyspnea episode. He is on effective inhaler molecules (LAMA, LABA, and ICS); however multiple separate devices may be complicating the ability to adhere to the medication schedule. He has also never participated in a Pulmonary Rehabilitation program. Comprehensive pharmacologic and non-pharmacologic interventions will help to optimize disease and symptom management, maintain independence at home and promote as high a quality of life for as long as possible.

In the setting of known hand osteoarthritis, his possible dexterity issues and in order to reduce the burden of polypharmacy, a single device containing a LAMA, a LABA; and an ICS (taken as one single inhalation, once daily) was prescribed. The inhaler device was chosen for ease of use in terms of hand dexterity and hand-mouth coordination and was appropriate for his measured peak inspiratory flow.

Although caution is advised in a patient known for atrial fibrillation in the past since bronchodilators have been described as pro-arrhythmic agents, he was also prescribed a short-acting beta-2 agonist (rescue inhaler) with a spacer device; he was instructed on the importance of rescue inhaler use when indicated for severe acute dyspnea episodes, and he will monitor for symptoms of side effects (such as heart palpitations) during use. Available evidence suggests an acceptable safety profile for long-acting beta-2 agonists, anti-muscarinics, and inhaled corticosteroids in this setting.

In order to prevent future severe acute exacerbations, he was provided with a Written Action Plan (which serves as an instructional guideline for the patient) comprising of an oral antibiotic and oral corticosteroid in the event of an exacerbation, and he received directed teaching on when and how to appropriately use it with a COPD Case Manager (who also acts as his ongoing liaison/ connection with the clinic). In anticipation for the possible future need of a chronic macrolide to reduce further exacerbations and given subjective symptoms of hearing loss, a baseline audiometry test was arranged as well as a baseline ECG. He was encouraged to continue to adhere to age-appropriate vaccination schedules including receiving his annual influenza vaccine.

He was promptly referred to and successfully completed his first Pulmonary Rehabilitation program. The exercise component improved his physical conditioning, his ability to perform his activities of daily living, his lower limb strength, and his balance, which may reduce the risk of future falls and will further support his ability to continue living independently at home. The education and self-management components of the program provided him with important information about his disease that he can integrate into his daily life, including how to use his controller therapies, his rescue therapies and his Action Plan, and energy utilization/conservation strategies and breathing techniques such as pursed lip breathing when performing demanding tasks such as navigating stairs. The social aspect provided a welcomed support network and camaraderie during and well after completion of the Pulmonary Rehabilitation program. Further refining his self-management skills with ongoing follow-up visits will also increase the likelihood that making positive decisions about adequate medical treatments and/or a healthy lifestyle can continue long after the Pulmonary Rehabilitation program is completed.

Following pharmacological and non-pharmacological optimization, and armed with valuable knowledge about his disease, with adaptive behaviours and newly developed positive physical activity habits, the patient's symptoms of chronic dyspnea were better controlled. He continued to live well and independently at home.

REFERENCES AND RESOURCES

2022 Global Strategy for Prevention, Diagnosis and Management of COPD. https://goldcopd.org/2022-gold-reports/ and https://goldcopd.org/gold-teaching-slide-set/

Canadian Cohort Obstructive Lung Disease (CanCOLD) Study. www.cancold.ca

Incalzi RA, Scarlata S, Pennazza G et al. Chronic obstructive pulmonary disease in the elderly. Eur J Intern Med 2014;25:320–328.

Bourbeau J, Bhutani M, Hernandez P et al. Canadian thoracic society clinical practice guideline on pharmacotherapy in patients with COPD-2019 update of evidence. Can J Respir Crit Care Sleep Med 2019;3:4,210–232.

Nici L, Mammen MJ, Charbek E et al. Pharmacologic management of chronic obstructive pulmonary disease. An official American Thoracic Society clinical practice guideline. Am J Respir Crit Care Med 2020;201:e56–e69.

2019 American Geriatrics Society Beers Criteria® Update Expert Panel. American Geriatrics Society 2019 updated AGS Beers Criteria® for potentially inappropriate medication use in older adults. J Am Geriatr Soc 2019;67:674–694.

Usmani OS. Choosing the right inhaler for your asthma or COPD patient. Ther Clin Risk Manag 2019;15:461–472.

Canadian Thoracic Society Video Resource: "How to Properly Use an Inhaler". https://cts-sct.ca/covid-19/how-to-properly-use-an-inhaler/

Living Well with COPD (LWWCOPD) Online Platform. https://www.livingwellwithcopd.com/

23 How Do I Manage My Patient with Peripheral Arterial Disease?

Oren K. Steinmetz, MDCM, FRCSC, FACS and Anna Eva Kinio, MD, MSc

CONTENTS

CLINICAL VIGNETTE

A 78-year-old man with a past medical history of diabetes, coronary artery disease, and smoking complains of severe pain in his right foot at night. The pain began one month ago and prevents him from sleeping. He only experiences relief when he dangles his leg out of bed. Despite taking large amounts of acetaminophen, the pain persists and his quality of life has deteriorated. More recently, he has noticed that the tip of his right 5th toe has turned black. On questioning the patient describes previously experiencing pain in both calves when walking which resolved with rest. However, since the pain in his foot developed, he has become almost entirely sedentary.

Physical exam reveals palpable femoral pulses bilaterally without any palpable popliteal, dorsalis pedis, or posterior tibial pulses bilaterally. As the patient sits on the side of the bed, the foot becomes a deep red. The toes are painful on light palpation and the tip of the right 5th toe is necrotic, without any palpable fluctuance or pus.

An ankle-brachial index (ABI) is ordered which reveals an ABI of 0.32 at the right posterior tibial artery with a dampened monophasic waveform. Toe pressure is 22 mmHg.

BACKGROUND AND EPIDEMIOLOGY

Peripheral arterial disease (PAD) is defined as chronic occlusive disease of the lower extremities secondary to atherosclerosis. While the majority of patients with PAD are asymptomatic, disturbance in oxygen delivery to tissues below the level of occlusion can result in tissue hypoxia. This can result in lower extremity muscular pain during exercise, intermittent claudication, but can also progress to severe limb-threatening ischemia.

The aging population, increased prevalence of smoking, hypertension, dyslipidemia, and diabetes have contributed to PAD becoming a major global health concern. Estimates from epidemiologic studies suggest that globally more than 200 million individuals are affected by PAD.[1] There is also a strong age-dependent increase in prevalence, with a prevalence of 25% in individuals over the age of 80 years.[2] As the population grows older, the prevalence of PAD is therefore expected to rise dramatically. Currently, PAD is already the leading cause of disability in patients greater than 50 years of age, largely due to pain, limb loss, and associated increased risks of cardiovascular and cerebrovascular events. Many patients will progressively lose independence due to physical

DOI: 10.1201/9781003344476-26

limitations caused by the disease and will require home care or institutionalization to meet their care requirements. Despite this high social and economic cost, PAD remains significantly under-diagnosed and under-treated, with half of patients receiving no medical risk management.[3] With the global population aging and PAD prevalence expected to double in some countries, it will be imperative to aggressively address risk factors and to limit progression of disease whenever possible.

RISK FACTORS FOR PERIPHERAL ARTERIAL DISEASE

PAD is a local manifestation of the systemic atherosclerotic disease process, and so shares the same risk factors as coronary artery disease and cerebrovascular disease. This is highlighted by the high incidence of myocardial infarction, stroke, and vascular-related death in the PAD population.

Demographic Risk Factors

Advanced age is the strongest risk factor for PAD. Prevalence increases with increasing age, and up to 25% of individuals above age 80 years were found to have PAD in one epidemiological study.[2] Other demographic risk factors include race, low socioeconomic status, and male sex.

Modifiable Risk Factors

Cigarette smoking is strongly associated with PAD prevalence and disease progression. Conversely, smoking cessation has been found to limit the progression of PAD to critical limb ischemia, while also reducing the risk of cardio- or cerebrovascular events and related deaths.

Hypertension, diabetes, and hyperlipidemia are all associated with PAD and medical management can result in improved outcomes.

Although elevated serum *homocysteine* has also been significantly associated with PAD, reduction of homocysteine levels with folic acid and vitamin B6 and B12 has not been shown to limit disease progression.

DIAGNOSIS OF PERIPHERAL ARTERIAL DISEASE

Classification systems such as the Rutherford classification (Table 23.1) have previously been used to stage patients with PAD based on clinical presentation and physiologic measurements and can assist with treatment decisions and limb prognosis.

Population-based studies have demonstrated that most patients with a reduced ankle-brachial index indicative of PAD are asymptomatic. Patients may not experience symptoms due to low burden of disease or the anatomic location of disease, sedentary lifestyle, or collateralization.

Table 23.1 Rutherford Classification of Chronic Limb Ischemia

Grade	Category	Clinical Description	Objective Criteria
0	0	Asymptomatic	Normal treadmill or reactive hyperemia test
	1	Mild Claudication	Able to complete treadmill exercise; AP after exercise > 50 mmHg but at least 20 mmHg lower than at rest
I	2	Moderate Claudication	Between Rutherford 1 and 3 categories
	3	Severe Claudication	Cannot complete treadmill exercise and AP after exercise < 50 mmHg
II	4	Rest Pain	Resting AP < 40 mmHg and/or TP < 30 mmHg, PVR barely pulsatile or flat
III	5	Minor tissue loss (non-healing ulcer, focal gangrene with diffuse pedal ischemia)	Resting AP < 60 mmHg and/or TP < 40 mmHg, PVR barely pulsatile or flat
	6	Major tissue loss extending beyond the transmetatarsal level, functional foot no longer salvageable	Same as category 5

Note: AP: Ankle Pressure; TP: Toe Pressure; PVR: Pulse Volume Recording

However, even in asymptomatic individuals, presence of PAD is associated with physical decline and carries a high risk of cardiovascular events and mortality. While a minority of these patients are believed to progress to intermittent claudication, they should nevertheless be assessed for medical management of their risk factors and counselled on smoking cessation, a healthy diet and regular exercise to reduce their risk of PAD progression, MI, stroke, and vascular-related death.

Intermittent claudication occurs when arterial disease causes disturbances in downstream muscle perfusion during exercise. Depending on the anatomic level of disease it is characterized by a reproducible buttock, hip, thigh, or calf pain or fatigue which occurs at exercise and is relieved by rest. A detailed history should be taken from the patient to distinguish this syndrome from neurogenic, musculoskeletal, or venous disorders which also present with lower extremity pain. While the risk of major amputation remains low at less than 1% per year, a significant percentage of patients will progress to critical limb ischemia.[4] Additionally, these patients are at significant risk of functional decline and cardio- or cerebrovascular mortality. First-line therapy consists of supervised exercise programs, smoking cessation, and medical risk factor management with statins, blood pressure control, and antiplatelet therapy. In select circumstances open or endovascular revascularization may be considered if quality of life is severely impaired and the patient is a low-risk surgical candidate.

Progression to chronic limb-threatening ischemia (CLTI) is characterized by presence of rest pain in the affected limb with or without tissue necrosis (Rutherford Grade II and III), indicating that baseline limb perfusion is severely compromised and unable to meet resting tissue requirements. CLTI represents a broad class of PAD and has been further categorized based on clinical presentation and non-invasive measurements in the Rutherford classification (Table 23.1). However, compared to asymptomatic disease or intermittent claudication, CLTI patients are at a higher risk of major amputation and should be assessed for revascularization. Benefits of revascularization must be tailored to each patient based on anatomic and patient characteristics, especially given the higher burden of cardiovascular and cerebrovascular disease in this population. Notably, advanced age and increased frailty have been associated with poorer survival and limb outcomes post-intervention and so should be considered in the pre-operative planning for CLTI patients.[5]

Patient Interview

A detailed history and physical exam are vital components of the vascular assessment. Outlines of a focused vascular history and physical exam are found in Tables 23.2 and 23.3.

Table 23.2 Vascular Clinical History Guide

Components of Vascular History	Documentation Pertinent to Vascular History
Reason for Referral	Asymptomatic disease, claudication, rest pain, tissue loss
Past Medical History	CAD, CVA, diabetes, renal disease
Past Surgical History	Previous revascularization, CABG, determine if/which saphenous vein has been used
Medications	Anticoagulation, antiplatelets, statin, blood pressure control
Allergies	Iodine-based contrast, antibiotics
Habits	Smoking history
Social History	Ambulatory/activity status, level of independence with ADLS and IADLS, level of family/social assistance available
History of Presenting Illness	Presence of lower extremity pain: • Use OPQRST acronym to characterize pain—onset, provocative factors, progression, quality, relieving factors, severity, timing • Determine which limb experiences pain and at what level (if both limbs affected, is one worse?) • Pain present at rest or with exercise? If so, how much exercise/what distance causes pain onset? • Quality of life or work affected? • Questions can be asked to differentiate claudication from other potential causes of lower extremity pain (i.e. neurogenic, venous, musculoskeletal causes) Presence of lower extremity wounds/tissue loss

Note: CAD: Coronary artery disease; CVA: Cerebrovascular Accident; CABG: Coronary Artery Bypass Graft; ADL: Activities of Daily Living; IADL: Instrumental Activities of Daily Living

Table 23.3 Physical Examination for PAD

Initial Inspection	Vital signs?
	Presence of mobility devices?
Inspection of Leg	Skin changes?
	Muscle atrophy?
	Hair distribution?
	Mottling/Erythema/Pallor?
	Temperature?
	Edema?
	Ulcerations?
	Motor and sensory function?
	Positive Buerger test?
	Major amputations?
	Previous saphenous vein harvest?
	Previous bypass surgeries?
	Other surgical scars?
	Comparison to ipsilateral limb?
Inspection of Foot	Foot deformity?
	Abnormalities in nail growth?
	Presence of ulcers/gangrene?
	Discolouration of foot?
	Temperature?
	Motor and sensory function?
	Digital/metatarsal amputations?
	Comparison to other foot?
Inspection of Ulcers/Tissue Loss	Ulcer/dry gangrene/wet gangrene?
	Site of tissue loss?
	Proximal extent of tissue loss?
	Presence of odour?
	Presence of exudate?
	Palpable collection?
	Appearance of wound bed?
Vascular Exam	Palpable femoral, popliteal, posterior tibial, and dorsalis pedis pulses?
	If not palpable, audible signals on doppler?
	Palpable calcified arteries?
	Bounding pulses?
	Capillary refill time?
	Palpable pulses or audible signals in previous bypass grafts?

Investigations

Ankle-Brachial Index

The ankle-brachial index (ABI) is a fast and non-invasive test that is often the first-line investigation ordered when PAD is suspected. It is obtained by positioning the patient supine and using a doppler to measure both brachial, posterior tibial, and dorsalis pedis systolic blood pressures. The higher of the two readings for each limb is then divided by the higher brachial pressure to obtain the index for each lower extremity. An interpretation of ABI pressures is found in Table 23.4.

Toe brachial pressures (TBI) are frequently measured in conjunction with ABI and will may provide additional information in patients with incompressible tibial arteries. A TBI less than 0.70 is indicative of PAD and a toe systolic pressure of less than 30 mmHg may indicate healing impairment.

Table 23.4 Interpretation of ABI Results

ABI	Interpretation
> 1.30	Non-compressible vessels
0.90–1.29	Normal
0.70–0.89	Mild PAD
0.40–0.69	Moderate PAD
< 0.40	Severe PAD

Duplex Ultrasound Imaging

Duplex ultrasound is another non-invasive imaging modality with excellent sensitivity and specificity for arterial disease. Brightness mode, or B-mode, imaging can be used to assess arterial anatomy and measure diameter, wall thickening, and plaque morphology.

Colour doppler, or duplex, can be used to assess direction and velocity of flow. Increases in velocity, presence of colour aliasing, and changes in flow lumen diameter are suggestive of arterial stenosis.

Computed Tomography Angiography

Computed tomography angiography (CTA) is performed by injecting an intravascular iodine-based contrast agent to more clearly visualize arterial anatomy compared to conventional computed tomography. It has excellent sensitivity and specificity for arterial disease while providing information on surrounding anatomy. Given the potential nephrotoxic side effects of the contrast agent, use of CTA in patients with renal insufficiency should be limited.

Digital Subtraction Angiography

Digital subtraction angiography (DSA) is considered the gold-standard for arterial imaging. It is performed by obtaining arterial access, most commonly via the femoral arteries, and injecting intra-arterial contrast to assess arterial anatomy and contrast flow under fluoroscopy.

DSA may be performed in conjunction with endovascular treatment. Risks of the procedure include pseudoaneurysm formation, access-site bleeding, arterial dissection, distal embolization, or acute kidney injury from the contrast agent. In patients with underlying renal insufficiency, it may be performed with carbon dioxide in lieu of the contrast agent.

DSA and CTA are generally reserved for assessment and planning in patients who require intervention.

TREATMENT

Treatment for PAD is decided on a case-by-case basis, taking patient characteristics, burden of arterial disease, clinical presentation, and patient wishes into account. Goals of treatment vary based on these factors but are generally aimed at reducing the risk of vascular-related events and death, improving quality of life and limb-salvage. Therefore, surgical or endovascular revascularization is generally reserved for patients with chronic limb-threatening ischemia or for select patients with severe claudication. Patients who undergo revascularization will require long-term follow up and can often benefit from the expertise of a multidisciplinary team to assist in wound care and management of comorbidities. In particularly comorbid and frail patients, less invasive options for revascularization are often preferred to maximize patient quality of life while minimizing the risk of perioperative complications.

Lifestyle and Risk Factor Modification

Any patient with suspected PAD should be medically managed to reduce their risk of cardiovascular and cerebrovascular events and mortality. Patients should be counselled on smoking cessation, regular exercise, and a healthy diet. Blood pressure, hyperlipidemia, and blood glucose should be controlled with medication and lifestyle modification.

In addition to measures mentioned earlier, supervised exercise programs have been shown to increase walking distance and reduce functional decline in patients with intermittent claudication. Exercise should consist of walking for at least 30 minutes in duration, at least three times a week for a minimum of 12 weeks. When being counselled, patients should be instructed to walk until limited by pain, rest until pain subsides, before recommencing until a total exercise time of 30 minutes is attained.

Lastly, proper foot hygiene should be maintained with care to avoid injury. Chiropodists (podiatrists) may be employed for nail care to avoid trauma. Patients with wounds may require home wound care and should be regularly assessed by their wound care and vascular specialists.

Antiplatelet Agents and Anticoagulation

Single-agent antiplatelet therapy (ASA or clopidogrel) should be initiated in patients with PAD to reduce the risk of major adverse cardiac events and cardiovascular death. While dual antiplatelet therapy (DAPT) been found to reduce the risk of major adverse cardiac and major adverse limb events in several studies, the benefit is minimal and is accompanied by an increase in bleeding.[6] Dual antiplatelet therapy use for PAD is therefore generally limited to patients who undergo infrainguinal endovascular stenting in the 1–3 months following their procedure.

In the WAVE trial, the addition of warfarin to antiplatelet therapy increased the risk of life-threatening bleeding from 1.2% to 4% without conferring a reduction in adverse cardiac or limb events.[7] There have not been any studies assessing the impact of full anticoagulation with non-vitamin K antagonist oral anticoagulants (NOACs) and ASA in patients with chronic PAD. However, the COMPASS trial examined the effect of adding low-dose rivaroxaban to ASA in patients with stable PAD and found that this combination did confer a relative risk reduction in major adverse limb events, stroke, myocardial infarction, and cardiovascular death.[8] There was an associated increased risk of bleeding; however the majority of bleeding events were gastrointestinal and there was no increased risk of fatal or symptomatic bleeding into an organ.[8] Low dose (2.5 mg) rivaroxaban combined with aspirin could therefore be considered in select patients with both PAD and CAD.

Endovascular Treatment

Percutaneous angioplasty and or stent can be a viable option for revascularization in select patients. This minimally invasive option can usually be performed without hospital admission even in frail patients and is particularly attractive for patients with short-segment disease, those with many comorbidities or who lack autologous options for a bypass conduit. Despite several shortcomings, the BASIL-1 trial demonstrated that a "balloon-angioplasty first" approach could be considered in patients with a life expectancy of less than two years to reduce patient morbidity and procedure cost in patients who were unlikely to enjoy the longer-term benefits of bypass surgery. While endovascular treatment generally carries a low risk profile, post-operative complications of this procedure can include access site hemorrhage, pseudoaneurysm formation, arterial injury, or dissection and distal embolization.

Open Surgical Revascularization

There are multiple options for open surgical revascularization. The surgical plan is developed after proper assessment of patient comorbidities, extent of PAD symptoms and vascular anatomy. In general terms, open surgical interventions such as endarterectomy and bypass are needed with patients with a higher disease burden.

Risks of open surgery are generally higher and include wound infections or wound dehiscence, bleeding, cardiopulmonary complications, distal embolism, and graft thrombosis.

Amputation

Amputation is reserved for patients with extensive tissue loss, wet gangrene, bed-bound or non-ambulatory patients or for pain palliation in patients without options for revascularization due to extensive arterial disease or with very low life expectancy. Minor amputation is defined as digital amputation while major amputation denotes a below knee or more proximal amputation. Patients may learn to walk on a prosthesis following a below-knee amputation despite elevated cardiopulmonary fitness requirements. Ambulation after above-knee amputation is much less likely. This procedure should therefore be reserved for non-ambulatory patients.

RESOLUTION OF THE CLINICAL VIGNETTE

The patient's clinical history, physical exam, and ABI are consistent with Rutherford 5 chronic limb-threatening ischemia. He is referred to a vascular surgeon for evaluation. In the interim, a full review of his medical history and medications is performed (Figure 23.1).

Blood pressure is controlled and an Hb A1c is checked to assess adequate diabetic control. He is started on a low-dose aspirin and a statin. He is instructed to stop smoking to limit disease progression, to improve the efficacy of any attempted revascularization, and to reduce his risk of

Figure 23.1 Algorithm for PAD treatment

vascular events. Adequate pain control is prescribed while he awaits vascular assessment. He is also instructed to paint his necrotic toe daily with 10% proviodine to encourage autoamputation of necrotic tissue and to prevent superimposed infection.

At his vascular appointment the patient is assessed and deemed an appropriate candidate for angiogram. He undergoes a pre-operative medicine consultation prior to his procedure to ensure his medical comorbidities are appropriately managed prior to his surgery. Angiography demonstrates a diffuse and heavy burden of atherosclerosis extending down his superficial femoral artery and occlusion of the popliteal artery, with patent posterior tibial and peroneal artery run-off to his foot. The anatomy of disease is considered unfavourable for endovascular intervention. He is found to have an adequately sized and good quality right greater saphenous vein and is scheduled for right femoral to posterior-tibial bypass.

REFERENCES

1. Fowkes FG, Rudan D, Rudan I, et al. Comparison of global estimates of prevalence and risk factors for peripheral artery disease in 2000 and 2010: a systematic review and analysis. Lancet 2013;382:1329–1340.
2. Selvin E, Erlinger TP. Prevalence of and risk factors for peripheral arterial disease in the United States: results from the National Health and Nutrition Examination Survey, 1999–2000. Circulation 2004;110:738–743.
3. Stehouwer CD, Clement D, Davidson C, et al. Peripheral arterial disease: a growing problem for the internist. Eur J Intern Med 2009;20:132–138.
4. Sigvant B, Lundin F, Wahlberg E. The risk of disease progression in peripheral arterial disease is higher than expected: a meta-analysis of mortality and disease progression in peripheral arterial disease. Eur J Vasc Endovasc Surg 2016;51:395–403.

5. Kraiss LW, Beckstrom JL, Brooke BS. Frailty assessment in vascular surgery and its utility in preoperative decision making. Semin Vasc Surg 2015;28:141–147.
6. Cacoub PP, Bhatt DL, Steg PG, Topol EJ, Creager MA, Investigators C. Patients with peripheral arterial disease in the CHARISMA trial. Eur Heart J 2009;30:192–201.
7. Warfarin Antiplatelet Vascular Evaluation Trial I, Anand S, Yusuf S, et al. Oral anticoagulant and antiplatelet therapy and peripheral arterial disease. N Engl J Med 2007;357:217–227.
8. Anand SS, Eikelboom JW, Dyal L, et al. Rivaroxaban plus aspirin versus aspirin in relation to vascular risk in the COMPASS Trial. J Am Coll Cardiol 2019;73:3271–3280.

24 How to Manage Type 2 Diabetes in Frail Elderly Patients

Young-Sang Kim, MD, PhD and José A. Morais, MD, FRCPC

CONTENTS

CLINICAL VIGNETTE

Mrs. Sweet is an 86-year-old widow. She was admitted with a hip fracture consecutive to a fall. She is known for type 2 diabetes of 15 years duration. She also has a history of hypertension, dyslipidemia, coronary artery disease and arthritis. She uses a walker to ambulate but has no memory issues. Her medications include glyburide 5 mg bid, metformin 500 mg bid, perindopril 4 mg die, metoprolol 25 mg bid, ASA 80 mg die, atorvastatin 10 mg die and acetaminophen 500 mg tid, on needed basis. She has a good appetite. Her body mass index (BMI) is 31 kg/m^2 and her BP is 140/90 mmHg, sitting. According to the results of initial laboratory tests, the concentration of morning fasting blood glucose was 9 mmol/L, hemoglobin A1c level 9.2%, creatinine clearance 55 mL/min/1.73m^2 and the concentration of LDL cholesterol 3 mmol/L. What could be the objectives in treating type 2 diabetes in this frail patient?

BACKGROUND

Type 2 diabetes (T2D) is highly prevalent in older adults afflicting 25% of those > 75 years old, which is double that of a middle-aged population. In long-term care settings, these figures reach one-third of residents who carry a very high comorbidity burden. Unfortunately, in the community, only half of the individuals are aware of the diagnosis and therefore cannot benefit from lifestyle advice and treatments available to reduce the morbidities associated with this medical condition. The reason for a high percentage of elderly people with T2D is that aging is associated with adipose tissue accumulation especially intra-abdominally, sedentary lifestyle, low-grade inflammation, abnormal secretion of insulin and the effects of certain drugs. T2D increases the risk of micro and macro vascular complications that contribute to an acceleration of the manifestations of aging and predispose the elderly to geriatric syndromes. In more advanced age, T2D is associated with decreased weight, loss of independence, falls, cognitive impairment and depression. It has been estimated that T2D by these complications increases the risk of hospitalization in acute care by 43% and placement in long-term care by more than 52%. This population has particular characteristics, including a great heterogeneity of insulin secretion according to body composition. It has been found that in older adults with BMI < 27 kg/m^2, the main mechanism contributing to hyperglycemia is defective insulin secretion whereas in those with BMI > 27 kg/m^2 it is insulin resistance. These characteristics are good to keep in mind to guide in the selection of the most appropriate antidiabetic medications.

RISK OF HYPOGLYCEMIA

Another important aspect to consider in this population is their propensity to develop hypoglycemia. The rate of emergency room visits for hypoglycemia has been estimated at 54 vs 19/1000 diabetic visits in those ≥ 75 y compared with those 45–64 y. Hypoglycemia tends to be less perceived in older adults with T2D as both autonomic (e.g., sweat) and neuroglycopenic (e.g., slowness of thought); symptoms of hypoglycemia are vague in older patients, especially in those who are

DOI: 10.1201/9781003344476-27

Table 24.1 General Treatment Objectives

Maintain adequate caloric intake

Set appropriate A1c targets

Avoid hypoglycemia

Consider kidney function of the elderly patient

Consider the cardiovascular health risk of the elderly patient

Maintenance of quality of life

frail. These frail patients also are more frequently malnourished. Therefore, in the frail elderly with T2D, it is more important to prevent hypoglycemia than to control hyperglycemia intensively. Hypoglycemia itself carries detrimental consequences including cardiovascular disease, fall, fracture, physical deconditioning and progressive neuroglycopenia (psychomotor slowness). Of interest, frailty has been found to be a better predictor of complications and death in older adults with diabetes than chronological age or burden of comorbidity. When treating older adults with diabetes one has to keep in mind the objectives presented in Table 24.1 that are relevant to this population. Further, the determination of the presence of frailty is of utmost importance as vigorous older adults with T2D should be treated similarly to middle-aged individuals whereas those with frailty require special consideration.

ASSESSMENT OF FRAILTY

Frailty is the manifestation of impairment in multiple organ systems that results in increased susceptibility to poor health outcomes and reduced physical function. Please refer to Chapter 3 for further information on this syndrome. The most used definitions of frailty include the Frailty Phenotype and the Frailty Index. The former is based on five criteria that include shrinking (i.e., weight loss), weakness (i.e., loss of muscle strength), exhaustion, slowness (i.e., decreased walking speed) and low levels of physical activity. Having > 3 criteria defines frailty, having 1–2 criteria is considered pre-frailty and none is a normal state. The Frailty Index is calculated based on the deficit of any variable one wishes to apply to assess frailty with a minimum of ten to be included. Frailty is considered when a quarter of the variables show a deficit. These and other methods of assessing frailty requiring measurements can be cumbersome in a busy clinical practice. The Clinical Frailty Scale is a frequently employed tool that can overcome this limitation by simply recognizing a patient's vulnerability. The CFS uses clinical descriptors and pictographs that provide clinicians with an easily applicable tool to stratify older adults according to level of vulnerability. It ranges from very fit (stage 1) to terminally ill (stage 9), in which the first 3 stages are considered non-frail or functionally independent, stage 4–7 as frail with increasing dependency, whereas stage 8–9 individuals are totally dependent, which implies that they are disabled and therefore more than frail. A patient suffering from dementia is, by definition, classified as being frail.

SUGGESTED HEMOGLOBIN A1C TARGETS, BLOOD PRESSURE AND LIPIDS OUTCOMES

In the frail elderly with T2D, since it is difficult to maintain adequate caloric intake and to avoid hypoglycemia, clinicians need to set appropriate hemoglobin A1c targets and to re-evaluate the patients on a regular basis. As presented in Table 24.2, these targets are slightly different between national or international societies according to the criteria retained to ascertain frailty, but all societies propose less stringent A1c targets to prevent hypoglycemia. While the target for most adults with T2D is below 7.0%, for functionally dependent patients it is better to aim at 7.1–8.0%. For those patients clearly considered as frail, the target should be further eased to < 8.5%, whereas for end-of-life patients one should aim at avoiding symptomatic hyperglycemia with no hypoglycemia.

As for blood pressure control (Table 24.2), the Canadian guidelines are the most stringent, aiming at values < 130/80 mmHg until a person with diabetes becomes dependent. Both the ADA and the IDF guidelines are more liberal by setting the goal for BP control to < 140/80–90 mmHg and comprising intermediary stages with acceptable BP up to 150/90 mmHg, depending on the severity of the functional impairment. Finally, recommendations for lipid control are an LDL-C value < 2 mmol/L, with the exception of the ADA, which recommends < 1.8 mmol/L.

Table 24.2 Recommendations for Clinical Outcomes for Older Adults with Type 2 Diabetes

Outcome	Diabetes Canada	American Diabetes Association	International Diabetes Federation
A1c	Functionally independent: ≤ 7.0% Functionally dependent: 7.1–8.0% Frail and/or dementia: 7.1–8.5% End of life: A1c measurement not recommended. Avoid symptomatic hyperglycemia and any hypoglycemia.	Healthy: < 7.5% Complex/Intermediate: < 8.0% Very Complex/Poor Health: < 8.5%	Functionally independent: 7.0–7.5% Functionally dependent: 7.0–8.0% Sub-level frail: < 8.5% Sub-level dementia: < 8.5% End of life: avoid symptomatic hyperglycemia
Blood Pressure	Functionally independent with life expectancy > 10 years: < 130/80 mmHg Functionally dependent, orthostasis or limited life expectancy: individualize BP targets	Healthy: < 140/80 mmHg Complex/Intermediate: < 140/80 mmHg Very complex/Poor health: < 150/90 mmHg	Functionally independent: < 140/90 mmHg Functionally dependent: < 140/90 mmHg Sub-level frail: < 150/90 mmHg Sub-level dementia: < 140/90 mmHg End of life: strict BP control may not be necessary
LDL-C	< 2.0 mmol/L or > 50% reduction	< 1.8 mmol/L from baseline	< 2.0 mmol/L and adjusted based on CV

Note: A1c: glycated hemoglobin; BP: blood pressure; CV: cardiovascular; LDL-C: low density lipoprotein cholesterol
Source: Adapted from Diabetes Canada

PHARMACOTHERAPY IN THE FRAIL OLDER ADULT WITH TYPE 2 DIABETES

In frail older people with T2D, sulfonylureas should be used with caution and some products avoided (e.g., glyburide) because the risk of hypoglycemia increases substantially with age. Hence, some classes of antidiabetic medications with low risk of hypoglycemia are preferred to them. Available oral agents include biguanides such as metformin, dipeptidyl peptidase-4 inhibitors (DPPi-4), and if used carefully, insulin secretagogues such as meglitinides, and the sulfonylureas gliclazide and glimepiride. DPPi-4 should be used over sulfonylureas as second-line therapy to metformin, because of a lower risk of hypoglycemia. To use sulfonylureas in older persons, the initial doses should be started at the half of those commonly used for younger people, then the doses could be increased slowly. Gliclazide, gliclazide MR and glimepiride should be used instead of glyburide, as they have evidences of lower frequency of hypoglycemic events than glyburide. Meglitinides (Repaglinide, Nateglinide) may also be used instead of glyburide to reduce the risk of hypoglycemia, keeping in mind that they have a rapid onset of action with a short duration. In those patients with erratic eating behavior, one should offer the meglitinide after having been assured that the patient has eaten half of her/his meal.

In frail persons, some other classes of medications are to be avoided. These include thiazolidinediones (TZDs) due to the concern of fluid retention and heart failure. Sodium-glucose co-transporter protein-2 (SGLT-2) inhibitors carry a risk of dehydration with hypotension and urinary tract infections. Alpha-glucosidase inhibitors commonly cause enteric symptoms and possibly reduce appetite. Among the parenteral agents, insulin can be used with careful monitoring, but glucagon-like peptide-1 (GLP-1) receptor agonists are not recommended due to suppression of appetite.

Of note, decreased serum albumin is commonly observed in persons with severe malnutrition, in cancer, heart failure and other systemic illness. If the albumin-bound drugs decrease in circulation, this implies that the free portion is elevated and so is the risk of adverse or toxic effects. In the presence of malnutrition, due to concerns with adverse effects, some antidiabetic medications including repaglinide, gliclazide and glimepiride should be discontinued.

REDUCED KIDNEY FUNCTION

Reduced kidney function is common in the frail elderly. When the kidney function is impaired, one needs to avoid certain antidiabetic medications, and to make dosage adjustments according to the kidney function impairment. A key value of estimated glomerular filtration rate (eGFR) to

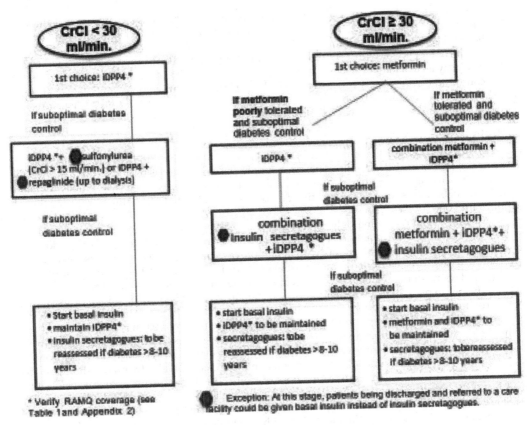

Figure 24.1 Drug treatment algorithm in the elderly diabetic based on renal function.

retain is 30 ml/min/1.73 m² as several antidiabetic medications are required to be stopped. These include metformin (risk of lactic acidosis), sulfonylureas and most GLP-1 analogues, except for liraglutide. DPPi-4 are safe, except for saxagliptine when eGFR is < 15 but all require dose adjustments when eGRF is below 50–60. In a non-frail patient and although not recommended, liraglutide can be used without dose adjustment when eGFR > 15 mL/min/1.73 m². In patients with an eGFR < 60, dapagliflozin is not recommended, and when an eGFR is below 45, the other SGLT-2 inhibitors also need to be avoided or used only with caution. Due to a concern of fluid retention, TZDs are less preferred in patients with chronic kidney disease.

Figure 24.1 presents a guide to select safe antidiabetic classes for frail older adults with T2D in the presence of kidney dysfunction. When the eGFR is less than 30, DPPi-4 are recommended as the initial choice, then one can progress to insulin therapy or to the insulin secretagogue, repaglinide, that is safe in kidney failure. When the eGFR is greater than 30, metformin should be used as the first choice, then one can add or change to DPPi-4. If glucose control requires further adjustments, insulin secretagogues (except glyburide) and sub-cutaneous insulin may be used consecutively.

REMARKS ABOUT CARDIOVASCULAR SAFETY AND HEART FAILURE

In older diabetic patients with clinical cardiovascular disease and with an eGFR > 30 mL/min/ 1.73 m², clinicians can choose or add an agent with demonstrated cardiovascular outcome benefit to reduce the risk of major cardiovascular events. Among the DPPi-4 which are preferred in the frail elderly with T2D, all have demonstrated to be cardiovascular safe, from the ischemic heart perspective.

As for congestive heart failure, each 1% increase in hemoglobin A1c is associated with 8% increased risk of heart failure. Antidiabetic treatment has been expected to lower the risk of the complication of heart failure in diabetic patients. However, rosiglitazone and other TZDs are known to precipitate congestive heart failure in susceptible patients. Among the DPPi-4 inhibitors, saxagliptine significantly increased the risk of hospitalization for heart failure in post hoc analyses of SAVOR-TIMI 53 study. Alogliptin, sitagliptin and linagliptin were confirmed not to increase the risk of hospitalization for heart failure.

To treat the older patient with T2D and heart failure, clinicians should approach heart failure in the same way as in a patient without diabetes. Concurrently with the diabetes treatment and unless contraindicated, clinicians need to carefully use inhibitors of the renin angiotensin aldosterone system or the combination of sacubitril/valsartan, known to increase the B-type natriuretic hormone. TZDs and saxagliptin need to be avoided.

INSULIN

If oral agents are contraindicated or glucose control is suboptimal, insulin is an inevitable choice in the frail elderly with T2D. Insulin types are roughly classified into bolus and basal insulins. Bolus insulins are rapid-acting analogues and regular human insulins, which are usually used at prandial time. Basal insulins are long-acting analogues and intermediate-acting human insulins, administered once or twice a day.

Because of the high risk of hypoglycemia, insulin should be used with caution. In fact, insulin is the second leading cause of emergency visits for adverse drug events. The frequency of dosages needs to be minimized in patients with a high prevalence of cognitive disorders, dexterity problems (e.g., arthritis, neuropathy, and movement disorders), vision problems, irregular eating patterns and so on. In many instances, a system of surveillance or assistance to administer insulin needs to be put in place to help maintain the older person safely at home. These involve use of pens, providing daily pre-filled syringes or having a nurse visit on a daily basis. Patients whose clock-drawing ability is deficient are at risk of having problems with insulin regimen.

Insulin may be used temporarily in short-term geriatric care units. Insulin use is required in diabetic patients who have erratic eating patterns, have to remain fasting, or are suffering from an acute episode leading to uncontrolled glycemia. In these cases, insulin treatment should not be based on a sliding scale. Instead, a morning dose of long-acting basal insulin analogue needs to be calculated. Patients in whom oral agents are no longer effective would be candidates for a permanent insulin regimen. When adding basal insulin to oral agents, insulin secretagogues are not recommended, and the combination of DPPi-4 with basal insulin should be preferred. If insulin therapy is the sole antidiabetic treatment, a regimen of long-acting basal insulin analogue combined with fast-acting bolus insulin analogue is the best choice.

RESOLUTION OF THE CLINICAL CASE

Soon after her admission, we should plan to improve the diabetic treatment of Mrs. Sweet. The initial target of hemoglobin A1c should be 7–8% since she is moderately frail as evidenced by using a walker. Her renal function is slightly below normal and therefore there is no contraindication to raise the dosage of metformin. We would increase metformin to 850 mg bid. Meanwhile, glyburide should not be used in a frail elderly, because of the concern of hypoglycemia, and in her case one could hypothesize that it may be related to the fall. Hence, we should stop glyburide. At this point, there are two options in the selection of an oral agent. The first option would be to start gliclazide MR 30 mg PO die for a week, and then increase to 60 mg PO die if no adverse event occurs, including hypoglycemia. The second option is to switch the sulfonylureas altogether to a DPPi-4. For this purpose, we could choose sitagliptin 100 mg PO die instead of glyburide. After 3 months on a stable dose and good control based on an A1c at the target value mentioned earlier, the oral antidiabetic regimen could be simplified into Janumet 50/850 mg bid or Janumet XR 50/1000 mg die.

The BP control is appropriate for her age and functional capacity level. There is room to improve the lipid values by increasing atorvastatin to 20 mg die. No attempt should be made to reduce caloric intake in this patient. During her stay in the hospital or rehabilitation, one should evaluate the gastric or digestive tolerance of higher metformin doses, the stability of blood glucose level and the presence of muscle symptoms possibly caused by the higher dose of atorvastatin. There is also an opportunity to teach her how to monitor blood glucose with capillary measurements, and how to recognize and manage the symptoms of hypoglycemia. Eventually, one should be able to discharge her and plan the next outpatient visit. We should ask her to measure and record capillary blood glucose at home twice a day on a cycle of morning with once at lunch time, next day at supper and the following day at night time, and to restart the cycle. Eventually, if glucose values are very stable, the intensity of monitoring can be reduced to twice a week at different times of the day. Recommendation to ambulate using the walker should be made to prevent further falls. Finally, the patient should be referred to home care services and advised to receive influenza vaccination.

CONCLUSION

The approach to the frail elderly patient with T2D is different in several ways from that of an older robust patient or a middle-aged person. Optimized strategies are required to cope with the more frequent hypoglycemia, reduced kidney function, poor appetite, comorbidities and shorter life expectancy. In the frail elderly, the previously mentioned situations and the frequently encountered cognitive deficits compel the physician to allow a less tight hemoglobin A1c control and to define a more personalized approach. The diet need not be controlled; a healthy diet plan will suffice. The simplest drug regimen should be proposed to facilitate patients' compliance.

REFERENCES

1. Lee PG, Halter JB: The Pathophysiology of Hyperglycemia in Older Adults: Clinical considerations. *Diabetes Care* 2017, 40(4):444–452.
2. Bremer JP, Jauch-Chara K, Hallschmid M, Schmid S, Schultes B: Hypoglycemia Unawareness in Older Compared with Middle-Aged Patients with Type 2 Diabetes. *Diabetes Care* 2009, 32(8):1513–1517.
3. Moorhouse P, Rockwood K: Frailty and Its Quantitative Clinical Evaluation. *J R Coll Physicians Edinb* 2012, 42(4):333–340.
4. Meneilly GS, Berard LD, Cheng AYY, Lin PJ, MacCallum L, Tsuyuki RT, Yale JF, Nasseri N, Richard JF, Goldin L *et al*: Insights Into the Current Management of Older Adults With Type 2 Diabetes in the Ontario Primary Care Setting. *Can J Diabetes* 2018, 42(1):23–30.
5. American Geriatrics Society Beers Criteria Update Expert Panel: American Geriatrics Society 2015 Updated Beers Criteria for Potentially Inappropriate Medication Use in Older Adults. *J Am Geriatr Soc* 2015, 63(11):2227–2246.

25 Hepatobiliary Considerations, Including Cancer

Erica C. Roth, MD, Sunil Karhadkar, MBBS, FACS and Antonio di Carlo, MD, CM, FRCSC, FACS

CONTENTS

CLINICAL VIGNETTE

At age 79, Ms. Smith began experiencing some abdominal pain with different meals. Since the death of her husband, she had been eating less and had lost some weight. Her primary care physician ordered an ultrasonogram of the abdomen. Relevant findings were multiple gallstones and a poorly defined 2 cm cyst in the head of the pancreas. An HPB surgeon saw her in consultation. A CT scan was performed and extensive laboratory tests were completed. The laboratory tests (liver panel, CBC, CA 19.9, amongst others) were deemed unremarkable. The CT scan showed multiple partially calcified gallstones and a 2.3 cm cyst in the head of the pancreas. The rest of the pancreas was relatively atrophic and the pancreatic duct was not dilated. Ms. Smith's history includes diabetes, osteoporosis and CKD 3 (Stage 3 chronic kidney disease). She lives in an assisted living facility and ambulates with a cane and sometimes a walker. On further discussion, when evaluating the required testing and likely benign diagnosis of the pancreatic cyst at this time, it was decided not to pursue the pancreatic lesion. However, Ms. Smith felt that the gallbladder problems were preventing her from eating and that she would prefer an operation. Ms. Smith underwent an uncomplicated laparoscopic cholecystectomy and was observed for 2 days as an inpatient before returning home.

INTRODUCTION

As the life expectancy of the general population continues to increase, physicians are increasingly caring for older patients. With the evolution of perioperative care, minimally invasive techniques and the improved health in older patients, considering an octogenarian for a major HPB operation is

DOI: 10.1201/9781003344476-28

not that unusual. With a multidisciplinary approach, the surgical candidacy of an older patient can be better determined. Equally importantly, the time frame of disease progression can be assessed in comparison to the impact on life expectancy of the individual patient. This requires knowledge of the unique problems that arise with age, as well as the different disease pathologies. Many different hepatobiliary diseases, which encompass diseases of the gallbladder, biliary tract, liver, and pancreas, increase in prevalence with age. Knowledge of these common diseases, including their clinical presentation, work-up and treatment, are essential in caring for older patients. The purpose of this chapter is to recognize different hepatobiliary diseases, understand the nature of each disease and its management, and consider the unique aspects of care within the elderly population.

Immune-Related Changes

There are several physiologic changes that occur within our immune function and hepatobiliary system as we age. Immunity declines with age, increasing the likelihood of sepsis and postoperative infections. This is due to a decrease in skin barrier functions, macrophage presentation of antigens, cell-mediated innate immunity and humoral B cell responses. There are fewer numbers of T and B cells with increasing age and increasingly impaired functions of the cells that are present.

Hepatobiliary Changes

Within the gallbladder, there is an increased propensity for gallstone formation, likely due to changes in bile constitution. There is also a trend for decreased responsiveness of the gallbladder to cholecystokinin (CCK), leading to decreased gallbladder contractility and overall increased hypomobility. Within the liver, the number of hepatocytes decreases with age, accompanied by decreases in hepatic blood flow and overall liver volume. This decrease in liver volume is thought to be associated with a decrease in drug metabolism, likely due to less cytochrome P450. Although liver function tests tend not to change with age, bilirubin levels can occasionally be lower due to less muscle mass and a lower baseline hemoglobin concentration. There are a variety of age-related changes within the pancreas, although not all have clinical significance. There is fatty replacement of acinar parenchyma with aging, but this does not appear to cause pancreatic insufficiency. There are several cell-related changes that may contribute to increased neoplastic changes within the aging pancreas. Replacement of normal non-mucinous, cuboidal ductal cells with mucinous tall columnar epithelial cells has been associated with increased prevalence of pancreatic intra-epithelial neoplasia. The overall accumulation of genetic mutations, telomere shortening and fibrosis all contribute to increasing incidence of pancreatic cancer with age.

GALLBLADDER

Cholelithiasis

The presence of gallstones increases with age due to physiologic changes in the biliary system. The presentation of cholelithiasis can vary from asymptomatic and incidentally found to severe complications. When gallstones are found incidentally with no symptoms, there is no indication for further diagnostic work-up or prophylactic cholecystectomy, except for a few rare circumstances, such as after cardiac transplantation.

Biliary colic refers to pain associated with contraction of the gallbladder against the cystic duct. Patients often present with pain in the epigastrium or right upper quadrant. The pain tends to be severe, constant, with occasional radiation to the back or scapula. Patients usually describe pain developing after meals and at night, which can awaken them from sleep. In elderly patients, presentations tend to be more variable and can include altered mental status and incontinence. Lab work usually does not reveal significant abnormalities. Ultrasound is often the diagnostic imaging modality of choice, with greater than 90% sensitivity for identifying gallstones, which will appear as acoustic shadowing. There are several medical therapies for biliary colic that have been tried for stone dissolution, such as bile acid therapy with ursodeoxycholic acid or extracorporeal shock-wave lithotripsy. These options tend to be reserved for poor surgical candidates. If an elderly patient is deemed to be of acceptable surgical risk, elective cholecystectomy is the treatment of choice for persistent biliary colic given the increased likelihood of developing complications, such as acute cholecystitis and pancreatitis.

Acute Cholecystitis

Acute cholecystitis is the acute inflammation of the gallbladder. This most commonly occurs due to a gallstone becoming lodged in the cystic duct. Patients generally present with epigastric or right upper quadrant pain with tenderness to palpation in that area. Murphy's sign, which is inspiratory arrest during gallbladder palpation, may also be present. Patients may also report fevers, nausea or vomiting. Laboratory markers tend to show mild leukocytosis and abnormal liver function tests. In the elderly, there tends to be a higher variability in presenting symptoms. Some older patients can present without pain or leukocytosis, making the diagnosis more difficult. In addition, the diagnosis of acute cholecystitis may also be confounded by other comorbid conditions, such as peptic ulcer disease. The diagnostic test of choice remains ultrasonography. Ultrasound of acute cholecystitis characteristically shows pericholecystic fluid, gallbladder sludge, distension, gallbladder wall thickness greater than 4 mm, gallstones and a positive Murphy's sign. If the clinical picture remains unclear, computed tomography (CT) and hepatobiliary iminodiacetic acid (HIDA) scan may be useful adjuncts.

In addition to intravenous hydration and antibiotics, the standard treatment of acute cholecystitis is cholecystectomy. Laparoscopic cholecystectomy is generally performed within 72 hours of symptoms. There have been higher rates of perioperative morbidity associated with cholecystectomy in the elderly, thus careful patient selection is key. Elderly patients tend to have more comorbidities and tend to present with more severe forms of cholecystitis compared to younger patients. In addition, there are higher rates of conversion to an open cholecystectomy in older patients, which is associated with an increased risk of complications and longer hospitalization. Amongst patients older than 80 years old, there is an even higher risk of in-hospital mortality as well as greater likelihood of discharge to an institutional care facility rather than to home.

An alternative to cholecystectomy in high-risk patients is percutaneous drainage. Percutaneous cholecystostomy tubes can be used to avoid general anesthesia in patients with severe comorbid conditions or when a patient has become clinically unstable. This procedure is generally performed with sedation or local anesthesia and involves placing a tube directly into the gallbladder under radiographic guidance. Duration of tube placement remains a topic of debate. In general, cholecystostomy tubes are left in place for 3–6 weeks to allow for a tract to form. A contrast tube study is generally performed after several weeks to ensure patency of the cystic duct before tube removal. Delayed interval cholecystectomy remains the treatment of choice in appropriate patients. Approximately half of patients can be managed with percutaneous drainage alone without recurrence, while others have subsequent episodes of acute cholecystitis. In extremely high-risk elderly patients, it may be a definitive treatment rather than a bridge to surgery.

Choledocholithiasis

Choledocholithiasis refers to gallstones within the common bile duct. Presentation may range from asymptomatic to persistent right upper quadrant pain to signs of obstructive jaundice. This includes scleral icterus, dark urine and acholic stools. There is an increased incidence of common bile duct stones in the elderly, thought to be secondary to increased gallstone prevalence. Work-up includes laboratory studies and ultrasonography. Lab work may indicate a cholestatic pattern of liver function tests, with an elevated total bilirubin and alkaline phosphatase, although these are not specific for choledocholithiasis. Imaging may show the presence of a stone within the common bile duct or evidence of common bile duct dilation (>6 mm) without stones. However, common bile duct size tends to be increased in patients over 50 years of age. Thus, a higher cut-off of 8.5 mm among the elderly has been suggested.

Management includes endoscopic retrograde cholangiopancreatography (ERCP), sphincterotomy, intra-operative cholangiography (IOC) and common bile duct exploration. ERCP involves endoscopically clearing stones within the common bile duct. This is often paired with balloon dilation or sphincterotomy, which entails incision through the muscular layers of the sphincter of Oddi to facilitate stone passage. IOC is used during laparoscopic cholecystectomy if common bile duct stones are suspected. IOC involves placement of an angiocatheter directly into the cystic duct and injection of a water-soluble dye. Fluoroscopy is then used to identify potential filling defects within the ducts. Common bile duct exploration, which can be done laparoscopically or open, can be an option to surgically remove stones within the common bile duct, although this tends to be associated with a higher morbidity. If the etiology is gallstones, interval cholecystectomy within two weeks of ERCP is generally recommended to prevent recurrence.

Acute Cholangitis

Acute cholangitis refers to acute bacterial infection of the biliary tract usually secondary to cholestasis. This often occurs due to obstruction of the common bile duct from stones, strictures or tumors, although it can also be caused by interventions involving the biliary tree. Patients often present with right upper quadrant pain, fevers and occasionally septic shock. Charcot's triad refers to the presence of right upper quadrant pain, fever and jaundice; Reynold's pentad adds hypotension and altered mental status. Elderly patients may present with only hypotension or altered mental status and may quickly progress to sepsis and multi-organ dysfunction. Work-up often shows leukocytosis, elevated liver enzymes and elevated bilirubin levels. Ultrasonography may show biliary dilatation, but location will depend on where the obstruction is located. Stones within the gallbladder or common bile duct may or may not be present. Management involves fluid resuscitation, empiric antibiotics and additional supportive measures, including ICU management in severe cases. Biliary drainage mostly via ERCP, should occur promptly to relieve the obstruction and provide source control. Older patients have a similar rate of complications, about 6–7%, from emergent ERCP compared to younger patients. Complications include pancreatitis, bleeding, duct perforation, worsening cholangitis and recurrence. If ERCP is unsuccessful, additional treatment options include percutaneous transhepatic biliary drainage (PTBD) and common bile duct exploration as a last resort.

Gallbladder Cancer

Gallbladder cancer is a rare but aggressive malignancy that tends to occur in older patients. Although some cases are found incidentally in an early stage, most are discovered in advanced stages. Incidental gallbladder cancer is often found during cholecystectomy for gallstone disease. When patients present with symptomatic gallbladder carcinoma, they often present with weight loss, biliary colic symptoms, jaundice or vague abdominal pain. Lab work may show elevated CA 19–9 or carcinoembryonic antigen (CEA). Ultrasonography may show a mass within the gallbladder, irregular gallbladder wall thickening, biliary obstruction and possible involvement of adjacent structures. If gallbladder cancer is suspected, a staging CT scan may be performed to reveal distant or peritoneal metastases, lymphadenopathy, vascular involvement, and assist in preoperative planning. For very early-stage cancer, simple cholecystectomy is sufficient. However, as most gallbladder carcinomas are discovered later, radical resection with negative margins becomes the treatment of choice. This extended cholecystectomy involves an en bloc resection of the gallbladder, partial hepatectomy, portal lymphadenectomy of more than six lymph nodes, and potential bile duct resection. Age is not a contraindication to radical resection as it has been shown to prolong survival in the elderly. If surgical resection does not appear feasible, patients should be considered for neoadjuvant chemotherapy.

LIVER

Benign Liver Lesions

There are a wide variety of benign liver lesions that can be seen in older patients. These most often are found incidentally as most patients are asymptomatic. The most important consideration for these lesions is the ability to distinguish them from primary malignancies and metastases. The most common benign liver lesions include hepatic adenomas, focal nodular hyperplasia, cysts, hemangiomas and biliary cystadenomas. Hepatic adenomas and focal nodular hyperplasia tend to be diagnosed in younger patients, while cysts, hemangiomas and cystadenomas are more likely to be encountered in older patients.

Cysts

Hepatic cysts are common and range from simple to complex. Benign liver cysts are the most common liver pathology and can be seen in up to 20% of patients. Most of these are asymptomatic in presentation and do not require any further intervention. They are often found incidentally when patients are undergoing imaging for other reasons. They tend to contain serous fluid and are spherical in nature. Most liver cysts do not communicate with the biliary system. Ultrasonography is usually the first line diagnostic modality and shows a well-circumscribed lesion with a thin wall and simple homogenous fluid inside. If there are other signs of a more complex cyst, such as nodules, enhancing wall or solid components, CT or magnetic resonance imaging (MRI) may be indicated. If the patient is asymptomatic, no further interventions are required if the lesion is still deemed to be benign. Symptomatic patients may present with vague abdominal pain, fullness or early satiety. One treatment option involves aspiration with sclerotherapy to destroy the cyst lining, but this approach is associated with high recurrence. This approach is preferred for high-risk operative patients. The standard of care is now laparoscopic cyst fenestration, which involves excising and de-roofing the extrahepatic cyst wall and ablation of the intrahepatic portion in appropriately selected patients. This is routinely performed as ambulatory surgery.

Hemangiomas

Hemangiomas are benign liver tumors comprising blood-filled cavities. They tend to present in ages 30–50 years old and more often in females. Most patients are asymptomatic, and these are found incidentally on imaging. Larger lesions are associated with increased symptomatology including vague abdominal pain, early satiety, nausea, vomiting and bloating. Very large hepatic hemangiomas could present with obstructive symptoms, spontaneous rupture and rarely thrombocytopenia (Kasabach-Merritt syndrome). Diagnostic imaging often begins with ultrasound. Ultrasound will show a homogenous, hyperechoic nodule with well-defined borders and posterior acoustic enhancement. On contrast CT, a hemangioma appears as a well-defined, hypodense lesion with peripheral nodular enhancement on arterial phase and progressive centripetal homogenous filling on portal venous phase. If ultrasonography or CT are inconclusive, MRI or tagged red blood cell scintigraphy scans may also be used. Biopsy of suspected hemangiomas is contraindicated given the bleeding risk and low likelihood of obtaining adequate tissue. For asymptomatic patients, no surgical intervention is indicated. In symptomatic patients, surgical management includes enucleation and both anatomic and nonanatomic resections. These can be performed laparoscopically or open, with the approach varying based on size and location of the hemangioma as well as surgeon preference. Intra-arterial embolization and external beam radiation may also be considerations, especially in a symptomatic patient with concerns for an operation.

Biliary Cystadenoma

Biliary cystadenoma is a premalignant liver cystic lesion that can occur both in intrahepatic and extrahepatic portions of the biliary tree. Approximately 20% will progress to malignant biliary cystadenocarcinoma. Patients tend to be asymptomatic, but some will present with vague abdominal symptoms. On ultrasound, biliary cystadenoma appears anechoic with highly echogenic internal septations. CT scan shows a well-circumscribed thick-walled cyst with internal septations. Formal surgical resection is the treatment of choice given the malignant potential and high recurrence with alternative methods, even in asymptomatic patients.

Cholangiocarcinoma

Cholangiocarcinoma refers to cancers arising from the biliary tract and are the second most common cause of liver cancer after hepatocellular carcinoma. They tend to present in the sixth and seventh decade of life and are associated with hepatitis B and C, parasite infections, inflammatory bowel disease, primary sclerosing cholangitis and choledochal cysts. There are three major categories based on anatomic location. Intrahepatic cholangiocarcinoma refers to a cancer located within the liver parenchyma. Hilar cholangiocarcinoma is between the extrahepatic biliary tree to cystic duct, while distal cholangiocarcinoma refers to the ductal area from the cystic duct to the ampulla of Vater.

Intrahepatic Cholangiocarcinoma

Patients may be asymptomatic or may present with weight loss, abdominal pain, poor appetite, jaundice and fatigue. Labs often show elevated liver enzymes with elevated direct bilirubin and alkaline phosphatase. On imaging, intrahepatic cholangiocarcinomas tend to show a homogenous hypodense mass with irregular borders and biliary duct dilation. On contrast-enhanced CT, they tend to show irregular peripheral enhancement on late arterial phases and central hyperenhancement on delayed phases. Biopsy is not always required. Prior to resection, liver function and volumes should be checked. Preoperative functioning should be assessed in the elderly population as well, as surgical resection is associated with high morbidity and mortality. Few of these tumors tend to be amenable to surgical resection given the technical location of resection and need for negative margins. Survival has been associated with the ability to achieve a negative margin resection. Surgical resection of these tumors is associated with increased severe postoperative complications in the elderly. Despite increased perioperative mortality, older patients can still benefit from long-term outcomes after resection compared to younger patients. For patients with unresectable disease, chemotherapy, stereotactic body radiotherapy, transarterial chemoembolization (TACE), and liver transplantation are additional options.

Hilar Cholangiocarcinoma

Hilar cholangiocarcinoma tends to grow along the bile duct, resulting in strictured or dilated ducts, usually without formation of a mass. Patients often present with jaundice and pruritus, but may also have weight loss, abdominal pain and fatigue. Lab work-up should include liver function tests and tumor markers. Imaging often shows bile duct wall thickening with enhancement, irregular margins and asymmetric narrowing or dilation of the intrahepatic bile ducts. For patients with obstructive jaundice, preoperative biliary drainage is indicated. Surgical resection and biliary reconstruction are technically difficult and are associated with high morbidity. Thus, surgery may only be offered to healthy older patients with few comorbidities. Chemotherapy and radiation may also be used as adjuvant or palliative treatments. In carefully defined cases, liver transplantation may be an option. However, these are not very common and age restrictions are likely to apply depending on the transplant hospital.

Distal Cholangiocarcinoma

Distal cholangiocarcinomas tend to present with painless jaundice, weight loss, abdominal pain and fatigue. Labs tend to show a very elevated bilirubin and elevated liver enzymes. Imaging tends to show biliary ductal dilation in both the intrahepatic and extrahepatic ducts. These tumors can be small and difficult to see on imaging. ERCP may be useful to obtain a tissue sample and better characterize the bile duct pathology. The main treatment is surgical resection with a pancreaticoduodenectomy; however, chemotherapy and radiation may be offered if the disease is deemed unresectable or the patient prohibitive.

Hepatocellular Carcinoma

Hepatocellular carcinoma (HCC) is the most common malignant liver tumor. Approximately 80% of cases arise from a cirrhotic liver, while approximately 20% occur in non-cirrhotic livers. Major risk factors include underlying liver disease, such as chronic hepatitis B and C, alcoholic liver disease, and non-alcoholic fatty liver disease. There are also genetic diseases that increase risk, such as alpha-1 antitrypsin deficiency and hemochromatosis. Most patients are asymptomatic, but some may present with vague right upper quadrant pain, fatigue and weight loss. Lab work-up should include alpha-fetoprotein, which is usually elevated. Imaging via contrast-enhanced CT scan or MRI generally shows hyperenhancement on the arterial phase with washout and subsequently hypoenhancement on the venous phase. Biopsy is generally not indicated as imaging is able to accurately diagnosis HCC in most circumstances.

Treatment of HCC includes ablation, TACE, resection and liver transplantation. Radiofrequency ablation (RFA) is a potential treatment for patients who are not able to tolerate a liver resection or transplant. The heat directly at the tumor leads to necrosis and is particularly effective with small tumors less than 4 cm. TACE is another option for poor surgical candidates. It involves injection of chemotherapy followed by embolization beads to occlude the tumor blood supply. This has been shown to improve survival and progression-free survival in advanced HCC cases among elderly patients without serious adverse events. Surgical resection of HCC is indicated in the appropriately selected patient and is the primary curative treatment. Factors to consider include liver function, position of tumor that would allow for enough future liver remnant and ability to achieve negative resection margins. Recurrence rates can be high, especially in cirrhotic patients. Several poor prognostic indicators include lymphovascular invasion, size greater than 5 cm, multiple tumors and capsular absence. Large resections for HCC are not contraindicated in elderly patients if they have well-controlled health conditions otherwise. Older patients do tend to have a longer postoperative recovery and may be at higher risk of both cardiac and pulmonary postoperative complications. In select cases, when tumors are not amenable to resection, liver transplantation may be considered. The options are transplantation from living or deceased donors. Again, older patients may face age restrictions and more difficulty in finding a potential living donor.

PANCREAS

Pancreatitis

Acute pancreatitis is characterized by acute inflammation of the pancreas secondary to several different causes. These include cholelithiasis, post-ERCP, alcohol, medications, and hyperlipidemia. The prevalence of acute pancreatitis has been steadily increasing in the elderly population, thought to be partly due to increased prevalence of cholelithiasis. Patients may present with acute abdominal pain of variable intensity. Among older patients, symptoms may be non-specific and can overlap with symptoms of other intra-abdominal pathology, such as peptic ulcer disease, gallstone disease or mesenteric ischemia. Older patients also tend to present later and with more severe forms of pancreatitis. A diagnosis of acute pancreatitis is made based on two of the following three criteria: 1) acute abdominal pain, 2) an increase in blood amylase or lipase of threefold and 3) imaging characteristic of pancreatitis. Imaging may show inflammation surrounding the pancreas, peripancreatic fluid collections, necrosis, infarction and vascular abnormalities. Treatment involves fluid resuscitation, early introduction of enteral intake as tolerated and adequate pain control. For pancreatitis caused by gallstone disease, ERCP is indicated within 72 hours. Antibiotics are indicated when there is concern for infected pancreatic necrosis but are not indicated prophylactically. A step-up approach is the standard of care for pancreatic necrosis, beginning with percutaneous drainage, followed by surgical drainage and necrosectomy (debridement of necrotic tissue) if failure with less invasive approaches.

Complications of pancreatitis include abscesses, pseudocysts, pseudoaneurysms, necrosis, ascites and abdominal compartment syndrome. Older patients tend to have more systemic complications, such as pleural effusions, acute respiratory distress syndrome (ARDS), renal failure, vascular complications and multi-organ failure. Older patients tend to have longer hospital length of stay and progression of the disease compared to younger patients. They tend to suffer from more severe forms of the disease and have a higher mortality, especially in patients over 80 years of age. This can be attributed to medical comorbidities, less physiologic reserve and more severe complications.

Pancreatic Cancer

Pancreatic cancer is an aggressive cancer associated with poor outcomes. It is often diagnosed in older patients, with a median age of diagnosis of 70 years. Patients may present with a variety of symptoms, which vary based on tumor location and size. These include epigastric pain with radiation to the back, jaundice and pruritus from biliary obstruction, nausea and vomiting from duodenal obstruction, and ascites from carcinomatosis. Unfortunately, most patients present with cancers that are inoperable or metastatic. Work-up includes basic lab work and CT imaging. Imaging helps reveal the tumor location, vascular involvement, biliary obstruction and ascites. Initial management may involve mediating presenting symptoms, such as ERCP with stent placement for obstructive jaundice.

Treatment is surgical resection, which is the only curative option, for appropriately selected patients with resectable disease. The type of resection depends on location of the tumor. Tumors in the pancreatic head are resected via pancreaticoduodenectomy (Whipple procedure), while pancreatic tail tumors are resected via partial distal pancreatectomy. Older patients overall are less likely to be offered an operation. Pancreatic surgery is associated with high morbidity and mortality, with almost half of patients experiencing perioperative complications, such as fistula, bile leak, infection and pancreatitis. Age alone is not a contraindication to surgery, but medical comorbidities play an important role in consideration for surgery.

For older patients presenting with metastatic or inoperable disease at presentation, palliative chemotherapy may be an option. Older patients are overall less likely to receive chemotherapy compared to younger patients. The determination of chemotherapy treatment for older patients is difficult, in part because older patients were excluded from most chemotherapy clinical trials. Previously the standard of care was single agent gemcitabine, which has been demonstrated to be safe and mostly tolerated in older patients. More recently, FOLFIRINOX (5-fluorouracil, leucovorin, irinotecan, oxaliplatin) has showed increased median overall survival, but at the expense of more adverse side effects. It is generally not recommended for older patients with numerous comorbidities or poor baseline performance status.

Intraductal Papillary Mucinous Neoplasms of Pancreas

Intraductal mucinous neoplasms of the pancreas (IPMNs) are the most common cystic neoplasm of the pancreas. They are further classified into three groups based on histologic features and anatomy: main duct IPMN, branch duct IPMN and mixed-type IPMN. Main duct IPMN is characterized by dilation, segmental or diffuse, of the main pancreatic duct by 5 mm and has the highest association with malignancy compared to the other two types. Almost half of patients present with symptoms. Branch duct IPMN is characterized by a cystic lesion that is over 5 mm and in direct communication with the main pancreatic duct. This has a lower association of malignancy and is more common than the other two types. Mixed-type IPMN is characterized by a multiloculated cystic lesion involving both the dilated main pancreatic duct and its branches.

Most patients are asymptomatic on presentation. Symptomatic patients tend to present most commonly with abdominal pain, but may also have weight loss, jaundice or pancreatitis. Although most lesions are found incidentally on imaging, the best diagnostic modality is CT or MRI abdomen and pelvis with pancreas protocol. Having proper imaging is key in differentiating benign cystic pathology from IPMNs, as well as identifying suspicious features that suggest malignancy. Suspicious imaging features include mural nodules, cyst size over 3 cm, main pancreatic duct size of 5–9 mm, thick cyst walls with enhancement and presence of lymphadenopathy. Given that IPMNs are premalignant lesions, it is critical to weigh options of surveillance vs early resection based on malignancy risk and patient surgical risk. Endoscopic ultrasound (EUS) can be a useful adjunct in risk stratification and biopsy, especially in branch duct IPMNs. EUS with fine needle aspiration (FNA) can be used to sample cyst fluid and help characterize IPMNs from other cystic lesions.

Guidance for the surveillance of IPMN lesions without high risk or worrisome features is provided by the Fukuoka guidelines and the AGA (American Gastroenterological Association). However, in older patients an assessment of surgical candidacy and life expectancy may serve to determine the benefit of continued surveillance. For example, with branch duct IPMN, the annual rate of progression to malignancy is less than 7%. Continued annual surveillance in an 85-year-old patient may have limited value.

Surgery is generally indicated for all IPMNs when obstructive jaundice, mural nodules or main pancreatic duct dilation over 10 mm is present in appropriate surgical candidates. The location of the IPMN will determine the type of pancreatic resection, which can vary from Whipple resection, total pancreatectomy, central pancreatectomy, to distal pancreatectomy. Older patients should be carefully considered, based on functional status and comorbidities, to determine if they would be able to tolerate a large pancreatic surgery.

PERIOPERATIVE CARE

Older patients require specialized care in the perioperative period. In addition to optimizing comorbidities preoperatively, care extends to the increased likelihood of postoperative complications and potential loss of functional independence. Best practices guidelines identify nine areas of assessment, which include cognitive and behavioral disorders, cardiac evaluation, pulmonary evaluation, functional status, frailty index, nutritional status, medication management, patient counseling and preoperative testing.

Preoperative Care

There are several areas of preoperative care that are particularly important in caring for older patients. Polypharmacy can lead to medication interactions and potentially adverse drug events. Review of essential medications and discontinuation of nonessential medications is key. It is important to consider potential withdrawal and whether the patient is not able to take medications by mouth for several days if undergoing major abdominal surgery. Malnutrition is more common in older patients. If an older patient is considered malnourished prior to surgery, additional supplements should be started given the higher risk of adverse outcomes postoperatively associated with malnutrition. Supplements and close nutritional monitoring can be continued in the postoperative setting. Mobility should also be assessed. Patients with poor mobility should be considered for mobility training or physical therapy prior to major surgery due to increased fall risk postoperatively. Patients' values and quality of life should be discussed preoperatively as well given that many hepatobiliary surgeries are considered high risk. Discussion of possible functional outcomes, loss of independence, long-term symptoms and survival is important before proceeding with surgery.

Frailty Index

Frailty is a syndrome characterized by decreased physiologic reserve and functional status. It has generally been associated with the elderly population, although it can be used to describe younger patients with chronic illnesses. It has been used to assess a patient's preoperative risk, but also has been used as a prognostic indicator for worse postoperative outcomes. Patients who screen positive for frailty tend to have higher rates of postoperative mortality, pneumonia, pulmonary embolism, myocardial infarction, sepsis, hospital readmission, length of stay, higher likelihood of discharge to a facility and higher cost of care. Numerous frailty scores exist. An 11-point modified frailty index (mFI) has been used to identify patients at risk for postoperative complications and mortality. This includes comorbid conditions such as diabetes, chronic obstructive pulmonary disease (COPD), congestive heart failure (CHF), peripheral vascular disease, stroke, hypertension, as well as functional status. For patients with a positive frailty screen prior to elective surgery, preoperative participation in a rehabilitation program has been shown to decrease negative postoperative outcomes.

Postoperative Care

Postoperative care for older patients should include the management of standard postoperative problems, such as pain control, but also focus on problems specific to older patients. Delirium is a common postoperative complication and can be managed by good sleep hygiene tactics, minimizing certain psychoactive medications, and encouraging frequent redirection. Older patients are at higher risk of pulmonary complications, especially after major surgery, due to pain control and aspiration risk. Encouragement of early ambulation when appropriate and incentive spirometer use, as well as adequate pain analgesia, are useful prevention strategies. Fall risk assessment should be performed and universal fall precautions applied if indicated. Older patients who have undergone major hepatobiliary surgery have been shown to have higher rates of postoperative delirium, pneumonia, and 90-day mortality compared to younger patients, although these differences were negligible after propensity score matching. Among postoperative liver resections, patients who were considered frail based on a frailty index score did have increased risk of morbidity and mortality postoperatively. Another aspect of good postoperative care is providing written detailed instructions for discharge. This includes medication changes, clear follow-up with surgeons and primary care doctors, and any relevant labs or imaging.

CONCLUSION

As patients continue to live longer, doctors will increasingly encounter a wide range of hepatobiliary diseases in older patients. It is important to be familiar with the diagnosis and pathophysiology of common hepatobiliary diseases, as well as understand the next steps in work-up and management. Hepatobiliary surgery can be associated with high morbidity and mortality among older patients. Thus, optimization of medical comorbidities and perioperative care is paramount. Multidisciplinary discussions between primary care doctors, medical subspecialists, hepatobiliary surgeons and patients are key to providing individualized patient-centered care.

SUGGESTED ADDITIONAL READINGS

1. Kahng KU, Roslyn JJ. Surgical issues for the elderly patient with hepatobiliary disease. Surg Clin North Am. 1994 Apr;74(2):345–373. PMID: 8165472.
2. Chhoda A, Mukewar SS, Mahadev S. Managing gallstone disease in the elderly. Clin Geriatr Med. 2021 Feb;37(1):43–69. doi: 10.1016/j.cger.2020.08.005. Epub 2020 Oct 29. PMID: 33213774.
3. Tajiri K, Shimizu Y. Liver physiology and liver diseases in the elderly. World J Gastroenterol. 2013 Dec 14;19(46):8459–8467. doi: 10.3748/wjg.v19.i46.8459. PMID: 24379563; PMCID: PMC3870491.
4. Matsuda Y. Age-related morphological changes in the pancreas and their association with pancreatic carcinogenesis. Pathol Int. 2019 Aug;69(8):450–462. doi: 10.1111/pin.12837. Epub 2019 Jul 24. PMID: 31339204.
5. Cobden I, Lendrum R, Venables CW, James OF. Gallstones presenting as mental and physical debility in the elderly. Lancet. 1984 May 12;1(8385):1062–1064. doi: 10.1016/s0140-6736(84)91462-4. PMID: 6143985.
6. Trowbridge RL, Rutkowski NK, Shojania KG. Does this patient have acute cholecystitis? JAMA. 2003 Jan 1;289(1):80–6. doi: 10.1001/jama.289.1.80. Erratum in: JAMA. 2009 Aug 19;302(7):739. PMID: 12503981.
7. Shea JA, Berlin JA, Escarce JJ, Clarke JR, Kinosian BP, Cabana MD, Tsai WW, Horangic N, Malet PF, Schwartz JS, et al. Revised estimates of diagnostic test sensitivity and specificity in suspected biliary tract disease. Arch Intern Med. 1994 Nov 28;154(22):2573–2581. PMID: 7979854.
8. Gurusamy KS, Samraj K, Fusai G, Davidson BR. Early versus delayed laparoscopic cholecystectomy for biliary colic. Cochrane Database Syst Rev. 2008 Oct 8;(4):CD007196. doi: 10.1002/14651858.CD007196.pub2. Update in: Cochrane Database Syst Rev. 2013;6:CD007196. PMID: 18843746.
9. Parker LJ, Vukov LF, Wollan PC. Emergency department evaluation of geriatric patients with acute cholecystitis. Acad Emerg Med. 1997 Jan;4(1):51–5. doi: 10.1111/j.1553-2712.1997.tb03643.x. PMID: 9110012.
10. Loozen CS, van Ramshorst B, van Santvoort HC, Boerma D. Early cholecystectomy for acute cholecystitis in the elderly population: a systematic review and meta-analysis. Dig Surg. 2017;34(5):371–379. doi: 10.1159/000455241. Epub 2017 Jan 18. PMID: 28095385.
11. Ambe PC, Weber SA, Christ H, Wassenberg D. Primary cholecystectomy is feasible in elderly patients with acute cholecystitis. Aging Clin Exp Res. 2015 Dec;27(6):921–936. doi: 10.1007/s40520-015-0361-0. Epub 2015 Apr 24. PMID: 25905472.

12. Kuy S, Sosa JA, Roman SA, Desai R, Rosenthal RA. Age matters: a study of clinical and economic outcomes following cholecystectomy in elderly Americans. Am J Surg. 2011 Jun;201(6):789–796. doi: 10.1016/j.amjsurg.2010.04.018. PMID: 21741511.

13. Zarour S, Imam A, Kouniavsky G, Lin G, Zbar A, Mavor E. Percutaneous cholecystostomy in the management of high-risk patients presenting with acute cholecystitis: Timing and outcome at a single institution. Am J Surg. 2017 Sep;214(3):456–461. doi: 10.1016/j.amjsurg.2017.01.030. Epub 2017 Feb 14. PMID: 28237047.

14. Bachar GN, Cohen M, Belenky A, Atar E, Gideon S. Effect of aging on the adult extrahepatic bile duct: a sonographic study. J Ultrasound Med. 2003 Sep;22(9):879–82; quiz 883–5. doi: 10.7863/jum.2003.22.9.879. PMID: 14510259.

15. Tohda G, Ohtani M, Dochin M. Efficacy and safety of emergency endoscopic retrograde cholangiopancreatography for acute cholangitis in the elderly. World J Gastroenterol. 2016 Oct 7;22(37):8382–8388. doi: 10.3748/wjg.v22.i37.8382. PMID: 27729744; PMCID: PMC5055868.

16. Chen C, Geng Z, Shen H, Song H, Zhao Y, Zhang G, Li W, Ma L, Wang L. Long-term outcomes and prognostic factors in advanced gallbladder cancer: Focus on the advanced T stage. PLoS One. 2016 Nov 15;11(11):e0166361. doi: 10.1371/journal.pone.0166361. PMID: 27846279; PMCID: PMC5112857.

17. Onoyama H, Ajiki T, Takada M, Urakawa T, Saitoh Y. Does radical resection improve the survival in patients with carcinoma of the gallbladder who are 75 years old and older? World J Surg. 2002 Nov;26(11):1315–1358. doi: 10.1007/s00268-002-6163-5. Epub 2002 Sep 26. PMID: 12297924.

18. Pitchaimuthu M, Duxbury M. Cystic lesions of the liver-A review. Curr Probl Surg. 2017 Oct;54(10):514–542. doi: 10.1067/j.cpsurg.2017.09.001. Epub 2017 Sep 28. PMID: 29173653.

19. Bajenaru N, Balaban V, Săvulescu F, Campeanu I, Patrascu T. Hepatic hemangioma -review. J Med Life. 2015;8(Spec Issue):4–11. PMID: 26361504; PMCID: PMC4564031.

20. Newhook TE, LaPar DJ, Lindberg JM, Bauer TW, Adams RB, Zaydfudim VM. Morbidity and mortality of hepatectomy for benign liver tumors. Am J Surg. 2016 Jan;211(1):102–108. doi: 10.1016/j.amjsurg.2015.06.010. Epub 2015 Jul 31. PMID: 26307421.

21. Lee DH, Lee JM. Primary malignant tumours in the non-cirrhotic liver. Eur J Radiol. 2017 Oct;95:349–361. doi: 10.1016/j.ejrad.2017.08.030. Epub 2017 Aug 31. PMID: 28987692.

22. Vitale A, Spolverato G, Bagante F, Gani F, Popescu I, Marques HP, Aldrighetti L, Gamblin TC, Maithel SK, Sandroussi C, Bauer TW, Shen F, Poultsides GA, Marsh JW, Pawlik TM. A multi-institutional analysis of elderly patients undergoing a liver resection for intrahepatic cholangiocarcinoma. J Surg Oncol. 2016 Mar;113(4):420–426. doi: 10.1002/jso.24148. Epub 2016 Jan 12. PMID: 27100027.

23. DeOliveira ML, Cunningham SC, Cameron JL, Kamangar F, Winter JM, Lillemoe KD, Choti MA, Yeo CJ, Schulick RD. Cholangiocarcinoma: thirty-one-year experience with 564 patients at a single institution. Ann Surg. 2007 May;245(5):755–762. doi: 10.1097/01.sla.0000251366.62632.d3. PMID: 17457168; PMCID: PMC1877058.

24. Orcutt ST, Anaya DA. Liver resection and surgical strategies for management of primary liver cancer. Cancer Control. 2018 Jan-Mar;25(1):1073274817744621. doi: 10.1177/1073274817744621. PMID: 29327594; PMCID: PMC5933574.

25. Tang Q, Huang W, Liang J, Xue J. Efficacy and safety of transarterial chemoembolization in elderly patients of advanced hepatocellular carcinoma with portal vein tumor thrombus: a retrospective study. Front Oncol. 2021 Jul 7;11:646410. doi: 10.3389/fonc.2021.646410. PMID: 34307128; PMCID: PMC8293292.

26. Wu FH, Shen CH, Luo SC, Hwang JI, Chao WS, Yeh HZ, Jan YG, Yen Y, Cheng SB, Wu CC, Lin YL, P'eng FK. Liver resection for hepatocellular carcinoma in oldest old patients. World J Surg Oncol. 2019 Jan 3;17(1):1. doi: 10.1186/s12957-018-1541-0. PMID: 30606220; PMCID: PMC6317186.

27. Koziel D, Gluszek-Osuch M, Suliga E, Zak M, Gluszek S. Elderly persons with acute pancreatitis—specifics of the clinical course of the disease. Clin Interv Aging. 2018 Dec 21;14:33–41. doi: 10.2147/CIA.S188520. PMID: 30613137; PMCID: PMC6306050.

28. Kayar Y, Dertli R, Konur S. Clinical outcomes of acute pancreatitis in elderly patients: An experience of single tertiary center. Pancreatology. 2020 Oct;20(7):1296–1301. doi: 10.1016/j.pan.2020.06.006. Epub 2020 Jun 19. PMID: 32900631.

29. He F, Zhu HM, Li BY, Li XC, Yang S, Wang Z, Zhang M. Factors predicting the severity of acute pancreatitis in elderly patients. Aging Clin Exp Res. 2021 Jan;33(1):183–192. doi: 10.1007/s40520-020-01523-1. Epub 2020 Mar 17. PMID: 32185694.

30. Corrigan LR, Bracken-Clarke DM, Horgan AM. The challenge of treating older patients with pancreaticobiliary malignancies. Curr Probl Cancer. 2018 Jan-Feb;42(1):59–72. doi: 10.1016/j.currproblcancer.2018.01.015. Epub 2018 Jan 31. PMID: 29459178.

31. Jung HA, Han BR, Kim HY, Kim HJ, Zang DY, Jung JY. Treatment and Outcomes of Metastatic Pancreatic Cancer in Elderly Patients. Chemotherapy. 2021;66(4):107–112. doi: 10.1159/000517245. Epub 2021 Aug 4. PMID: 34350854; PMCID: PMC8619775.

32. Hoshi H, Zaheer A, El Abiad RG, Maxwell JE, Chu LC, Gerke H, Chan CH. Management of pancreatic intraductal papillary mucinous neoplasm. Curr Probl Surg. 2018 Apr;55(4):126–152. doi: 10.1067/j.cpsurg.2018.03.001. Epub 2018 Mar 14. PMID: 29753366.

33. Tanaka M, Fernández-Del Castillo C, Kamisawa T, Jang JY, Levy P, Ohtsuka T, Salvia R, Shimizu Y, Tada M, Wolfgang CL. Revisions of international consensus Fukuoka guidelines for the management of IPMN of the pancreas. Pancreatology. 2017 Sep-Oct;17(5):738–753. doi: 10.1016/j.pan.2017.07.007. Epub 2017 Jul 13. PMID: 28735806.

34. Hirono S, Yamaue H. Surgical strategy for intraductal papillary mucinous neoplasms of the pancreas. Surg Today. 2020 Jan;50(1):50–55. doi: 10.1007/s00595-019-01931-5. Epub 2019 Dec 5. PMID: 31807871; PMCID: PMC6923258.

35. Mohanty S, Rosenthal RA, Russell MM, Neuman MD, Ko CY, Esnaola NF. Optimal perioperative management of the geriatric patient: a best practices guideline from the American college of surgeons NSQIP and the American Geriatrics Society. J Am Coll Surg. 2016 May;222(5):930–947. doi: 10.1016/j.jamcollsurg.2015.12.026. Epub 2016 Jan 4. PMID: 27049783.

36. Velanovich V, Antoine H, Swartz A, Peters D, Rubinfeld I. Accumulating deficits model of frailty and postoperative mortality and morbidity: its application to a national database. J Surg Res. 2013 Jul;183(1):104–110. doi: 10.1016/j.jss.2013.01.021. Epub 2013 Feb 1. PMID: 23415494.

37. Panayi AC, Orkaby AR, Sakthivel D, Endo Y, Varon D, Roh D, Orgill DP, Neppl RL, Javedan H, Bhasin S, Sinha I. Impact of frailty on outcomes in surgical patients: A systematic review and meta-analysis. Am J Surg. 2019 Aug;218(2):393–400. doi: 10.1016/j.amjsurg.2018.11.020. Epub 2018 Nov 27. PMID: 30509455; PMCID: PMC6536365.

38. Gani F, Cerullo M, Amini N, Buettner S, Margonis GA, Sasaki K, Kim Y, Pawlik TM. Frailty as a risk predictor of morbidity and mortality following liver surgery. J Gastrointest Surg. 2017 May;21(5):822–830. doi: 10.1007/s11605-017-3373-6. Epub 2017 Mar 6. PMID: 28265844.

39. Takagi K, Umeda Y, Yoshida R, Nobuoka D, Kuise T, Fushimi T, Fujiwara T, Yagi T. The outcome of complex hepato-pancreato-biliary surgery for elderly patients: a propensity score matching analysis. Dig Surg. 2019;36(4):323–330. doi: 10.1159/000489826. Epub 2018 Jun 26. PMID: 29945139; PMCID: PMC6604258.

26 Abdominal Organ Transplantation in the Older Person

Antonio di Carlo, MD, CM, FRCSC, FACS and Sunil Karhadkar, MBBS, FACS

CONTENTS

CLINICAL VIGNETTE

At age 78 Mr. Smith initiated hemodialysis and was referred for kidney transplant evaluation. His kidney disease was attributed to chronic non-steroidal analgesic use. Mr. Smith remained active, and his only comorbidity was hypertension. He lived with his wife of 50 years and had good support from his children and friends. He underwent standard peri-operative testing including a cardiac stress test (negative for ischemia), trans-thoracic echocardiogram and CT of the abdomen and pelvis which other than kidney cysts showed mild calcifications of the distal aorta and bilateral iliac arteries. He was deemed to be a suitable candidate and placed on the deceased donor waitlist for a kidney transplant. He was encouraged to find a potential living donor, but Mr. Smith felt that at his age he did not want a living donor. Four years later, at age 82, a potential deceased-donor kidney became available. The deceased donor was a 67-year-old male who died of isolated head trauma. The donor did not have diabetes or hypertension but had an elevated terminal serum creatinine. Mr. Smith underwent a successful kidney transplant and was discharged to outpatient follow-up with an improving serum creatinine on post-operative day 5.

INTRODUCTION

In North America there are no unified criteria or guidelines for transplanting older patients for any organ. Literature discusses "older patients" starting at 65 but most centers would consider 70 as genuinely older and potentially an upper limit for consideration for most organs. Nonetheless, while certain centers will not consider evaluating a 70-year-old for a kidney transplant, others have performed lung transplants on 70-year-olds. Of all the potential abdominal organs that can be transplanted, the kidney is the one that older patients need most. There have been anecdotal reports of kidney transplantation in octogenarians, with the oldest patient in personal experience being 85 years old. Pancreas and intestinal transplantation is usually limited to recipients younger than 60 to 65 and liver transplantation to those below 70 years.

When being considered for an organ transplant, older patients frequently encounter discrimination and selection bias. Organ transplantation for end-stage disease is limited by a global shortage of organs in the face of rising demand leading to a long waitlist to receive life-saving therapy. Hence, allocation of scarce organs to older recipients raises ethical questions that arouse significant debate. As donor organs are a societal gift, when allocating an organ the impact on recipient longevity must be considered. Certain countries like Israel have made strict age cutoffs. Other countries have implemented older organs for older patients. A general consideration is making the most usage of a donor organ and trying to decrease "death with functioning graft". However, there is more than just the age of a recipient that determines how long a transplant will last and how much benefit it can provide. Sometimes, age is just a number.

Another bias and at times pressure that older patients may face is only being considered if they can find a living donor. Kidney transplantation from living donation is a well-established modality and living donor liver transplantation is proliferating. The rationale for this bias and pressure

DOI: 10.1201/9781003344476-29

is that living donors do not deny somebody else the opportunity of receiving a deceased donor transplant. From a more practical perspective, a living donor will significantly shorten the wait time for a transplant and allow the transplant to happen when the recipient is "healthier". Waiting times for deceased donor kidneys can range from 2 to 9 years and the allocation of deceased donor livers is based on who is the sickest and least likely to survive without a transplant.

Kidney Transplantation

In comparison to staying on dialysis, there is compelling data to suggest that the life expectancy of an older patient is better with a transplant. This increase in life expectancy is observed even with organs from older donors and organs from what were called extended criteria donors. The challenge is in the proper selection of candidates beyond any defining age.

Candidate Evaluation

The evaluation process for an organ transplant is quite rigorous and thorough. The spheres that are assessed include: will the patient benefit from a transplant, will the patient survive the operation and will the patient be able to take care of the organ?

WILL THE PATIENT BENEFIT FROM A TRANSPLANT?

The goals of abdominal organ transplantation include increasing longevity and improving quality of life. In the older patient this is especially relevant. The recovery after an organ transplant is 3 to 6 months. In an older patient, the goal would be to get at least 5 years of life post transplantation. The expected longevity of a deceased donor kidney transplant is at least 10 years for the general population. Hence, when evaluating an older patient, the prediction of life expectancy needs to account for not only the impact of end-organ disease but also all other comorbidities. The older patient with end-stage kidney disease is likely to have diabetes, hypertension, coronary artery disease and peripheral atherosclerosis. Moreover, the calculation of life expectancy needs to include the prediction of wait time until an organ becomes available. With a 5 year wait until transplant and aiming for 5 years of post-transplant survival, the question becomes: will this older patient survive 10 years independently of their disease? This is where the age of 70 becomes relevant: 70 at time of transplant becomes quite different than 70 at time of initial evaluation.

Another important consideration in an older patient is quality of life. If the patient has physical or cognitive restrictions, many centers will hesitate to consider an older patient. The limiting factor remains that with a shortage of organs, will the older patient genuinely benefit? There is hesitation to transplant a debilitated or bed-ridden older patient. Similarly, cognitive decline and early dementia will be considered as contra-indications in the older patient. This is likely due to the impression that such conditions are predictive of decrease of life expectancy and that organ transplantation would be expected to make little impact on quality of life. Cognitive impairment and immobility are overlooked in younger patients if there is sufficient support of the patient.

WILL THE PATIENT SURVIVE THE OPERATION?

Many tools have been developed to predict surgical outcomes and tools with assessment of frailty play an important role in patient selection. There is no standard-of-care tool to evaluate an older patient's candidacy for organ transplantation. However, certain factors have been historically validated: cardiac status considering coronary artery disease, pulmonary function including oxygen dependence, nutritional status and obesity. Peripheral arterial disease also becomes a major limiting factor as the organ to be transplanted needs appropriate vascular sites for implantation. With increasing age and with the comorbidities associated with end-stage renal disease, there is an increased incidence of arterial disease in the common and external iliac arteries. In younger patients, there may be an option for vascular reconstruction or bypass to facilitate the implantation; these options will not be considered on the older patient out of concern of too much surgery.

WILL THE PATIENT TOLERATE IMMUNOSUPPRESSION?

Organ transplantation cannot be a consideration if there are contra-indications to immunosuppression. Obvious contra-indications are the presence of malignancy and sepsis. Different malignancies have different recommended wait times prior to proceeding with a transplant. This wait time does not preclude listing the patient and allowing the patient to accumulate time on the list. Hence, when evaluating the older patient, consideration must also be made to the age the patient will be when the period of recurrence-free observation will end.

The standard of care for immunosuppression for organ transplantation includes two phases: an induction phase at the time of implantation and a maintenance phase that usually lasts the patient's lifetime. Induction regimens include steroids and antibodies that can be either monoclonal or polyclonal and cytotoxic or non-cytotoxic. Maintenance regimens utilize a combination of drugs that block signaling in lymphocytes such as an antibody, a calcineurin inhibitor (tacrolimus or cyclosporine), an anti-metabolite and steroids. The most commonly used calcineurin inhibitor, tacrolimus, has side effects especially relevant to older patients—namely, neurotoxicity. While it can induce seizures at higher levels, the more common problem at standard therapeutic levels is tremor. Even in younger patients, tacrolimus can induce a tremor for the first few months that impacts the ability to write and perform tasks requiring manual dexterity. In the older patient this can be very debilitating such as when tremors prevent the ability to use silverware for eating. The anti-metabolites (mycophenolate compounds) can cause gastrointestinal distress to varying degrees. This may present as a reluctance to eat due to upper gastrointestinal symptoms of bloating, heartburn or lack of appetite. Alternatively, it can present as significant diarrhea. In the older patient these side effects are significantly more impactful and alter the quality of life. The diarrhea is easier to recognize but may still require a hospital admission due to dehydration and electrolyte imbalance. The upper gastrointestinal symptoms may be more subtle and the first indication may be weight loss as the patients may not self-report the loss of appetite. The treatment for gastrointestinal side effects is dose reduction or discontinuation.

Immunosuppression increases the risk of infection due to bacteria and viruses such as cytomegalovirus and BK virus (polyoma virus). The older patient is more prone to viral infections. Induction protocols are often modified for the older recipient utilizing monoclonal antibodies (basiliximab) with a lower risk profile for immunosuppression as opposed to using cytotoxic antibodies (anti-thymocyte globulin, alemtuzumab). Older patients may also have increased risk factors for urinary tract such as poor bladder motility and prostate enlargement. Hence, there needs to be increased vigilance for urinary tract infections.

Upon discharge the transplant recipient may be overwhelmed by the transplant-induced polypharmacy. In the older patient, this may exacerbate an already existing list of medications. This is further exacerbated by frequent dosing changes to achieve therapeutic range of calcineurin inhibitors. While the transplant programs can assist with preparing pill boxes, these changes may also be necessary outside of clinic hours.

WILL THE PATIENT BE ABLE TO TAKE CARE OF THE ORGAN?

The routine follow-up after kidney transplantation requires two to three clinic visits per week for the first month. This poses a logistic challenge in the older patient and often taxes the social support available to autonomous older patients. Inherently, their limiting disability may preclude driving to the clinic. Lack of easy access to medical transportation makes it difficult for the older patient to be able to take care of the transplanted organ.

The social worker plays an important role in the evaluation of the older patient. An extensive assessment of the social support and the living conditions of the older patient becomes crucial. Often this involves family meetings and evaluating the commitment of family or friends.

Psychological Impact

In-center dialysis is a 3 day per week event with over 4 hours spent per session. The wait times for a kidney transplant exceed 4 years and are closer to 6 in many areas. For some older patients, the nursing staff and other patients at the dialysis center become friends and family and the focus of their social network. A successful kidney transplant eliminates the need for dialysis and dismantles social support. Depression from transplant-induced social isolation has been observed in older patients. Moreover, a form of survivor guilt is also seen. The older patient sometimes ponders if they have deprived a younger person from benefiting from a transplant. Inherent to this is the feeling that the organ is being wasted on them. This depression can be impactful and may need intervention.

Liver Transplantation

Livers are being increasingly allocated to the sickest patients first. The physiological ravages caused by end-stage liver disease are significant. By the time of transplant the patient with end-stage liver disease is extremely debilitated. For this reason, many centers will not consider an older patient with decompensated liver disease for transplantation. With advances in the field of liver transplantation the age-limit consideration for an older patient requiring liver transplantation has become 70 years. The patients aged 65 and older who do receive liver transplants are often those with relatively compensated liver cirrhosis who receive priority allocation for other reasons—mostly hepatocellular carcinoma. The challenges with liver transplantation are larger than those encountered with kidney transplantation. The intra-operative cardiopulmonary stressors are significant. The post-operative course invariably requires a longer ICU stay. The recovery time is closer to 6 months. The large incision makes post-operative mobility difficult at first. When evaluating a patient for a liver transplant, there is less room for significant comorbid conditions. Even with liver transplant, the older patient is often highly encouraged to consider a living donor. The pressure for livers for transplant is quite significant. Whereas hemodialysis exists as a survival option for patients with renal failure, the inability to receive a liver transplant in a timely fashion can often result in death. Hence, the selection bias in liver transplant candidacy is stronger towards maximizing the impact of liver transplantation. However, there is data to support that older patients can do well and have similar 5-year survival rates. There are isolated reports of patients receiving a liver transplant in their late 70s. Hence, while 70 years of age may be a general guideline for liver transplantation, with selective evaluation this life-saving therapy may be available to certain older patients.

CONCLUSION

With improvement in the care of transplant patients, this life-saving therapy is being offered to older patients. However, end-stage organ disease is damaging and easily depletes the physiological reserves of the older patient. The careful and individualized assessment is essential to obtaining good outcomes and making meaningful use of donor organs. With the increasing need in younger patients, it will prove to be increasingly challenging to allocate organs to more older patients.

REFERENCES

1. Halloran PF. Immunosuppressive Drugs for Kidney Transplantation. N Engl J Med 2004; 351:2715–2729.
2. Gavara CG, Esposito F, Gurusamy K et al. Liver Transplantation in Elderly Patients: A Systematic Review and First Meta-Analysis. HPB 2019; 21(1):14–25.
3. Sutherland AI, Ijzermans JNM, Forsythe JLR, Dor FJMF. Kidney and Liver Transplantation in the Elderly. Br J Surg 2016; 103(2):e62–72.
4. Pinter J, Hanson CS, Chapman JR, et al. Perspectives of Older Kidney Transplant Recipients on Kidney Transplantation. Clin J Am Soc Nephrol 2017; 12(3):443–453.
5. Arcos E, Perez-Saez MJ, Comas J, et al. Assessing the Limits in Kidney Transplantation: use of Extremely Elderly Donors and Outcomes in Elderly Recipients. Transplantation 2020; 104(1):176–183.

PART IV

CANCER

27 Cancer in Older Adults

Doreen Wan-Chow-Wah, MD, FRCPC

CONTENTS

CLINICAL VIGNETTE

An 87-year-old woman living in a seniors' residence is referred by the oromaxillofacial surgeon to assess suitability for surgery for a squamous cell carcinoma of the tongue which will involve a resection under general anesthesia. Her comorbidities include hypertension, diabetes mellitus type 2, gastroesophageal reflux disease, osteoarthritis, and osteoporosis. Her medications include amlodipine 7.5 mg qd, acetaminophen 650 mg TID, lorazepam 1 mg qHS, metformin 500 mg TID, enteric coated ASA 80 mg qd, pantoprazole 40 mg qd, vitamin D 10 000 units qweek, calcium 500 mg qd, and alendronate 70 mg qweek. She is an ex-smoker, and denies alcohol consumption or recreational drugs.

She is independent for her activities of daily living and the residence provides meals and medications. Her daughter assists her with her finances. She uses no walking aids, and does not drive. She has lost 10 lbs over the last 6 months, unintentionally. She is a retired seamstress with an elementary school level of education.

On examination, BP 133/81, pulse 64, weight 61.9 kg, BMI 23, grip strength 24 kg (normal for her gender and BMI), gait speed 0.74 meter/second (normal is ≥ 1 meter/second). Her general physical examination was unremarkable. MMSE Folstein was 23/30. Her creatinine clearance was calculated as 55 ml/min, and the rest of her blood test results were within normal limits.

EPIDEMIOLOGY OF CANCER IN OLDER ADULTS

Geriatric oncology is a relatively young subspecialty. Originally well established in the United States and Europe, it has been developing in Canada over the past 10 years, starting with the Geriatric Oncology Clinic established at the Segal Cancer Center of the Jewish General Hospital in Montreal. Since then, other centers across Canada have followed, recognizing the unique needs of older cancer patients.

Aging is the number one risk factor for developing cancer. With the growth and aging of the population, we are seeing an increasing cancer burden. Cancer is the leading cause of mortality in the country, surpassing cardiovascular disease. Forty-four percent of new cancer cases are diagnosed in patients aged ≥ 70, and 62% of deaths due to cancer occur in those aged ≥ 70. Lung, colorectal, prostate, and breast cancers are the most common cancers diagnosed in the older population. Half of all newly diagnosed lung and colorectal cancer cases will occur in those aged 70 and older. More deaths from breast cancer occur in those ≥ 80 than any other age group.

PARTICULARITIES OF OLDER PATIENTS WITH CANCER

The elderly constitute a heterogeneous population, meaning that a group of 80-year-old individuals will differ significantly in terms of their health and functional status, as compared to a group of 40-year-old adults. With aging comes various physiological changes (increased fat, decreased muscle mass, decreased renal function, and hepatic metabolism) that impact cancer and its treatment. There are age-based disparities in the provision of cancer care. We know that the elderly are understaged, undertreated, and overall receive suboptimal care. A certain proportion of patients are also overtreated, and suffer the consequences of treatment toxicities which impact significantly on their quality of life.

Important questions to ask ourselves are: will the patient die with or from the cancer, will they suffer from the cancer, will they tolerate the treatments, and are there factors (medical, functional,

DOI: 10.1201/9781003344476-31

social) which may interfere with the cancer treatment but are potentially reversible? Because the elderly are underrepresented in clinical trials, there is a lack of guidelines on how to best treat this population.

Older patients may be socially isolated or have limited social support which increases their vulnerability. Some patients are caregivers for their spouse. Many suffer from various degrees of cognitive impairment which has important implications on their ability to adhere to treatments (e.g. medication adherence) and recognize side effects of treatments. Seemingly trivial logistical issues such as transportation to and from medical appointments can actually be significant barriers to older patients receiving adequate cancer treatments.

DETERMINING FITNESS FOR CANCER TREATMENTS

Patients may undergo one or more of the following treatment modalities: surgery, chemotherapy, radiotherapy, and, increasingly, targeted treatments that can involve immunotherapy (see Glossary: cancer, immunotherapy, checkpoint inhibitor, receptor site, T-lymphocyte, vaccine). Cancer treatments can be administered with curative or palliative intent. Alternatively, patients may also be referred to palliative care to receive end-of-life care and adequate management of symptoms. Guidelines put forth by scientific organizations such as SIOG (International Society of Geriatric Oncology) and the NCCN (National Comprehensive Cancer Network) recommend a comprehensive geriatric assessment (CGA) for patients aged 70 years and older for whom chemotherapy is considered. Studies have confirmed the usefulness of the CGA in oncology. A CGA can help detect impairment not identified on routine history or physical examination, predict severe treatment-related toxicity, predict overall survival in a variety of tumors and treatment settings, and influence treatment choice and intensity. Treatment must be tailored to patients' health and functional status rather than their chronological age.

Given oncologists' busy practice, it has been proposed that older cancer patients should first be screened for potential vulnerabilities, and that those who screen positive should subsequently be referred for a comprehensive geriatric assessment.

There exist several screening tools to choose from; the G8 (Oncodage) and Vulnerable Elders Survey (VES-13) have been well validated in geriatric oncology.

In the Geriatric Oncology Clinic, the following domains are evaluated as part of a comprehensive geriatric assessment (CGA): comorbidities, medications, functional status, mood, cognition, nutritional status, social support, life expectancy, and patient's goals. We describe a patient's functional status based on their ability to perform activities of daily living (ADLs) and instrumental activities of daily living (IADLs). Cognitive screening tools such as the Mini-Cog (3 word delayed recall + clock drawing), mini mental state examination (MMSE), and/or Montreal Cognitive Assessment test (MoCA) are used to evaluate cognitive function. In order to better detect potential vulnerability, we also measure grip strength and gait speed which are sensitive markers of frailty.

Polypharmacy

About one-third of community dwelling older adults take ≥ 5 prescription drugs. A study looking at the prevalence of polypharmacy and inappropriate drug use in ambulatory older adults with cancer found that 41% of seniors took more than 5 medications, 43% took more than 10 medications, and 51% took potentially inappropriate medications. Taking multiple medications increases the risk of drug-drug interactions and drug-disease interactions.

Older patients with cancer often already take multiple prescribed drugs for pre-existing comorbidities. The addition of cancer treatments such as chemotherapy or molecularly targeted therapies and their potential side effects and/or toxicities constitutes an added challenge. Certain chemotherapy drugs such as taxanes or platinum agents can cause painful peripheral neuropathy. Aromatase inhibitors prescribed for hormone receptor positive breast cancer decrease bone mineral density and can cause arthralgias and myalgias, which can be debilitating in older women. Many systemic cancer treatments, as well as radiotherapy, can cause significant fatigue which interferes with daily function.

Another potential side effect of cancer treatments is "chemo brain", which is now referred to as cancer and/or cancer therapy-related cognitive changes. Cognitive changes are not solely related to getting chemotherapy. They can occur after receiving a cancer diagnosis, or after surgery or radiotherapy (particularly but not restricted to the brain). The exact pathophysiology remains unclear but the cognitive impacts are described as difficulties in concentration, multitasking, attention and short-term memory amongst others. The evolution of these cognitive changes is also unknown; they may resolve after the cancer treatment ends, or may persist over a more prolonged period.

Patients are also often prescribed supportive therapies in conjunction with their chemotherapy to minimize side effects. Supportive drugs such as antiemetics and potent steroids such as dexamethasone can cause unwanted side effects, or interact with pre-existing conditions (drug-disease interactions). For example, prochlorperazine (Stemetil) use on a regular basis can lead to extrapyramidal side effects, causing parkinsonism. Dexamethasone (Decadron) in diabetic patients can cause significant hyperglycemia requiring adjustments of oral hypoglycemic agents or insulin.

It is important to frequently re-evaluate medications at each medical visit. Given the potential for one's health condition to change especially while undergoing cancer treatments, prescription drugs which may have been appropriate prior to the cancer diagnosis may actually be detrimental as the patient's health changes along their cancer care trajectory. For example, antihypertensives in the context of dehydration will further lower blood pressure and cause orthostatic hypotension and subsequent falls. In another scenario, a diabetic patient taking gliclazide may become hypoglycemic if their oral intake decreases significantly because of chemotherapy-induced nausea and vomiting. Hypoglycemia can lead to mental status changes, weakness, and even syncope and falls if severe.

Life Expectancy

It is possible to estimate one's life expectancy, based on the number and severity of comorbidities and functional status (degree of autonomy); these are stronger predictors than age alone. A patient with severe congestive heart failure, severe obstructive lung disease, end stage renal disease or who is very dependent for their basic activities of daily living will have a life expectancy much below average; on the other hand, a patient with few comorbidities who is autonomous in their daily activities will have a life expectancy much above average.

There exists a useful online prognostic tool called ePrognosis (www.eprognosis.org) which was developed to help clinicians estimate their patients' mortality risk based on various indices. Knowing a patient's life expectancy can assist in the treatment decision-making process. The CARG (Cancer and Aging Research Group) predictive chemotherapy toxicity tool can help clinicians estimate a patient's risk of developing toxicity from chemotherapy. It has shown that factors such as age >72, a gastrointestinal or genitourinary cancer, standard chemotherapy dose, polychemotherapy, decreased hemoglobin (<11 g/Dl in males and <10 g/Dl in females), decreased creatinine clearance (<34 ml/min), impaired hearing, falls in the past 6 months, requiring help to take medications, inability to walk one block, and limitations in social activities increase the risk of toxicity from chemotherapy.

GOALS OF CARE AND ADVANCED CARE PLANNING

When facing a potentially fatal disease like cancer, the goal of treatment is often to cure and prolong survival. However, for many older adults, the most important reason to undergo treatment is preservation or improvement of quality of life. Older patients favor quality of life over quantity, and wish to maintain their independence. It is important for clinicians to establish early on in the therapeutic relationship the goals of care of the older patient and whether they have discussed advanced care planning which involves expressing their wishes based on their values and ensure they have a designated substitute decision-maker in case of incapacity. It is imperative to determine "what matters most" to the patient.

RESOLUTION OF THE CLINICAL VIGNETTE

The comprehensive geriatric assessment revealed that our 87-year-old patient with a squamous cell carcinoma of the tongue has certain frailty markers including cognitive impairment (Major Neurocognitive Disorder), diminished gait speed, and weight loss. She has a 59% risk of mortality at 4 years according to the Lee index (eprognosis.org). Given her baseline dementia, she is at a higher risk for post-op delirium and therefore, preventative measures for delirium should be implemented such as early mobilization and reorientation, early removal of IVs and catheters, adequate pain control, avoidance of anticholinergic drugs, and ensuring adequate bladder and bowel hygiene. Particularly in her case, one must not forget to represcribe her regular nighttime dose of lorazepam to prevent withdrawal symptoms and delirium. At a later stage one could consider a tapering of this medication. Despite the frailty markers, we recommended to proceed with the surgery since not having the surgery would translate into further morbidity and limited life expectancy. Knowing the information obtained from the CGA allows the treating team to put measures in place to prevent delirium as well as post-op complications and deconditioning.

REFERENCES

1. Canadian Cancer Society—Canadian cancer statistics 2016. https://cancer.ca
2. Walter LC and Covinsky KE. Cancer screening in elderly patients: A framework for individualized decision making. JAMA 2001; 285: 2750–2756.
3. Extermann M. Basic assessment of the older cancer patient. Current Treatment Options in Oncology 2011; 12: 276–285.
4. Hurria A. Predicting chemotherapy toxicity in older adults with cancer: A prospective multicenter study. JCO 2011; 29: 3457–3465.
5. Nightingale G et al. Evaluation of a pharmacist-led medication assessment used to identify prevalence of and associations with polypharmacy and potentially inappropriate medication use among ambulatory senior adults with cancer. JCO 2015; 33 (15):1453–1459.
6. www.SIOG.org

28 Cancer Screening in the Older Adult

Catalina Hernandez Torres, MD, FRCPC and Tina Hsu, MD, FRCP(C)

CONTENTS

CLINICAL VIGNETTE

Mrs. Smith is a 77-year-old female who has a past medical history of hypertension, diabetes, coronary artery disease and osteoarthritis. She presents to her family doctor for her regular follow-up visit. Her medications include hydrochlorothiazide, metformin, metoprolol, aspirin, acetaminophen as needed. She reports overall doing well with no new significant concerns. She continues to live by herself, and she is independent for all her instrumental activities of daily living. She wants to discuss with her family physician whether she should continue to have cancer screening for breast and colon cancer. She has two close friends who were recently diagnosed with cancer. One friend was diagnosed with early breast cancer and another one with colorectal cancer. She has had regular mammograms with no prior abnormalities; the last mammogram was three years ago. She also had screening for colorectal cancer with fecal occult blood testing that was negative four years ago. She does not have any family history of cancer.

INTRODUCTION

Cancer is a common diagnosis and age is a major risk factor. When diagnosed late, it can be associated with significant morbidity and mortality. Older adults are often diagnosed at more advanced stages. Furthermore, older adults are more likely to be under-treated when diagnosed, which can result in worse outcomes in some older patients. The role of cancer screening in older adults, however, is controversial. This chapter provides an approach to cancer screening in older adults, in particular for breast, colorectal, lung, prostate and cervical cancer.

CONSIDERATIONS IN CANCER SCREENING

Early diagnosis of cancer through cancer screening before a patient becomes symptomatic can improve morbidity and mortality associated with cancer. As per the World Health Organization (WHO), "Screening refers to the use of simple tests across an apparently healthy population to identify individuals who have risk factors or early stages of disease, but do not yet have symptoms". For a screening test to be beneficial several criteria must be met (Table 28.1).

The benefit of screening can be expressed as the number of subjects needed to be screened over a period of time to prevent one death associated with the specific disease. This is

DOI: 10.1201/9781003344476-32

Table 28.1 Characteristics of an Effective Screening Test

Disease Characteristics	Screening Test Characteristics	Diagnostic and Treatment Characteristics
• Prevalent disease. • Natural history well understood. • Long time between the presence of risk factors or subclinical disease and overt disease. • Early intervention improves clinical and public health outcomes.	• High sensitivity and specificity. • Simple, reliable and affordable test. • Acceptable to patient and staff.	• Access and availability to diagnostic facilities. • Accessible and effective treatment options. • Cost-effective and sustainable treatment. • The benefit of treatment outweighs the harm.

Source: Adapted from the World Health Organization

known as the number needed to screen (NNS). The larger the benefit, defined as the absolute risk reduction (ARR), the smaller the number needed to screen to prevent one death. The NNS is the inverse of the ARR, which is calculated by subtracting the mortality associated with non-screened population (CER) event rate from the screened population event rate (SER) (Equation 1). The NNS also depends on the prevalence of the disease in the screened population.

ARR: Absolute risk reduction. SER: Screened Event Rate. CER: Control Event Rate.

Screening and early detection can also be associated with negative outcomes or risks. Risks associated with screening include:

- False positives: a test result that indicates that a disease is present when there is no disease, leading to unnecessary investigations and anxiety.

- False negatives: a negative test result when the person has the disease. This results in false reassurance and can delay treatment.

- Overdiagnosis: the diagnosis of a disease that will never cause symptoms or death. Overdiagnosis results in patients receiving treatment that they otherwise did not need (overtreatment) and/or psychological distress from diagnosis of disease.

For example, out of 1000 adults screened for lung cancer with low dose CT, only three will benefit from screening (i.e. not die from lung cancer due to screening). However, seven will be diagnosed with lung cancer that would not have affected their life expectancy (overdiagnosis leading to overtreatment). Furthermore, 351 will require further testing that ultimately reveals no cancer (false positives), of which three will have major complications from invasive testing, and one will die from invasive testing.

The implementation of cancer screening has resulted in earlier diagnosis of cancer and improved outcomes for some cancers. However, an understanding of its potential risks is important to help individualize the decision of whether to initiate or stop screening.

CANCER SCREENING RECOMMENDATIONS

Both Canada and the United States have organizations that issue clinical practice guidelines for preventive health care. Table 28.2 provides a summary of current cancer screening guidelines in Canada and the United States. Recommendations are based on a systematic review of scientific evidence from which consensus recommendations are developed. However, older adults, over the age of 75, are rarely included in the studies upon which these guidelines are based. Although these guidelines provide specific ages when screening for cancer should be discontinued, data to decide at what age to discontinue screening is limited. For this reason, a discussion with those older adults interested in continuing screening about the benefits and harms of screening is recommended.

Table 28.2 also has links to patient decision aids that illustrate the performance of each screening test demonstrating how many patients benefit or are harmed by the test.

Table 28.2 Summary Screening Recommendations from the Canadian Task Force on Preventive Health Care and the United States Preventive Services Task Force

Cancer	Screening Modality/ Frequency	Age to Start Screening	Age to Consider Stopping Screening	Comments
Breast cancer	Screening mammography every 2 years	50 years old	74 years old	Breast Cancer 1000-Patient Tool*
Colorectal cancer	Stool based tests: Gfobt and FIT every year (Canada and U.S.) Direct visualization tests: Flexible sigmoidoscopy every 5 (Canada) to 10 years (U.S.) or colonoscopy every 10 years (U.S.) or CT colonography every 5 years (U.S.)	50 years old	75 years old	Colorectal Screening Decision Aid Tool*
Lung cancer	Low-dose CT scan for high-risk patients Canada: Annually for up to 3 years U.S.: Every year	55 years old	Canada: 75 years old U.S.: 80 years old, has not smoked in the last 15 years, or develops a health problem that limits life expectancy	For patients at high risk of lung cancer (30 pack-year smoking history who currently smoke or quit less than 15 years ago) Lung Cancer 1000-Person Tool*
Prostate cancer	PSA—no routine screening schedule.	Do not routinely screen at any age	Do not routinely screen at any age	U.S.: Individualized decision starting at age 55 Prostate Cancer Screening 1000-Person Tool*
Cervical cancer	Pap smear cervical cytology every 3 years (Canada and U.S.) or hrHPV testing every 5 years in women age 30–65 (U.S.)	Canada: 25 years old U.S.: 21 years old	Canada: 70 (if the last 3 Pap tests for the last 10 years were negative) U.S.: 65 (if adequate prior screening)	Adequate prior screening: 3 consecutive normal cytologies or 2 consecutive normal hrHPV tests. Cervical screening clinician algorithm. Cervical screening FAQ*

Note: Gfobt: guaiac fecal occult blood test; FIT: Fecal Immunochemical Test; PSA: Prostate Specific Antigen; CT: computed tomography; hrHPV: high-risk Human Papillomavirus
* Decision aid screening tools from CTFPHC available online at https://canadiantaskforce.ca/tools-resources/

FACTORS TO CONSIDER WHEN DISCUSSING SCREENING FOR CANCER IN OLDER ADULTS

Cancer screening decisions in older adults are complex, and screening guidelines provide only a baseline to initiate these conversations and ultimately make shared decisions with patients. This section provides a general approach to cancer screening in older adults.

Cancer Risk Assessment

Reviewing prior screening history may play a role in deciding if screening should be considered in older adults. For instance, in cervical cancer, a one-time screening is recommended for women 65 and over that have incomplete or no prior screening for cervical cancer, as data shows that most women aged 65 and over who are diagnosed with cervical cancer did not have prior appropriate cervical cancer screening. Similarly, some studies suggest that older adults who benefit most from colorectal screening are those who have never had any prior screening.

The information provided in this chapter pertains to cancer screening for those at average risk of breast, colorectal, cervical or prostate cancer. Lung cancer is the only cancer screening program focused on patients at high risk, defined as patients with a 30 pack-year smoking history who currently smoke or who quit less than 15 years ago. If patients have a prior history of any of these malignancies, extensive family history or recent abnormal screening tests results, these recommendations do not apply. Recommendations for these patients are beyond the scope of this chapter.

Life Expectancy

There is often a lag period between the detection of cancer through screening and when it results in a cancer death. For this reason, life expectancy, more so than absolute age, is important to consider when deciding about the benefits of continuing cancer screening. Studies of breast and colorectal cancer have demonstrated that this lag time is approximately 10 years. For instance, it takes about 10 years before one death from colorectal cancer was prevented for 1000 patients screened.

Many different factors influence life expectancy, including current age, the year a person was born, gender, comorbidities, function, social supports, economic status and geographical location. To improve a physician's ability to prognosticate life expectancy, multiple tools can be used. The following are two examples of prognostic tools in clinical practice:

- Life tables: These graphs provide median life expectancy by age group, gender and health status for the United States population. The quartiles differentiate subjects' overall health status. For instance, the upper percentile includes subjects with above average fitness for their age group.

- ePrognosis: Web-based tool that estimates life expectancy based on an evidence-based questionnaire that includes patient factors including health behaviours, comorbidities and functional status. Available free of charge at https://eprognosis.ucsf.edu.

Treatment Options

Benefit from screening presumes that a patient will be willing and able to undergo treatment for an early diagnosed cancer. Treatment options include surgical intervention, radiation therapy and/or systemic therapy. The type of surgical procedure and its inherent risks are greatly dependent on the tumour type. In breast cancer, lumpectomy and mastectomy are standard management options and are considered low risk for cardiac complications. In women with multiple comorbidities, resection of the breast tumour can sometimes be done under local anaesthetic depending on the size and location of the tumour. On the other hand, resection of a colonic or thoracic malignancy can be much riskier and may not be feasible or palatable in patients who are frail. For lung cancer, a rise in the use of stereotactic radiotherapy has expanded treatment options for patients with early stage non-small cell lung cancers with improvements in primary tumour control and overall survival in patients who are medically inoperable.

Given that the early detection of an asymptomatic malignancy is only potentially beneficial if a patient is eligible and willing to undergo treatment, consideration of patient willingness and fitness to undergo treatment is important when considering whether to continue with screening.

Patients' Values and Preferences

The decision about whether to continue cancer screening in older adults is challenging due to the increased risk of developing cancer with aging, increased risk of death due to non-cancer causes and lack of knowledge about the benefits and harms of screening in older adults. In this context, personal values and individual preference need to be considered even more when deciding whether to continue screening for cancer as patients age.

Ideally, screening decisions should be made within the primary care setting where there is an established patient-primary care provider relationship. The primary care physician often has a sense of the patients' values and preference and can establish rapport to discuss the benefits and risks of screening in the context of each patient's health status. For some patients, screening provides peace of mind; for others, it can cause increased anxiety.

Patients tend to focus on the benefits of screening that provide a sense of reassurance when the test is negative. However, they tend to be less well versed in the harms associated with cancer screening. This leads to an overestimation of benefit and underestimation of risk. When cancer screening is framed in terms of increasing harms in relation to decreasing benefit instead of citing the guideline recommendations' cut-off age as the reason to discontinue screening, most older adults find this approach acceptable, and it promotes the patient-physician relationship. Thus, a discussion that includes the benefits but also the limitations/risks associated with cancer screening to help older adults make an informed decision is essential.

DECISION AID TOOLS

To better understand the uncertainty and trade-offs of cancer screening, patient decision aids have been developed. Decision aids can be pamphlets, videos or web-based tools that outline the benefits and harms of a specific health care decision, in this case, cancer screening. These decision aids have shown to increase patients' knowledge of the decision at hand and help patients have an active role in decision making with a more accurate perception of benefits and harms. In turn, decision aids also help patients make decisions that are better aligned with their values.

Decision aids developed by the CTFPHC (Table 28.2) are an excellent tool to use with patients in clinic for a balanced discussion about cancer screening. Another decision tool for breast cancer and colorectal cancer screening is available on the ePrognosis website (http://cancerscreening. eprognosis.org/). It uses specific data about the patient's overall health to provide an estimate of the benefits and harms of screening. Figure 28.1 is an example of the breast cancer screening results provided for the case discussed at the beginning of this chapter using this tool.

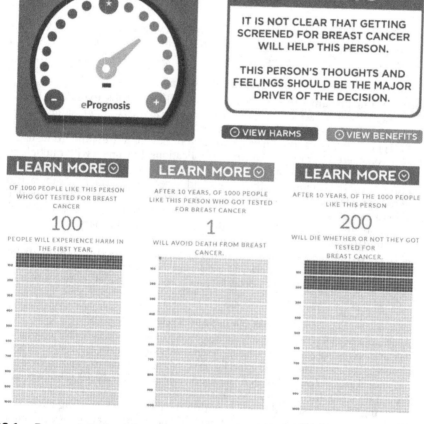

Figure 28.1 ePrognosis tool results sample for breast cancer screening in a 77-year-old female with minimal comorbidities.

Source: Reproduced with permission from ePrognosis.

SCREENING FOR BREAST CANCER IN OLDER ADULTS

Breast cancer is one of the most common cancers diagnosed, with a peak incidence occurring in those 80–84. This age group of women, however, has been generally excluded from trials about screening. Thus, despite the higher prevalence, there remains an uncertainty about whether screening in this population will result in improved outcomes, specifically survival.

The discovery of an abnormality on mammography typically results in a call back for further imaging, including compression mammogram views and targeted ultrasound, to better characterize these findings. If the lesion still appears suspicious, then a biopsy is arranged. Even if testing ultimately rules out the presence of cancer, indicating a false-positive result, these tests can result in anxiety about the possibility of cancer and pain related to biopsies. For older women, the burden of screening may be increased due to difficulties with mobility and transportation. Many studies have shown that the risk of false positives increases with more frequent (annual) screening compared to biennial screening. Thus, a recommendation of screening mammography no more than every two years would be suggested in those women who continue screening beyond the age of 74. This is consistent with the updated American and Canadian preventive screening guidelines.

The greatest potential harm of breast cancer screening in older women relates to the possibility of overdiagnosis and overtreatment of breast cancers that are ultimately not life limiting. The factors that increase overdiagnosis and overtreatment are decreasing life expectancy and a higher prevalence of slower growing disease. As a result, women may undergo treatment, typically surgery, for clinically asymptomatic tumours that are unlikely to affect their outcomes.

Standard treatment of breast cancer and pre-cancerous lesions, such as ductal carcinoma in situ (DCIS), involves surgical resection, either in the form of lumpectomy or mastectomy. Sampling of the axilla is also often conducted to help with prognosis and subsequent treatment decisions. In general, these surgeries are considered low-risk surgeries and, depending on the location of the tumour and the patient's comorbidities, can sometimes even be done under local anaesthetic. For this reason, many older women will still be offered and receive surgical intervention when diagnosed with breast cancer. However, this strategy can still expose women to a potentially unnecessary procedure and the risks inherent with any surgery. A prior retrospective study suggested that the odds of post-operative complications increased with age (OR 1.85 in patients over the age of 85) and multiple comorbidities (OR 1.71). However, overall survival was not adversely affected by experiencing post-operative complications. Those women with hormone sensitive breast cancers, who are not candidates for surgery or who refuse, can be considered for primary treatment with anti-estrogen agents such as tamoxifen or aromatase inhibitors. However, outcomes with these agents alone are not as robust as with surgery and thus patients with a life expectancy of more than two years should be strongly considered for surgery.

It is important to note that under-treatment of older women with breast cancer is also common. Several studies indicate that older women are more likely to be treated with surgery alone and less likely to receive radiation or systemic treatments. In those patients, age 80 and above, in whom under-treatment is common, this can result in poorer breast cancer outcomes, including increased death from breast cancer.

Although there are no firm recommendations in women age 75 and older, it is reasonable to continue screening every two years in women with a life expectancy of at least ten years who would be willing to undergo surgical resection. In those women with shorter estimated life expectancies, a discussion about the uncertainty of benefits and potential harms of screening is important. In these cases, patient preferences and values play a significant role in deciding whether to continue to undergo screening.

SCREENING FOR COLORECTAL CANCER IN OLDER ADULTS

More than half of all new cases of colorectal cancer are diagnosed in those 70 and over. There are several screening methods shown to decrease mortality from colorectal cancer, ranging from less invasive testing such as fecal occult blood testing and fecal immunochemical testing to more invasive tests such as sigmoidoscopy. Although several organizations recommend colonoscopy as a method to screen for colon cancer, it has not been prospectively shown to decrease mortality from colon cancer. These studies have been completed, but the results have yet to be reported.

In older adults, several factors need to be considered, including the potential benefits and harms from screening, and eligibility and willingness to undergo treatment. Colon cancers develop over a 10–15-year period from pre-malignant lesions. Thus, removal of pre-cancerous lesions (polyps) results in a decreased risk of colon cancer. Prior studies suggest that a life expectancy of ten years is warranted to benefit from colon cancer screening. Thus, patients with a shorter life expectancy may be less likely to benefit.

Despite the higher incidence of colorectal cancer in those 70 and over, there appears to be a smaller benefit from screening overall potentially due to a decrease in life expectancy. One study reported that although there was a higher prevalence of colorectal cancer detected using colonoscopy in those age 80 and over compared to those 50–54 (28.6% vs. 13.8%), on average there was a smaller improvement in life expectancy (0.13 years vs. 0.85 years) in older versus younger patients undergoing colonoscopy screening.

Although the absolute risk of complications is low, invasive testing with sigmoidoscopy and colonoscopy risks increased with age and comorbidities. Complications of colonoscopy include bleeding and perforation. This is even higher in those patients who have a polypectomy. Older adults with comorbidities that limit their mobility may also find the procedure and preparation more challenging. There are also higher risks related to the sedation given for colonoscopy in older compared to younger patients, including the potential of delirium. Given the higher risk of significant adverse events with invasive testing, older adults who choose to continue screening should undergo stool-based testing with fecal occult blood testing or fecal immunochemical testing. However, patients should be aware that a positive test warrants further testing with colonoscopy and should be willing and able to do so.

Lastly, patients should be aware of potential treatment recommendations if an asymptomatic malignant lesion is found. The standard treatment for colonic tumours is surgical resection, typically a hemicolectomy. The intent is to completely remove the tumour and to allow for nodal sampling, which influences prognosis and subsequent treatment decisions. In general, there are higher risks of surgical complications and mortality in older adults. There is a progressively increased rate of post-operative mortality with each decade of increasing age starting from age 65 onwards with those aged 75–84 experiencing a 3.2 times higher risk of post-operative mortality compared to those <65 years of age. Notably, however, the range of reported rates of complication varied greatly from lows of 0–5% and highs of 15–48.9%, suggesting that patient selection is key. Improvement in post-operative mortality has, however, been reported with time, with the greatest improvements seen in patients age 85 and over. This may be related to the greater use of laparoscopic procedures. Emergency or urgent need for surgical intervention is strongly associated with higher peri-operative risk in older adults. Overall, careful patient assessment and selection and planned elective surgeries may help mitigate some of the morbidity and mortality associated with colorectal surgery in this older population.

In early superficial cancers, there is a growing use of endoscopic submucosal dissection. Very few studies have looked at these outcomes and safety in older adults. However, some retrospective observational studies suggest that it can be performed safely, with a perforation rate of 3.1%. Overall, however, further studies are needed to better characterize which patients are ideal for these less invasive procedures and to characterize their long-term outcomes compared to more extensive surgery.

Resection of colon cancer can result in a cure for 85–90% of patients with stage I/II cancer and 40–50% cure in those with stage III (lymph node involvement). Although chemotherapy after surgery is considered standard of care in those with stage III disease, this can be decided on an individual basis with patients after surgery and an unwillingness or inability to undergo chemotherapy should not be a preclusion to definitive treatment of colon cancer or a decision to undergo screening.

Given these considerations, patient input is very important in the decision to offer or discontinue screening for colon cancer in patients over the age of 75. While the CTFPHC recommends against screening in adults age 75 and over, the United States Preventive Services Task Force (USPTF) recommends that in adults age 76 to 85, an individualized decision about colorectal screening be made taking in account patients' overall health and prior screening history.

LUNG CANCER SCREENING IN OLDER ADULTS

Lung cancer is the leading cause of cancer death in North America. About 80% of people diagnosed with lung cancer have non-curable disease at the time of diagnosis and most lung cancers when untreated are rapidly fatal. The median age for a diagnosis of lung cancer is 70 years old, affecting older adults disproportionately. Smoking is a well-known risk factor for lung cancer. Lung cancer screening should be offered only to those who are at high risk of developing lung cancer. At the same time, lung cancer differs from other solid malignancies by being known to be often an aggressive cancer that can cause significant morbidity and mortality in a short period of time.

The National Lung Screening Trial (NLST) was the first randomized study to show a benefit to lung cancer screening. This study compared low-dose computed tomography (CT) or chest x-ray annually for three years in patients 55 to 74 who had a smoking history of at least 30 pack-years or who had quit within the previous 15 years. This study showed a 20% relative reduction in mortality from lung cancer, with a number needed to screen of 320 to prevent one lung cancer death.

Lung cancer screening carries a high risk of false positive results. In the NLST trial, any nodule greater than 4 mm was considered a positive screening result and required further testing. After three years of yearly low dose CTs, 39% of study participants had positive findings, of those findings 95% were falsely positive. However, false positive results were ruled out by using serial CT scans to avoid unnecessary invasive investigations with thoracic biopsies. More recent data suggest that in the NLST trial about 18% of lung cancer detected by low-dose CT would otherwise not lead to significant morbidity or mortality and thus represented an overdiagnosis.

Extrapolating the findings of the NLST trial to older adults has been controversial as only 8.8% of patients in the NSLT trial were 70 and older. The incidence rate of lung cancer diagnosis was 2.2% in patients 65 and over; however, there was no benefit in mortality in the analysis restricted to patients 65 and over. Guideline recommendations to screen older adults come from statistical modelling designed to determine the least invasive screening program to prevent the highest percentage of cancer-related mortality. However, as most lung cancer cases occur in patients 70 years and older and due to the high morbidity and mortality associated with lung cancer, some guidelines recommend low-dose CT screening that extends to patients beyond the age of those included in the NLST trial. The US Preventive Task Force recommends screening patients aged 55 to 80 until patients have quit smoking for more than 15 years or until the patient develops a health problem that will limit their life expectancy or the ability to undergo curative treatment.

Finally, considerations for lung cancer screening should include discussions about diagnostic test (lung biopsy) and treatment options that need to be considered if lung cancer is diagnosed. Treatment of early-stage lung cancer typically includes surgical resection. This can range from a wedge resection, lobectomy or on occasion a pneumonectomy. Increasingly video-assisted thoracic surgery (VATS), rather than a thoracotomy, is being used, which can result in faster recovery and decreased hospitalization. Both of these procedures typically require patients to have adequate lung function to allow resection of the affected lung. There has also been a rise in the use of stereotactic radiotherapy in patients with early stage non-small-cell lung cancers with improvements in primary tumour control and overall survival in medically inoperable patients. Patients thus need to be willing and able to proceed with surgery or radiotherapy to benefit from lung cancer screening.

PROSTATE CANCER SCREENING IN OLDER ADULTS

Prostate cancer is the most common cancer affecting men age 70 and older, and the third leading cause of cancer-related deaths. The rate of high-risk prostate cancer increases with age, and older adults are less likely to receive local therapy once a diagnosis is made. Despite this, prostate cancer screening is controversial for all age groups as the harms of screening outweigh the benefits.

The main reason for this is due to the poor test characteristics of prostate-specific antigen (PSA) as a screening test. PSA has an estimated sensitivity of 21% for detecting any prostate cancer, meaning that of 100 people with prostate cancer 79 will have a false negative test result. Also, the specificity of the test is poor. The positive predictive value is only 30%, meaning that only 3 out of 10 men with an elevated PSA are diagnosed with prostate cancer. Abnormal PSA values lead to further diagnostic work-up with a prostate biopsy. Short-term risk of prostate biopsies includes anxiety, pain, hematuria, infection and hospital admission in up to 7% of patients.

Because of the indolent natural history of many prostate cancers, an estimated 40–60% of screen-detected prostate cancers are felt to be an overdiagnosis, in which the diagnosis of prostate cancer will never cause symptoms or death. The rate of overdiagnosis in prostate cancer is directly correlated to the age at diagnosis. Consequently, older adults are at increased risk of experiencing harm from prostate cancer screening. Overdiagnosis leads to psychological distress and unnecessary treatments. Primary treatment of prostate cancer can include either prostatectomy or radical radiotherapy plus or minus androgen deprivation therapy. Adverse effects of treatment with prostatectomy and radiotherapy include bowel dysfunction, urinary incontinence, erectile dysfunction and premature death, particularly in older men with poor functional status. Because a large proportion of prostate cancers are felt to be an overdiagnosis, current practice guidelines recommend active surveillance for men with clinically localized low-risk prostate cancer to minimize overtreatment in prostate cancer. This means curative intent treatment is deferred until there is evidence of disease progression. Even in the absence of treatment, however, diagnosis of a non-significant cancer can lead to undue anxiety.

In conclusion, PSA screening for prostate cancer should not be routinely performed in patients of any age and particularly in older adults in whom the harms of screening can significantly affect their quality of life without improving prostate cancer related morbidity and mortality.

CERVICAL CANCER SCREENING IN OLDER ADULTS

One-third of cervical cancer deaths occur in women age 65 and older. For average risk women, leading professional organizations recommend cervical cancer screening be discontinued in women 70 and older if they have had three consecutive negative cytologies in the last ten years. Nevertheless, many women approach age 65 without adequate screening for cervical cancer and catch-up screening may be needed to achieve adequate negative screening history.

Organized screening has reduced the incident rates of cervical cancer. Screening methods include Pap test and HPV testing either alone or in combination. Both tests require a gynecological exam with a speculum. A Pap test looks for abnormal cells in the cervix, and the HPV test detects HPV DNA viruses that could lead to cervical cancer. The risks associated with cervical cancer screening include a 14.4% rate of false positive cytology that resulted in unnecessary diagnostic tests and treatments. If cytology is abnormal, further testing with repeat cytology followed by colposcopy is required. This testing can lead to significant anxiety and discomfort in patients. For older post-menopausal women, the vaginal exam may be more uncomfortable given the hormonal changes associated with aging.

Cervical cancer is treated with a radical hysterectomy with pelvic lymph node dissection or pelvic external beam radiation therapy (EBRT). Depending on the stage of the cancer at diagnosis, EBRT is sometimes combined with chemotherapy or brachytherapy (localized radiation delivered directly to the cervix). Patients who have lymph node involvement or positive margins following surgery are also treated with EBRT and chemotherapy with or without brachytherapy. Data regarding risks of these treatments, specifically in older women, is unclear. However, older women are more likely to be treated with radiation rather than surgery. Those who do undergo surgery are less likely to have a lymph node dissection.

In summary, for women 70 and older who had a documented history of negative cervical cancer screening with 3 consecutive Pap test and/or HPV tests in the last 10 years, there is no evidence to support further screening. However, for older women who have never been screened a discussion about one-time screening may be considered.

RESOLUTION OF THE CLINICAL VIGNETTE

Mrs. Smith's health history was reviewed, and physical examination, including a normal breast exam, was completed. Using the ePrognosis tool (mortality risk for Lee Index), her median life expectancy was estimated to be 17.7–21.1 years with a ten-year mortality risk of 15–23%. In the context of her life expectancy, her physician decides it is reasonable to discuss the pros and cons of continuing cancer screening.

Mrs. Smith is provided with information regarding the benefits and harms of cancer screening, for breast and colorectal using the ePrognosis tool. After reviewing the data, she decides to continue with mammogram screening at this time given her overall good health and the fact that she would be willing to undergo treatment if needed.

For colorectal cancer, she decides against colorectal screening as she does not feel that she would be willing to undergo colonoscopy if stool-based testing was positive. She is educated on the signs and symptoms associated with colorectal cancer, including change in bowel habits and melena or hematochezia.

Given Mrs. Smith was not a smoker, lung cancer screening was not indicated. Further review of her history shows that she had 3 consecutive cytology results for cervical cancer screening that were normal. Thus, further cervical cancer screening is not recommended.

CONCLUSION

Cancer screening in older adults is a complex process that requires knowledge of the natural history of the specific malignancy, life expectancy estimates and understanding of a patient's values and preferences. It is reasonable to consider ongoing screening in those who are fit with a life expectancy of at least 10 years who are willing and able to undergo cancer treatment if a cancer diagnosis is confirmed.

REFERENCES

1. Bibbins-Domingo K, Grossman DC, Curry SJ, et al. Screening for Colorectal Cancer: US Preventive Services Task Force Recommendation Statement. JAMA. 2016;315(23):2564–2575. doi:10.1001/jama.2016.5989
2. Curry SJ, Krist AH, Owens DK, et al. Screening for Cervical Cancer: US Preventive Services Task Force Recommendation Statement. JAMA 2018;320(7):674–686.
3. Fenton JJ, Weyrich MS, Durbin S, Liu Y, Bang H, Melnikow J. Prostate-Specific Antigen–Based Screening for Prostate Cancer: Evidence Report and Systematic Review for the US Preventive Services Task Force. JAMA 2018;319(18):1914–1931.
4. Lee SJ, Boscardin WJ, Stijacic-Cenzer I, Conell-Price J, O'Brien S, Walter LC. Time Lag to Benefit After Screening for Breast and Colorectal Cancer: Meta-Analysis of Survival Data from the United States, Sweden, United Kingdom, and Denmark. BMJ. 2013;346:e8441. doi:10.1136/bmj.e8441
5. Moyer VA, U.S. Preventive Services Task Force. Screening for Lung Cancer: U.S. Preventive Services Task Force Recommendation Statement. Ann Intern Med. 2014;160(5):330–338. doi:10.7326/M13-2771
6. National Lung Screening Trial Research Team, Aberle DR, Adams AM, et al. Reduced Lung-Cancer Mortality with Low-Dose Computed Tomographic Screening. N Engl J Med. 2011;365(5):395–409. doi:10.1056/NEJMoa1102873
7. Siu AL, U.S. Preventive Services Task Force. Screening for Breast Cancer: U.S. Preventive Services Task Force Recommendation Statement. Ann Intern Med. 2016;164(4):279–296. doi:10.7326/M15-2886
8. Walter LC, Covinsky KE. Cancer Screening in Elderly Patients: A Framework for Individualized Decision Making. JAMA. 2001;285(21):2750–2756. doi:10.1001/jama.285.21.2750
9. Walter LC, Schonberg MA. Screening Mammography in Older Women: A Review. JAMA. 2014;311(13):1336–1347. doi:10.1001/jama.2014.2834
10. Wilson JMG, Jungner G. Principles and Practice of Screening for Disease. Geneva: World Health Organization. 1968.

29 Diagnosis and Management of Bowel Cancer

Jessica Holland, MD, FRCSC and Barry L. Stein, MDCM, FRCSC, FACS, FASCRS

CONTENTS

INTRODUCTION

Colorectal cancer (CRC) has the third highest cancer incidence worldwide, along with the second highest mortality behind lung cancer, and as we age our individual risk of CRC increases. In the United States, the average age of diagnosis for CRC is 67 years old and 56% of cases occur in patients that are 65 or older (1). However, older adults are less likely to receive the standard of care in treatment and are less likely to be included in clinical trials (2, 3). Clinicians caring for older adults need to understand the unique care needs of this population.

Caring for older adults with CRC requires a comprehensive review of the individual's co-morbidities, functional status, and values. Advanced age is associated with an increased risk of complications, short-term mortality, and short and long-term morbidity. Loss of quality of life (QOL) and functional independence after treatment is a major issue for older adults (3, 4). Chronologic age alone does not tell the entire story. Age is often a poor marker for physiologic frailty, which is a better composite marker of the individual's ability to tolerate stress and predictor of increased risk of morbidity and mortality following treatment (5). As a result, clinicians have increasingly moved away from strict age cut-offs as a criterion in decision making to a more complete look at the patient (5).

Case Examples

To illustrate some of the complexity of managing older adults with CRC, we will follow two common clinical scenarios throughout this chapter:

Mr. Davos is a 76-year-old man who lives at home with his partner of 30 years. He has a history of hypertension, high cholesterol, and mild chronic kidney disease (CKD). He has had regular colonoscopy-based screening since he turned 40 as his father and his older brother both died of CRC. He has a personal history of tubular adenomatous polyps. He has not had a colonoscopy since he turned 65 as he spent the last ten years as a caregiver to his partner.

Mrs. Alamitos is an 89-year-old woman who has been living in an assisted living facility for many years. She is independent with her personal care but requires help with preparing meals and managing her activities of daily living. Over the last three months she has been having worsening diarrhea, with new onset incontinence and rectal bleeding. Her past medical history includes osteoporosis, arthritis, diabetes currently controlled with an oral hypoglycemic, and mild cognitive impairment. She has never had a colonoscopy.

Screening:

Screening of older adults is controversial, and many guidelines do not recommend screening for patients 75 years or older due to a lack of demonstrated benefit in this population, although this is arguably due to systematic exclusion of these patients from trials rather than true evidence of the lack of benefit (6). National and society guidelines are designed for population-based applications

DOI: 10.1201/9781003344476-33

and by their nature do not always allow for consideration of individual circumstances. Screening should not be offered to patients who are expected to live less than five years or who would not be a treatment candidate. The screening recommendations apply only to asymptomatic older adults and should not be considered for the investigation of symptoms.

Most national CRC screening programs prioritize non-invasive options such as guaiac-based faecal occult blood testing (FOBT) or faecal immunochemical tests (FIT) (7). These tests are appropriate only for an average risk patient with no personal history of colorectal polyps or cancer, or visible rectal bleeding. They can be performed annually or biannually and are accepted as a solo screening method.

Invasive screening methods include flexible sigmoidoscopy and colonoscopy. Flexible sigmoidoscopy does not require a full bowel preparation or sedation and is useful in screening for left-sided colonic polyps and malignancy. It has the benefit of a less onerous preparation for the patient and fewer complications with regards to sedation but is limited in the area screened and is rarely used in practice in Canada. It is paired with non-invasive screening mechanisms in some guidelines (7).

Colonoscopy combines the full visualization of the colon with the ability to perform therapeutic interventions in one encounter. The procedure often requires some form of sedation. CT colonography is an alternative method of visualizing the colon without the need for sedation but does not permit therapeutic interventions or biopsies. Both investigations require full bowel preparation which can be challenging for a patient with limited mobility or swallowing difficulties. Low-volume preparations, such as sodium picosulfate (Pico-Salax®), require less liquid to be consumed pre-procedure but can result in significant fluid shifting and electrolyte imbalances and should be used judiciously in those with advanced kidney disease and heart failure. Large-volume preparations, such as 4 litres of polyethylene glycol (PEG) solutions may be safer to use in these patients because they do not cause loss of electrolytes or fluid shifts. Divided preparations which are completed over the course of two days can help the patient tolerate the preparation better.

The Canadian Task Force on preventative health currently recommends routine screening for the average-risk patient from 50 to 74 years old and does not recommend screening over 75 years old (8). The preferred screening modality for these patients is FIT testing every two years. Other methods such as capsule endoscopy and barium studies are rarely used as primary screening modalities.

This discussion of screening options does not apply to either Mr. Davos or Mrs. Alamitos. Mr. Davos has a personal history of colorectal polyps and would not be suitable for the non-invasive screening options described. His surveillance recommendation would be determined by the histology and number of previous polyps. Mrs. Alamitos has concerning symptoms. While rectal bleeding is often attributed to outlet bleeding from anorectal conditions such as hemorrhoids, the new onset of persistent symptoms warrant further investigation.

Diagnoses:
The symptoms of CRC can be subtle and insidious. Symptoms of CRC are often initially vague and can include abdominal pain, change in appetite, weight loss, rectal bleeding, iron deficiency anemia from chronic slow blood loss, and change in the calibre or pattern of stool. Older adults can experience a gradual change without seeking care. A patient with these symptoms should undergo investigation appropriate for their overall health. Non-invasive screening investigations like FIT or FOBT are inappropriate in the presence of symptoms.

Initial investigations should include a full medical history with particular attention to gastrointestinal symptoms and personal or family history of colorectal polyps or cancer. Genetic predispositions and hereditary colon cancer syndromes are less important in the older adult population as aggressive phenotypes present at a younger age. A physical exam including a digital rectal examination should be performed. A palpable rectal cancer will change the course and urgency of further investigations that should not be deferred to a specialist visit. Basic laboratory investigations include a complete blood count (CBC), electrolytes, and creatinine.

Carcinoembryonic antigen (CEA), a CRC tumour marker, is not useful as a screening or initial diagnostic tool. It is useful in surveillance, as a rising level can be an early indication of disease recurrence. A markedly elevated CEA can be a marker of liver metastases. Not all local recurrences of resected CRC raise CEA levels initially, but all will in a short time. Patients who smoke often have a slight baseline elevation in CEA (9).

Following an initial assessment, further investigations require a referral to an endoscopist. Colonoscopy is the primary and most accurate diagnostic tool for CRC. It is safe and well tolerated. Perforations in older adults from colonoscopy are rare, and the risk does not increase directly with age (10). The location of the lesion determines the treatment options available.

Mrs. Alamitos' symptoms are concerning and warrant an office visit which was arranged. She had no additional relevant history. On DRE, a distal rectal mass was palpable at the edge of the examiner's index finger. After a discussion with Mrs. Alamitos and her family, a decision was made to continue with staging investigations as her current symptoms were drastically reducing her QOL and increasing her daily care requirements.

After a brief discussion of his current health, Mr. Davos underwent a planned surveillance colonoscopy given his history of polyps and family history of CRC. In the ascending colon, a firm ulcerated non-obstructing mass was seen. Biopsies were taken and staging investigations ordered.

Staging Investigations for CRC

Once a CRC has been identified, full staging is required preceding treatment discussions. Computerized tomography (CT) of the chest, abdomen, and pelvis is recommended, although an ultrasound of the liver and radiograph of the chest may be acceptable in settings where CT scans are not accessible. Magnetic resonance imaging (MRI) of the rectum has become the gold standard of care for staging of rectal cancers (9, 11). For early rectal cancer, transrectal ultrasound may be the most appropriate for local staging.

For Mrs. Alamitos staging investigations were ordered by her primary care physician including a CT scan of the chest, abdomen, and pelvis, as well as an MRI of the rectum. She also ordered a CBC, electrolytes, creatinine required for the CT scan, and iron studies. A CEA was ordered for a baseline. A pre-albumin and albumin level were ordered to assess her nutritional status. She was referred to a colorectal surgeon for a colonoscopy to rule out a synchronous lesion and for discussion of treatment options. Her pelvic MRI demonstrated a rectal mass in the lower one-third of the rectum, bulky and significant upstream faecal loading. A colonoscopy was attempted but could not pass by the lesion. A virtual colonoscopy was ordered and did not demonstrate any other lesions.

Similar staging investigations were ordered for Mr. Davos. He has a history of moderate alcohol consumption and a liver panel including INR was ordered. The CT scan demonstrated a thickening of the ascending colon with no evidence of obstruction, and two lesions in the liver suspicious for metastatic disease. These were further characterized by an MRI and by morphology which were very consistent with metastatic disease. He was referred simultaneously to a colorectal and hepatobiliary surgeon.

TREATMENTS

Surgery remains the mainstay curative modality for the treatment of both colon and rectal cancer. The treatment of the latter, however, is increasingly complex and requires a multimodal approach. Treatment options include chemotherapy, radiation (short or long course), surgery (local and radical resections), and combinations of these. As such, all new rectal cancers should be referred to an experienced centre (3).

Prehabilitation: Process of improving the functional capacity of a patient prior to a surgical procedure. (See Glossary.)

Prehabilitation prior to colorectal surgery can positively affect the short- and long-term functional and oncologic outcomes of older CRC patients. This is especially true for frail patients. A multi-disciplinary team is essential for the success of these programs. Although the makeup of individual teams will vary, they often include geriatricians, internists, rehabilitation medicine physicians, physiotherapists, occupational therapists, geriatric nurse practitioners, social workers, a pharmacist, dietitians, and psychiatrists. Early identification of a frail patient will allow individual patients and their families to get the most out of the services provided (5). Where a specialized prehabilitation team is not available, a comprehensive geriatric assessment may help in many of the same ways, both with help on therapeutic decision making and reducing post-treatment complications (3). Without a multi-disciplinary team, unfortunately, there will be less support to the individual and their families to apply these recommendations than are available through a formal prehabilitation program.

Services can be tailored to the individual's needs. These can include nutritional support to deal with malnutrition, medical intervention to optimize cardiovascular and pulmonary health, medication revisions and modifications to improve glucose levels in diabetics, supplementation of iron stores for iron-deficiency anemia, and increasing stress tolerance and cardiovascular fitness through supervised exercise programs (e.g., stationary bicycles). Each of these interventions is designed to increase the patient's ability to withstand the physiologic stressor of CRC treatment. Minimizing polypharmacy and addressing risk factors for delirium can prepare patients and family for this common post-operative complication. Social workers may help the patient and family plan for the expected change in their functional capacity and independence during and following treatment.

Mrs. Alamitos was referred to the prehabilitation program at the time of her initial diagnoses. The first appointment, for a discussion of the functional outcome of surgery, was attended by her two children as well. She was counselled that she would need more support in her assisted living facility for at least the early post-treatment period. She was found to be moderately malnourished and met with the dietitian to begin a program of nutritional supplementation.

Mr. Davos was screened for frailty using the 10 min targeted geriatric assessment (TaGA) in the office (12). Investigation revealed significant iron-deficiency anemia and an elevated Hb A1c. He has also been on long-term benzodiazepines for help with sleep. He was referred to the prehabilitation program for medical optimization, a slow wean off his benzodiazepines and IV iron infusion for anemia in preparation for surgery.

Surgery

Oncologic colonic and rectal resections require segmental resections of the affected colon or rectum, along with the associated vascular pedicle and lymph node basin. Either an anastomosis is performed, or a stoma created with the distal small bowel (ileostomy) or colon (colostomy). Anastomotic leak remains the most devastating complication of CRC surgery with rate varying from 2% to 19% (13). Right-side anastomoses have a lower overall risk in comparison to left-sided anastomosis and the more distal the anastomosis, the higher the risk. Age is a minor risk factor for increased risk of anastomotic leak; however several co-morbidities which are increasingly prevalent with older age such as vascular, renal, and pulmonary disease are significant risk factors (13). Older adults have a lower physiologic reserve, making any surgical complication more devastating, and this contributes to their increased mortality in the post-operative period. Older adults who survive the first year have a similar CRC specific mortality to their younger counterparts (14).

There are ways to minimize the overall surgical risk in older adults. Laparoscopic surgery has been shown to be beneficial in the short term with reduced length of stay in hospital, reduced post-operative complications, and preserved functional status, without compromising overall survival or oncologic outcomes (15, 16). It has therefore become the standard approach in centres with the appropriate expertise. Emergency surgery has a significantly higher overall mortality in older adults in comparison to elective surgery, up to 30% vs 5%, and should be avoided whenever possible (14). This can be accomplished by an early discussion of the goal of treatment and establishing a plan for disease progression if surgery is declined upfront.

Curative intent treatment for metastatic disease in the older adult is more challenging as only complete resection of all gross disease provides significant oncologic benefit and these surgeries are often aggressive procedures with high morbidities. That is not to say that surgical resection cannot be pursued but the goal may be to focus on symptomatic management. Surgical diversion may provide the best QOL option for a patient with obstructing disease. Nonsurgical intervention such as endoscopic stenting can be considered. It is technically harder to do on the right than the left side. Local symptoms can worsen when a stent is placed too low in the rectum.

There are many different treatment algorithms for the treatment of rectal cancer (11). This is true in patients for whom the consequences of the removal of the rectum can have a profound effect on QOL (4). The need for neoadjuvant treatment with chemotherapy and radiation depends on multiple tumour- and patient-specific factors. Radiation treatment will decrease local recurrence but does not change overall survival and it can result in worse post-operative complications and functional impairment. Sphincter function and pre-operative continence needs to be carefully assessed prior to attempting an anastomosis low in the rectum. This procedure can affect the sphincter itself and removes the rectal reservoir which can result in debilitating symptoms including leakage, faecal urgency, and incontinence. The alternative, a permanent colostomy, has its own set of functional consequences. Considering the complexity of these discussions, it is recommended that all patients with rectal cancer be referred to a specialized centre and be reviewed by a multi-disciplinary tumour board (11).

Mrs. Alamitos' rectal tumour was low and near obstructing. Her frailty made her risk of complication high and the consequences of an anastomotic leak devastating. These factors along with her pre-operative incontinence, led her surgeon to recommend a resection with end-colostomy. She was presented to the tumour board and met with a radiation oncologist before deciding on treatment.

Mr. Davos has metastatic CRC. He was anemic because of chronic blood loss but has not had a clinically significant bleed. He was a good operative candidate for a laparoscopic right hemicolectomy given his overall functional status. The liver disease was localized to one lobe and was judged to be resectable with low morbidity by the hepatobiliary surgeon. He decided to proceed with a staged resection, and had his primary tumour removed initially followed by a liver resection, both of which went well.

Chemotherapy

Adjuvant chemotherapy is recommended for patients with high-risk stage II and stage III (node positive) CRC. It can also be used as a palliative treatment for metastatic CRC (17). In practice, older patients are less likely to receive chemotherapy and are less well represented in clinical trials, resulting in limited evidence on the benefit and risk of chemotherapy in this age group (17). Chemotherapy routines can include single agent oral capecitabine (a 5-Fluorouracil (5-FU) pro-drug), or combination therapies of 5-FU infusions, with or without leucovorin, and platinum-based agents such as oxaliplatin.

The combination regimes have demonstrated an overall and disease-free survival benefit when used as adjuvant therapy, but the benefit in patients over 70 is less clear and specifically the benefit of oxaliplatin in these patients is debated (14). Retrospective review of the SEER-Medicare database and ACCENT database found limited benefit of the addition of oxaliplatin in patients over 75 and 70 years of age, respectively. This lack of benefit was also seen in subset analyses of the NSABP C-07 and MOSAIC trial, but benefit was seen in other trials such as the NSABP C-08, XELOXA, X-ACT, and AVANT trials (18). There is an increased risk of acute and chronic toxicity from these combination regimes. Platinum-induced peripheral neurotoxicity is often the dose-limiting side effect of oxaliplatin, which is known to have a more chronic effect than other platinum-based agents. Oxaliplatin can result in prolonged or chronic pain, numbness, and cold sensitivity in the distal extremities, which can compound neuropathy from diabetes and peripheral vascular disease. This can result in difficulty with proprioception and fine motor skills. Frail patients with a poor performance status are not candidates for any adjuvant chemotherapy as the marginal survival benefits in these patients are offset by the upfront risks associated with the treatments.

In metastatic disease in the older adult, chemotherapy can be given with a palliative intent or a curative intent if the metastatic disease can be surgically resected. The goal of treatment is to improve overall survival while minimizing the toxicity and cost to a patient's QOL. Newer target agents, just as bevacizumab and cetuximab, should be considered in older patients if they are fit as the current limited evidence suggests that they have similar survival benefit in older adults as in their younger counterparts (3).

Mrs. Alamitos' overall health and functional status made her a poor candidate for systemic chemotherapy, and it was not offered. Mr. Davos had metastatic CRC and better functional status so he was offered chemotherapy with either a palliative intent to slow disease progression or neoadjuvant intent if surgical resection of his disease would be pursued.

Radiation Therapy

The use of radiation therapy is extremely limited in colon cancer due to injury to the radiosensitive small bowel, but it is part of the standard neoadjuvant treatment for locally advanced rectal cancer. It also has a role in the palliative treatment of bleeding rectal cancers. In practice, older adults are more often treated with radiation as part of a palliative approach than receive radiation in neoadjuvant setting (3). Neoadjuvant treatment can be delivered as a short course of 25 Greys over 5 days or a long course of 45 to 54 Greys over 25 to 28 days. Long course is usually given with concurrent radio sensitizing chemotherapy and followed by a delay of eight to ten weeks before surgery. Both treatment courses are well tolerated even in older adults, and anyone who would be considered a candidate for surgery is a candidate for radiation.

In a small percentage of rectal cancer patients, complete clinical response to radiation and chemotherapy may avoid surgery altogether. The 'watch and wait' approach to tumours which regressed and disappeared with neoadjuvant treatment is increasingly popular in older adults although they were excluded from early trials (14). The standard of care for 'watch and wait' requires regular surveillance every 3 months for the first 2 years with endoscopy and MRI, a schedule which can become onerous if attending appointments is difficult.

Given the bulk of her tumour, it would be reasonable to offer Mrs. Alamitos long-course radiation with chemo-sensitization. However, there was concern that she might develop worsening obstructive symptoms and getting back and forth for radiation treatment for a month was challenging for her and her family. They elected to proceed with short-course radiation to improve local control and facilitate proceeding to surgery without significant delay.

Metastatic Disease

Metastatic CRC is one of the few cancers in which limited disease is still curable. For fit older adults, there should be consideration of referral to a tertiary centre with expertise in the management of advanced disease where multi-disciplinary discussion of care is routine. With disease limited to the liver and/or the lungs, curative resections are still possible in up to 25% of patients. Palliation of symptoms can also involve a combination of treatments including surgical resection or diversion for obstructive symptoms, radiation for bleeding control, and chemotherapy for local and systemic disease control.

Mr. Davos has metastatic CRC and was offered chemotherapy. He had limited, surgically resectable disease and underwent upfront resection. Neoadjuvant treatment would have been a completely reasonable alternative. With all the gross disease resected, he has up to a 25% chance of achieving a long-term cure. He was therefore offered adjuvant chemotherapy and treated with three months of FOLFOX (5-FU, Leucovorin, and Oxaliplatin).

SURVIVAL AND SURVEILLANCE IN OLDER ADULTS

As more older adults receive successful treatment for CRC and survival increases, there is a large population of CRC survivors who require ongoing care. Survivorship care is often gradually transferred back to the primary care providers, and away from their surgeons and medical oncologists. Cancer survivorship does not necessarily mean a return to pre-treatment functional status and the morbidity of treatment often only becomes fully apparent over time (19).

In rectal cancer specifically, the restoration of bowel continuity is often one of the most important factors for patients when discussing treatment options. Older adults experience worse physical, cognitive, and social effects of treatment, but their overall QOL remains similar to young patients following treatment. Despite older adults being more likely to have a permanent ostomy, they maintain a high QOL score following treatment (20).

Managing with an Ostomy

Living with an ostomy presents a unique set of challenges and patients require active support while living in the community. Stoma-related complications are common and can have a devastating consequence on older adults' independence and QOL. All patients with an ostomy should be seen by an ostomy nurse specialist, also known as an enterostomal therapist (ET) or a wound, ostomy, and continence nurse (WOCN). These specially trained nurses are an essential support and guide to patients living with an ostomy. Caring for a stoma does require manual dexterity, and the inability to do so is an unfortunate but real reason for a patient to transition from independent living to an assisted living facility.

Diverting ileostomies are commonly placed to allow a distal rectal anastomosis to heal. The output from an ileostomy is semi-solid to liquid as it is small bowel contents. Moderate to high output can result in dehydration and electrolyte imbalances. Acute kidney injury is a common complication and careful monitoring of the output and aggressive management with anti-diarrheal agents, such as Lomotil and/or loperamide, are often required to prevent chronic kidney disease (CKD). The liquid contents are also irritating to the skin around the stoma and imperfect fitting of the stoma appliance can result in leakage, skin irritation, and peristomal dermatitis.

Long-term ostomies following CRC are more commonly colostomies and have a more solid output lessening the risk of acute kidney injury. Unfortunately, they have their own long-term complications including prolapse, stenosis, and peristomal hernia. Peristomal hernias occur in at least half of end-colostomies, although many surgeons would put that percentage much higher, and can interfere with proper pouch functioning, resulting in pain, obstruction, and large disfiguring bulges. Prevention of these hernias is difficult although some can be managed with appliance modifications and stoma belts. For the symptomatic hernia, the most lasting repair requires operative mesh placement as simply repositioning the stoma or suture-based repair inevitably led to short-term recurrence. Skin disorders are common, usually because of a poorly fitting appliance, but can also be a result of fungal infections or inflammatory disorders such as peristomal pyoderma gangrenosum. In patients with chronic stoma problems, there should be no hesitation in referring them back to their surgeon for discussion of management options if they are surgical candidates.

Low Anterior Resection Syndrome (LARS)

Low anterior resection syndrome (LARS) is a constellation of bowel symptoms which occurs following rectal cancer treatment, including variable unpredictable bowel function, increased frequency of bowel movements, urgency, clustering, incontinence, soiling, difficulty emptying, and pain with defecation (21). These symptoms have a well-characterized negative impact on a patient's QOL following sphincter sparing surgery (22, 23). These symptoms can be even more difficult to manage in older adults who have limited mobility and other functional limitations. A surgeon should be very hesitant to consider an anastomosis in a patient with any significant degree of pre-operative incontinence as their post-operative function will be debilitating. Management of LARS involved dietary measures including stool bulking with fibre supplementation, anti-diarrheal agents, and pelvic floor physiotherapy to improve pelvic floor strength. Other treatments like rectal irrigation and sacral neuromodulation require a highly motivated patient but can be tried if previous measures prove insufficient. The final treatment of unmanageable LARS is the creation of an end-colostomy (23). If a patient is unlikely to be able to manage the functional consequence of this common syndrome, early consideration should be given to proceeding with the end-colostomy at the time of initial resection. This approach also avoids the risk of anastomotic leak.

Surveillance

Following curative treatment, guidelines recommend an active surveillance program for the first five years (25). The benefit of surveillance is uncertain in stage I or IIA disease but has been clearly demonstrated in stage IIB and greater. History, physical exam, and CEA are recommended every 3 to 6 months for the first two years, then every 6–12 months for the following three years to complete a total of five years of surveillance. Colonoscopies are recommended at 1 year, 3 years, and 5 years post-operative. A full colonoscopy should be performed at 6 to 9 months post-operatively if the patient presented acutely obstructed and full colonic evaluation was not possible pre-operatively. CT scans of the chest, abdomen, and pelvis are recommended every 6 to 12 months for the first five years. For stage I disease, a less intensive surveillance schedule may be more appropriate. Surveillance should consider the overall health of the patient and should be pursued only if they are a candidate for further treatment.

Secondary Prevention

Secondary prevention for CRC is debatable. There is some data to suggest that daily aspirin may reduce the risk of recurrence and death as a results of CRC; however this must be balanced by the increased risk of bleeding complications. This is primarily based on observational data, and a randomized trial is ongoing (26).

REFERENCES

1. Howlader N NA, Krapcho M, Miller D, Brest A, Yu M, Ruhl J, Tatalovich Z, Mariotto A, Lewis DR, Chen HS, Feuer EJ, Cronin KA (eds). SEER Cancer Statistics Review, 1975–2018. National Cancer Institute Bethesda, MD.
2. Hurria A, Dale W, Mooney M, Rowland JH, Ballman KV, Cohen HJ, et al. Designing therapeutic clinical trials for older and frail adults with cancer: U13 conference recommendations. J Clin Oncol. 2014;32(24):2587–2594.
3. Papamichael D, Audisio RA, Glimelius B, de Gramont A, Glynne-Jones R, Haller D, et al. Treatment of colorectal cancer in older patients: International Society of Geriatric Oncology (SIOG) consensus recommendations 2013. Annals of Oncology. 2015;26(3):463–476.
4. Lapinsky E, Man LC, MacKenzie AR. Health-related quality of life in older adults with colorectal cancer. Curr Oncol Rep. 2019;21(9):81.
5. Saur NM, Davis B, Montroni I, Shahrokni A, Rostoft S, Russell M, et al. The American Society of Colon and Rectal Surgeons clinical practice guidelines for the perioperative evaluation and

management of frailty among older adults undergoing colorectal surgery. Dis Colon Rectum. 2022;65(4):473–488.

6. Arora A, Chadi SA, Chesney T. What should we recommend for colorectal cancer screening in adults aged 75 and older? Current Oncology. 2021;28(4):2540–2547.

7. Ebell MH, Thai TN, Royalty KJ. Cancer screening recommendations: an international comparison of high income countries. Public Health Rev. 2018;39:7.

8. Care CTFoPH. Recommendations on screening for colorectal cancer in primary care. Can Med Ass J. 2016;188(5):340–348.

9. Vogel JD, Felder SI, Bhama AR, Hawkins AT, Langenfeld SJ, Shaffer VO, et al. The American Society of Colon and Rectal Surgeons clinical practice guidelines for the management of colon cancer. Diseases Colon Rect. 2022;65(2):148–177.

10. Lippert E, Herfarth HH, Grunert N, Endlicher E, Klebl F. Gastrointestinal endoscopy in patients aged 75 years and older: risks, complications, and findings—a retrospective study. Int J Colorectal Dis. 2015;30(3):363–366.

11. You YN, Hardiman KM, Bafford A, Poylin V, Francone TD, Davis K, et al. The American Society of Colon and Rectal Surgeons clinical practice guidelines for the management of rectal cancer. Dis Colon Rectum. 2020;63(9):1191–222.

12. Aliberti MJR, Apolinario D, Suemoto CK, Melo JA, Fortes-Filho SQ, Saraiva MD, et al. Targeted geriatric assessment for fast-paced healthcare settings: Development, validity, and reliability. J Am Geriatr Soc. 2018;66(4):748–754.

13. McDermott FD, Heeney A, Kelly ME, Steele RJ, Carlson GL, Winter DC. Systematic review of preoperative, intraoperative and postoperative risk factors for colorectal anastomotic leaks. Brit J Surg. 2015;102(5):462–479.

14. Millan M, Merino S, Caro A, Feliu F, Escuder J, Francesch T. Treatment of colorectal cancer in the elderly. World J Gastrointest Oncol. 2015;7(10):204–220.

15. Fujii S, Tsukamoto M, Fukushima Y, Shimada R, Okamoto K, Tsuchiya T, et al. Systematic review of laparoscopic vs open surgery for colorectal cancer in elderly patients. World J Gastrointest Oncol. 2016;8(7):573–582.

16. Moug SJ, McCarthy K, Coode-Bate J, Stechman MJ, Hewitt J. Laparoscopic versus open surgery for colorectal cancer in the older person: A systematic review. Ann Med Surg (Lond). 2015;4(3):311–318.

17. Kim JH. Chemotherapy for colorectal cancer in the elderly. World J Gastroenterol. 2015;21(17):5158–566.

18. Network NCC. Colon Cancer https://www.nccn.org/professionals/physician_gls/pdf/colon.pdf2021 [Version 2.2021].

19. Kent EE, Park EM, Wood WA, Bryant AL, Mollica MA. Survivorship care of older adults with cancer: priority areas for clinical practice, training, research, and policy. J Clinic Oncol. 2021;39(19):2175–2184.

20. Manceau G, Karoui M, Werner A, Mortensen NJ, Hannoun L. Comparative outcomes of rectal cancer surgery between elderly and non-elderly patients: a systematic review. Lancet Oncol. 2012;13(12):e525–e536.

21. Keane C, Fearnhead NS, Bordeianou LG, Christensen P, Basany EE, Laurberg S, et al. International consensus definition of low anterior resection syndrome. Diseases Colon Rectum. 2020;63(3):274–284.

22. Sturiale A, Martellucci J, Zurli L, Vaccaro C, Brusciano L, Limongelli P, et al. Long-term functional follow-up after anterior rectal resection for cancer. Int J Colorect Disease: Clinic Molecul Gastroenterol Surg. 2017;32(1):83–8.

23. Battersby NJ, Juul, T., Christensen, P., Janjua, A. Z., Branagan, G., Emmertsen, K. J., Norton, C., Hughes, R., Laurberg, S. & Moran, B. J. Predicting the risk of bowel-related quality-of-life impairment after restorative resection for rectal cancer: a multicenter cross-sectional study. Diseases Colon Rectum. 2016;59(4):270–280.

24. Christensen P, IM Baeten C, Espín-Basany E, Martellucci J, Nugent KP, Zerbib F, et al. Management guidelines for low anterior resection syndrome—the MANUEL project. Colorectal Disease. 2021;23(2):461–475.

25. Liu SL, Cheung WY. Role of surveillance imaging and endoscopy in colorectal cancer follow-up: quality over quantity? World J Gastroenterol. 2019;25(1):59–68.

26. Elwood PC, Morgan G, Delon C, Protty M, Galante J, Pickering J, et al. Aspirin and cancer survival: a systematic review and meta-analyses of 118 observational studies of aspirin and 18 cancers. Ecancermedicalscience. 2021;15:1258.

30 Precision Medicine and Care of the Older Patient

Anne Croudass, RN, MSc and Donald White, PhD

CONTENTS

CASE STUDY PART I: Standard of Care Chemotherapy for NSCLC

Bill was a 79-year-old man with a diagnosis of stage III non-small-cell lung cancer (NSCLC). He lived independently at home with his wife of 57 years.

Bill was considered 'fit for his age' by his friends and family, still drove a car, played bowls once a week, and attended his local church every Sunday. For over 5 years Bill had been the main carer for his wife who had severe osteo-arthritis and limited mobility. He did all the shopping and enjoyed preparing their meals, claiming to have become a rather competent self-taught chef in his old age. Other than a daily aspirin and the occasional painkiller, Bill's only 'medication' was a small glass of whisky before bed to 'help him sleep'.

Sudden weight loss, increased breathlessness, and a general lethargy, however, prompted Bill to go to his GP, ultimately leading to his NSCLC diagnosis. A first-line treatment of six 21-day cycles of vinorelbine and cisplatin were subsequently prescribed and commenced shortly after diagnosis. To receive this treatment, Bill had to attend hospital for approximately 8 hours on day 1 and 3 hours on day 8 of each 21-day cycle.

In order to attend his hospital appointments, Bill had to arrange care for his wife. As they had no family nearby this involved a private care agency which involved financial outlay and emotional distress for his wife, who was not comfortable with different people coming in and out of their house.

Bill also suffered significant side effects from the chemotherapy. While the physiological side effects were managed pharmaceutically, the emotional, psychological, and social impact was considerable. Changes in taste and appetite, for example, meant that Bill lost all interest in cooking and eating. Severe fatigue resulting from the treatment, exacerbated by lengthy hospital visits, also prevented him driving and pursuing regular social activities. In addition, Bill required 2 blood transfusions during his course of chemotherapy, requiring him to sort out care for his wife at short notice. Sadly, both Bill and his wife were negatively impacted by the severity and nature of his side effects. Being dependent on Bill as her sole carer she, like Bill, experienced significant weight loss, social isolation, and depression, eventually requiring hospitalization from the combined effects of Bill's treatment.

Bill did eventually recover from the more acute side effects of his treatment, but only after his cycles of chemotherapy had finally ended. He and his wife, following her discharge from hospital, were then able to resume the activities they enjoyed prior to his diagnosis, with minimal external support. Unfortunately, Bill's cancer did eventually return 10 months after cessation of the chemotherapy. Since Bill and his wife had learned so much about the quality of time remaining rather than the quantity, they decided this time that they would rather pursue the palliative care option rather than undertake any further chemotherapy. Any success in temporarily shrinking the size of the tumour had been offset by the very significant negative impact on Bill's quality of life, as well as that of his wife. It was a path they did not wish to pursue again.

CASE STUDY PART II: Precision Medicine Option for NSCLC

Bill's case, to this point, is a classic example of the challenges facing cancer patients whose only option is chemotherapy. The toxic side effects and hospital visits that impacted Bill's health and ability to care for his wife ultimately led to the unfortunate choice of continuing treatment versus palliative care.

The toxicity of chemotherapy typically comes down to the mechanism of action of these medicines, which often target universal mechanisms of rapidly growing cells, such as cell division and

DOI: 10.1201/9781003344476-34

chromosome segregation pathways, which can indiscriminately target tissues such as blood, hair, and intestinal epithelium, as well as promote liver and kidney toxicity. Many of these compounds were initially identified through screening the effects of natural products on the growth of tumour cells in culture (ref 1). The natural origin of such compounds means that they often have large, complex chemical structures that require modification to increase absorption and distribution. Despite these efforts, the physiological barriers to absorption and distribution at various points along the way to reaching a tumour nonetheless necessitates intravenous administration, requiring prolonged hospital visits.

At the time of Bill's struggle with his cancer, however, another treatment option for NSCLC was emerging, one which held the promise of both reduced toxicity and relative ease of administration. Upon consultation with his oncologist and Clinical Nurse Specialist (CNS), Bill agreed to commence treatment with erlotinib, one of several examples of a relatively new class of compounds designed to target specific molecular changes within his cancer cells, rather than universal mechanisms of cell growth and division (ref 2). In Bill's case, the molecular target was the epidermal growth factor receptor (EGFR), suspected to be a common driver of tumour growth in NSCLC. A mutation in EGFR in Bill's tumour had been earlier identified by sequencing of DNA from his diagnostic biopsy. Central to Bill's decision was the fact that there was a strong likelihood that the treatment would provide benefit, in that his tumour was likely to respond to erlotinib, an inhibitor of the tumour-promoting EGFR kinase activity implied through sequencing of Bill's tumour. But perhaps more importantly for Bill and his wife, erlotinib could be self-administered orally at home, required fewer hospital visits, and had more manageable side effects. Lengthy turn-around time on the sequencing, however, combined with the urgency to start treatment for an aggressive disease like NSCLC, meant that Bill's oncologist initially chose standard of care chemotherapy over the more experimental strategy involving erlotinib. Bill eventually agreed to commence treatment on erlotinib on the understanding that he would stop the treatment if the side effects were too extreme and his quality of life was again affected.

The Emergence and Delivery of Precision Medicine

Bill's story was made possible through several simultaneous and complementary advances in DNA sequencing technology, chemical design, and synthesis of small molecule inhibitors, and the emerging field of molecular pathology. Advances in DNA sequencing technology in fact made possible the widespread analysis of tumour tissue across cancer types and subtypes, identifying mutations in genes—as well as copy number and structural rearrangements—associated with specific pathologies. The resulting field of molecular pathology slowly started to reveal specific underlying molecular features of individual cancers, within and between individual patients, which could not be identified by histology alone.

At first, these molecular profiles were used to classify individual cancers into subtypes which were useful for sorting patients into groups of those who responded well to standard therapy and those who did not. Relentless work by research scientists, however, started to separate out those genetic changes which played a direct role in tumour growth and development, versus those which had more of a bystander role. The result was a new industry designed to target pathologic or tumour-promoting 'driver' mutations, through the synthesis of small molecules which could inhibit the activity of a specific tumour-promoting gene product. Erlotinib is one such molecule, targeting aberrant protein kinases such as EGFR. Since the introduction of erlotinib, numerous small-molecule inhibitors have subsequently been synthesized which target a growing list of tumour-promoting kinases and aberrant proteins resulting from gene fusions and rearrangements, which are associated with specific indications and which can be identified through sequencing of the patient's DNA and RNA.

In contrast to bulky chemotherapeutic agents harbouring a large, complex chemical structure requiring IV administration, targeted small-molecule compounds like erlotinib are rationally designed at the minimal level of complexity and size, facilitating more efficient tissue distribution and allowing for formulations in pill form. For patients like Bill, this made a world of difference, being able to self-administer his medication while caring for his wife. And by targeting a specific tumour-promoting protein activity rather than a general feature of cell division, the widespread toxicity and malaise of chemotherapy can be circumvented.

Today, the challenge is to provide genetic testing at scale and in an affordable way. Providing a way to offer the advantages of targeted therapy, commonly known now as precision medicine, to a majority of cancer patients is certainly one objective. The other objective, however, is to offer repeated testing for each patient during the course of their therapy, to detect changes in the mutational landscape that may drive resistance and relapse. A further acquired change in EGFR, known as T790M, for example, resulted in resistance to erlotinib in a proportion of NSCLC patients. In line with the objectives of precision medicine, however, the compound osimertinib was subsequently developed specifically to target EGFR T790M, thereby offering a treatment option to those with NSCLC refractory to erlotinib (ref 3).

A recent addition to the precision medicine tool kit is the ability to follow disease progression and response to treatment through a simple blood test. The presence of residual disease, for example, can now be monitored through detection of DNA fragments released into the blood of patients by resident tumour cells (ref 4). More specifically, detection of DNA sequences and mutations associated with the initial assignment of patients into treatment modalities can be used to monitor the efficacy of the treatments. Local access to a general practitioner (family doctor) and nurse may be enough to facilitate treatment and monitoring, which is especially important for those older patients who live far from hospitals or large cancer care clinics, or who have dependents, such as in the case of Bill and his wife.

Precision medicine can be regarded as a subset of personalized medicine, a broad term taking into consideration the overall needs of a patient during the entire process from diagnosis through treatment, and any follow-up care and monitoring. The needs that are unique to any patient can include age, mobility, socioeconomic status, dietary restrictions, co-dependents, and so on. By addressing the needs of older patients in particular, precision medicine's place within the broader category of personalized medicine becomes more and more apparent.

But these needs include more than just finding the right treatment for a particular tumour, and one that can be delivered at home. An important and understated feature of precision medicine is in the ability to identify patients who would not benefit at all from existing therapies, whether targeted or otherwise. This last feature of precision medicine is worth highlighting, as overtreatment and treatment that has no benefit to the patient can worsen the quality of life while contributing to financial pressures and loss of work and time for family and other caregivers. In other words, precision medicine aims not only to identify patients who may benefit from a treatment, but also those who will likely not benefit from that same treatment. For older persons and their carers, precision medicine therefore provides another level of objective decision making to help families and patients make decisions that might otherwise be weighed down by doubt, uncertainty, and possibly regret.

CASE STUDY PART III: Bill's Journey

In contrast to the debilitating and disruptive effects of chemotherapy on him and his wife, Bill tolerated the erlotinib well, other than some gastrointestinal side effects which were controlled with regular loperamide and a mild skin rash which responded to emollients as required. Although Bill suffered from mild fatigue, he found that it did not impact his interest in his social activities. More importantly, his taste and appetite were not affected, and he was able to continue to act as the main carer for his wife.

Administration of erlotinib controlled the growth of Bill's cancer for a further 18 months, during which time he continued to enjoy his hobbies, spend quality time with his wife and even take short holidays. This was quality time that he was unlikely to have had if he had either embarked on further rounds of chemotherapy, or, as he initially planned, opted for supportive and palliative care.

CONCLUSION

Precision medicine is transformative, having the potential to revolutionize the impact of cancer treatments for elderly patients and their families, who often reside in fragile, co-dependent relationships, relying on each other for aspects of care and activities of daily living. While this chapter focused on the case of NSCLC and cancer in general, the potential of precision medicine applies to any disease where a patient can be matched to a drug or other intervention, based on a molecular profile specific to the patient and matching the molecular criteria for the treatment. Although we are still in the transitory stages of adopting precision medicine as a standard of care approach to disease, the approval of targeted therapies and companion diagnostics by the FDA (ref 5) and other regulatory bodies demonstrates the reality and inevitability of this approach. For patients like Bill and his wife, who valued their quality time together above all else, this will make all the difference.

REFERENCES

1. PMID: 20840315 https://pubmed.ncbi.nlm.nih.gov/?term=cancer+chemotherapy+annotated+history
2. PMID: 20530444 https://pubmed.ncbi.nlm.nih.gov/20530444/
3. PMID: 27885838 https://pubmed.ncbi.nlm.nih.gov/27885838/
4. PMID: 33049662 https://pubmed.ncbi.nlm.nih.gov/33049662/
5. https://www.cancer.gov/about-cancer/treatment/types/targeted-therapies/targeted-therapies-fact-sheet

31 Psycho-Oncology

Living with the Fear of Death

Norman Straker, MD, DLFAPA

CONTENTS

Psycho-oncology is a subspecialty of psychiatry that specifically addresses the emotional and psychiatric care of cancer patients and their families. While cancer is no longer a death sentence, much more frequently a treatable or chronic disease, the emotional experience of carrying a cancer diagnosis for some patients is terrifying and the most difficult part of the disease. However, many doctors and patients are inclined to avoid any discussion about their anxieties about cancer and their fears of dying.

My education as a medical student, intern, resident, and psychoanalyst left out the problem of how to help patients face death and how one can have a dialogue with a patient dealing with the patient's concerns about dying. In fact, to a large extent my experience is that for the most part the problem of avoiding the patient's concerns about dying is still true to the present time.

The longstanding avoidance of helping patients manage their fears and concerns about dying because of the discomfort of the doctor or therapist should no longer be accepted.

Psychotherapy with patients facing death requires a deep personal involvement in the patient's life and the angst that is facing all of us. It is a daunting task. The intimate connection with the dying person is an essential part of the therapeutic process. Usually the therapist is the singular person with whom the patient shares their daily suffering and their concerns about dying.

A wall of silence usually surrounds the patient and the family about such matters. The patient often wants to be remembered as stoic and brave and does not want to be a burden to the family. The family worries that any discussion with the patient about their declining health will lead to the patient feeling hopeless, and that he or she is dying. The therapist's openness to such discussions lessens the patient's aloneness and isolation and can be extremely helpful.

To some degree, depending on the personality of the oncologist, he or she may be involved to a greater or lesser degree in some of the same issues, although to a more limited extent. For some oncologists, however, the acknowledgement that the treatments are no longer working is experienced as a personal failure and is hard to accept. This denial may delay a referral for palliative or hospice care.

It has been my good fortune to benefit from some research on the natural defenses against death anxiety known as terror management (Solomon, 2011). These natural defenses include the individual's life achievements that will live on after a patient dies and an elevated self-esteem. I have incorporated and modified this research to lessen a patient's anxiety about dying. While dying, patients tell their life story, which they tend to do naturally. I suggest validating their achievements and attempting to find aspects of their life that can be complemented as contributing to the greater good. This will raise their self-esteem.

The availability of these interventions has helped me and others feel more comfortable and competent with patients facing imminent death. It has allowed for a detailed dialogue about patients' concerns about dying and death.

A more detailed account of my psychotherapeutic work with cancer patients who survived and those who died, along with detailed case presentations, is available in the bibliography that follows.

PSYCHIATRIC DISORDERS IN CANCER PATIENTS

Some psychiatric disorders in the cancer setting are responses to the cancer illness, while others are preexisting conditions that may be exacerbated by the cancer illness. Recent studies have observed that adjustment disorder, major depression, delirium, and anxiety disorders occur in between 10% and 34% of cancer patients (Zabora et al., 2001; Roth et al., 1998; Zabora and MacMurray, 2012).

DOI: 10.1201/9781003344476-35

Adjustment disorder is characterized by severe anxiety or depressive symptoms in response to a life stressor and causes undue interference with occupational, social, or school functioning. An initial diagnosis of adjustment disorder may be the beginning stages of a more severe anxiety or depressive disorder (Li et al., 2012).

Anxiety disorders can be associated with the diagnosis and treatment of cancer or can be related to preexisting chronic anxiety exacerbated during treatment (Noyes et al., 1998). The diagnosis of anxiety in cancer patients must be distinguished from medical problems such as inadequate pain control, delirium, steroids, respiratory distress from hypoxia or pulmonary embolism, withdrawal from alcohol, benzodiazepines, and narcotics, or akathisia (see Glossary).

Panic disorders and certain medical phobias can worsen in the medical setting (Miller and Massie, 2006) and can make medical treatment more difficult. Post-traumatic stress disorder (PTSD) is a specific type of anxiety disorder which can be caused by a life-threatening illness, like cancer. The prevalence of PTSD in cancer patients ranges from 5% to 19% (Rustad et al., 2012).

The diagnosis of depression in cancer patients can be difficult, because the physical symptoms of depression and cancer, and the symptoms caused by cancer treatment, often overlap. Identification of dysphoric mood, apathy, crying, anhedonia (see Glossary), feelings of helplessness, hopelessness, decreased self-esteem, guilt, social withdrawal, and thoughts of "wishing for death" or suicidal ideation are the hallmarks of depression (Snyderman and Wynn, 2009). Higher prevalence of depression in cancer patients is associated with a physical impairment, advanced stages of illness, inadequately controlled pain, and poor social support (Massie et al., 1989). Patients with pancreatic, oropharyngeal, gastric, and lung cancers also have higher rates of depression (Li et al., 2012). A few chemotherapeutic agents, such as prednisone, dexamethasone, vincristine, vinblastine, procarbazine, asparaginase, tamoxifen, interferon, and interleukin- 2, produce depressive symptoms. Depressive symptoms can also be produced by metabolic, nutritional, and endocrine disorders, such as electrolyte abnormalities; deficiencies of folate or vitamin B12; and hypothyroidism, hyperthyroidism, or adrenal insufficiency (Hall, 1978).

Cancer patients are two times more likely to commit suicide than individuals in the general population (Snyderman and Wynn, 2009). Those at a higher risk for suicide are those with a poor prognosis, advanced stage of illness, a psychiatric history or a history of substance abuse, previous suicide attempts, or a family history of suicide (Breitbart, 1989; Zweig and Hinrichsen, 1993; Dubovsky, 1978; Murphy, 1977) and those with lung, stomach, pharyngeal, or laryngeal cancers (Snyderman and Wynn, 2009).

Delirium presents with restlessness, confusion, disorientation and needs to be differentiated from anxiety. The initial management of delirium requires correction of the underlying medical or physiological causes and a reevaluation of the necessity of all medications that can cause mental status changes. Important nonpharmacologic interventions include providing a safe and supportive environment for patient, staff, and family. (See Chapter 8, How to Diagnose and Manage Delirium by Haibin Yin.)

SYMPTOMS OF CANCER AND THEIR RELATIONSHIP TO PSYCHIATRIC DISORDERS

Pain, fatigue, insomnia, sexual dysfunction, including side effects from chemotherapy, radiation, pain meds, and symptoms of the disease, contribute to psychiatric disorders and need to be differentiated from psychiatric disorders.

Uncontrolled pain often interferes with sleep, can cause insomnia, and contributes to psychiatric symptoms. Steroids often interfere with sleep and can cause psychiatric disorders (Howell et al., 2014). Sexual dysfunction and infertility can be the result of irradiation, surgery, and chemotherapy, or can be concomitant with a psychiatric disorder (Desimone et al., 2014).

BIBLIOGRAPHY

Breitbart W. (1989) Suicide in cancer patients. In: Holland J, Rowland J, eds. Handbook of Psycho-Oncology: Psychological Care of the Patient with Cancer. New York: Oxford University Press; 291–299.

Bukberg J, Straker N. (1982) The psychiatric consultant and the ambivalent surgical patient with cancer. Psychosomatics, October.

Desimone M, Spriggs E, Gass JS, Carson SA, Krychman ML, Dizon DS. (2014) Sexual dysfunction in female cancer survivors. J Clin Oncol.; 37:101–106.

DieTrill M, Straker N. (1993) Psychological adaptation to facial disfigurement in a female head and neck cancer patient Psycho-Oncology issue #4.

Dubovsky SL. (1978) Averting suicide in terminally ill patients. Psychosomatics.; 19: 113–115.

Hall RC, Popkin MK, Devaul RA, Faillace LA, Stickney SK. (1978) Physical illness presenting as psychiatric disease. Arch Gen Psychiatry.; 35:1315–1320.

Howell D, Oliver TK, Keller-Olaman S, et al. (2014) Sleep disturbance in adults with cancer: a systematic review of evidence for best practices in assessment and management for clinical practice. Ann Oncol.; 25:791–800.

Kissane DW, Clarke DM. (2001) Demoralization syndrome—A relevant psychiatric diagnosis for palliative care. J Palliat Care.; 17:12–21.

Li M, Fitzgerald P, Rodin G. (2012) Evidence-based treatment of depression in patients with cancer. J Clin Oncol.; 30:1187–1196.

Massie MJ, Holland JC, Straker N. (1989) Psychotherapeutic interventions. In: Holland JC, Rowland Eds. Oxford Press, NY: Handbook of Psycho-Oncology.

Miller K, Massie MJ. (2006) Depression and anxiety. Cancer J. 12:388–39734.

Mount BF, Boston PH. (2007) Healing connections: on moving from suffering to a sense of well-being. J Pain Symptom Manag.; Apr 33 (4):372–388.

Murphy GE. (1977) Suicide and attempted suicide. Hosp Pract.; 12:73–81.

Noyes R, Holt C, Massie M. (1998) Anxiety disorders. In: Holland J, ed. Psycho-Oncology. New York: Oxford.

Pao M, Kazak AE (2009) Anxiety and depression. In: Weiner LS, Pao M, Kazak AE, Kupst MJ, Patenaude AF, eds. Quick Reference for Pediatric Oncology Clinicians: The Psychiatric and Psychological Dimensions of Pediatric Cancer Symptom Management. Charlottesville, VA: IPOS Press.

Robinson Burney S, Kissane DW, Brooker J, Burney S. (2015) A systematic review of the demoralization syndrome in individuals with progressive disease and cancer: a decade of research. J Pain Symptom Manage.; 49:595–610.

Roth AJ et al. (1998) https:doi.org/10.1002(SICI)1097-0142(19980515)82:10<1904:AID-CNCR13>3.0. CO:2-X

Rustad JK, David D, Currier MB. (2012) Cancer and post-traumatic stress disorder: diagnosis, pathogenesis and treatment considerations. Palliat Support Care.; 10:213–223.

Snyderman D, Wynn D. (2009). Depression in cancer patients. Prim Care.; 36:703–719.

Solomon S. Greenberg J, Pyszczynski T., 2015 The Worm at the Core: On the Role of Life in Death. New York: House.

Solomon S, Lawlor K. https://doi.org/10.1007/978-1-4419-9440-0 9

Straker N. (1998) Psychodynamic psychotherapy for cancer patients. J Psychothe Pract Res.; 7:11–19.

Straker N. (2005) The courage to survive: facing the loss of your soul-mate. Video presentation (www.Internationalpsychoanalysis.net).

Straker N. (2008) Dynamic psychotherapy for cancer patients and their spouses. Psychiatric Times; 8(9):119–121.

Straker N. (2011) The courage to survive: facing the loss of your soul-mate. Palliative and Supportive Care.; 9(2).

Straker N. (2013) Facing Cancer and the Fear of Death: A Psychoanalytic Perspective on Treatment. Lanham, MD: Rowman and Littlefield.

Straker N. (2019a). Psychodynamic psychiatry for cancer patients, survivorship accepted for sept publication psychodynamic psychiatry.

Straker N. (2019b) Psychodynamic psychotherapy: the treatment of cancer patients who die accepted for sept publication psychodynamic psychiatry.

Straker N, Drazen R. (1990) On the edge of being: when doctors confront cancer. Video presentation (www.internationalpsychoanalysis.net).

Zabora J, MacMurray I. (2012) The history of psychosocial screening among cancer patients. J Psychosoc Oncol.; 30(6):625–635.

Zabora J et al. (2001) The prevalence of psychological distress by cancer site. Psycho-Oncology; 10(1):19–28.

Zweig RA, Hinrichsen GA. (1993) Factors associated with suicide attempts by depressed older adults: a prospective study. Am J Psychiatry.; 150:1687–1692.

PART V
CONSIDERATIONS

32 Incontinence in Older Adults

Samer Shamout, MD, MSc and Lysanne Campeau, MDCM, PhD, FRCS(C)

CONTENTS

CLINICAL VIGNETTE

An 83-year-old man with Alzheimer's disease is being cared for at home. During the past 2 months, his wife has noticed that it is increasingly difficult for him to make it to the restroom in time to urinate. He has stopped telling her when he needs to use the restroom, and she is unable to direct him to the restroom in the house quickly enough. This is causing significant caregiver stress. His wife believes his cognition has begun to worsen during the past 6 months, and she is considering placing him in a nursing home. His medication list includes terazosin 2 mg at bedtime, aspirin 81 mg daily, donepezil 10 mg at bedtime, lisinopril 5 mg daily, and venlafaxine extended release 75 mg daily. His Mini-Mental State Examination score is 15/30, and his Geriatric Depression Scale is 3/15. Standing blood pressure is 110/70 mm Hg.

The urinary incontinence is a significant problem for this patient and his caregiver, and should be addressed with appropriate workup and management plan.

WHY IS URINARY INCONTINENCE A REMARKABLE CLINICAL CONDITION IN ELDERLY POPULATION?

Urinary incontinence (UI) is a common and undertreated condition of morbidity in Canada and worldwide, with peak prevalence in the geriatric population. Approximately 3.3 million (10%) Canadians experience urinary incontinence, of whom 30% to 60% are over 65 years old. The prevalence of incontinence increases noticeably with age, affecting 19% of women and 10% of men above 60 years old. Urinary incontinence (UI) is defined as the complaint of involuntary leakage of urine.

The cost of UI in this population extends beyond monetary costs. It has a substantial negative impact on physical, psychological, and health-related quality of life. Moreover, UI has a great economic burden on society and on the healthcare system. It has been linked to many other critical health risks, including increased risk of hospitalization, frailty, fractures, functional disability, and depression. The social implications of incontinence include diminished self-esteem, restriction of social and sexual activities, and increased caregiver burden.

Unfortunately, elderly individuals encounter several obstacles in obtaining treatment for their problems. UI is rarely discussed by patients, many of whom are less likely to seek healthcare for this condition as they assume that UI is a part of aging process and there is no existing successful treatment.

WHAT ARE THE RISK FACTORS FOR UI?

The etiology of UI among the geriatric population is different and often multifactorial. As people age, physiological and functional changes in the lower urinary tract may contribute to the loss of continence in this population. Frail elderly people may have multiple comorbid medical illnesses, lifestyle, and medication changes that can cause or predispose to UI. Therefore, the evaluation and management of UI in older adults should be multidisciplinary with comprehensive understanding of the multidimensional concept of continence.

Risk factors for UI in women include changes related to anatomy, previous childbirth, hysterectomy, and menopause. Loss of estrogen at menopause and changes in the pelvic connective tissue

DOI: 10.1201/9781003344476-37

support may explain higher prevalence of UI in postmenopausal women. On the other side, factors associated with UI in men include prostatic enlargement or prostate surgery. Despite surgical advances, UI is frequently observed following prostate surgery, with reported estimates ranging from 6% to nearly 70%.

Multiple other conditions are also associated with UI in the frail elderly population. These include:

- Uncontrolled comorbid medical conditions that predispose to polyuria or increased nighttime urine production (e.g., congestive heart failure, peripheral venous insufficiency, diabetes mellitus, sleep apnea).

- Conditions resulting in impaired mobility and/or cognition (e.g., stroke, Parkinson's disease, degenerative joint disease, dementia).

- Constipation and fecal impaction that may contribute to double incontinence (urinary and fecal).

- Mental and cognitive disorders (e.g., depression and dementia).

- Medications: diuretics, calcium channel blockers, prostaglandin inhibitors, alpha-adrenoceptor blockers, selective serotonin reuptake inhibitors, cholinesterase inhibitors, opioid analgesics, psychotropic drugs, and systemic hormone replacement therapy.

- Environmental factors (e.g., inaccessible toilets or unavailable caregivers for toileting assistance).

In general, it is challenging to distinguish a single etiology responsible in the vast majority of geriatric population, as more often several factors interact. These possible causes of reversible UI can be summarized in a mnemonic DIAPPERS (Delirium, Infection, Atrophic vaginitis, Psychological, Pharmacologic, Excess urine output, Restricted mobility, and Stool impaction).

HOW IS THE DIAGNOSIS OF UI MADE?

There are different types of UI in elderly population: urgency urinary incontinence (UUI) (involuntary loss of urine associated with urgency), stress urinary incontinence SUI (involuntary loss of urine on effort or physical exertion, or on sneezing/coughing), and mixed UI (a combination of SUI and UUI). A concomitant related condition which is associated with UUI is called overactive bladder syndrome (OAB), defined as urinary urgency, usually accompanied by frequency and nocturia, with or without urgency UI, in the absence of urinary tract infection or other obvious pathology. Other distinct entities are nocturia (frequent nocturnal micturition), and 'functional' incontinence (incontinence caused by either physical or cognitive impairment, with no identifiable lower urinary tract disorder), all being associated with extensive patient and caregiver burden (Table 32.1).

Table 32.1 Common Types of Urinary Incontinences

Overactive Bladder	Stress UI	Mixed UI	Impaired Bladder Emptying	Functional Incontinence
Urinary urgency, with or without urgency incontinence, often with urinary frequency and nocturia	Urinary loss in association with exertion such as coughing, laughing, or lifting	Symptoms of both urgency incontinence and exertional incontinence (take a careful history as urgency or precipitancy is often reported by women with stress UI only)	Incomplete emptying is not well reported by men, but more so by women. A large post-void residual volume without symptoms (recurrent UTI, frequency, dribble, upper tract involvement) does not need treatment (a 250-ml residual volume may be acceptable in older people)	Incontinence unrelated to an underlying disorder or lower urinary tract function, perhaps related to either physical or cognitive impairment

Source: Modified from Urinary incontinence in older adults. *Medicine.* 2017;45(1):23–27.

HOW SHOULD PATIENTS BE INVESTIGATED?

Unlike urinary incontinence evaluation in younger adults, frail older persons often require a comprehensive approach (Table 32.2). The basic evaluation should primarily emphasize identification of transient and established causes of UI, assess the patient's environment and existing support, the degree of bother to the patient, and recognize other less common but serious entities that may trigger incontinence. The primary step is active screening for UI in the geriatric population, as more than 50% of elderly patients do not report their urinary symptoms to their healthcare providers. This could be due to numerous reasons, including social embarrassment, coping with symptoms, or misunderstanding that UI is a part of aging process and nothing can be done to improve this condition (grade A). The patient history is often the most important element in recognizing the type, severity, and burden of incontinence for those patients. Commonly, clinical evaluation requires numerous office visits for frail older individuals in order to perform the necessary tests and to avoid additional assessment in patients who respond to ordinary measures.

History

The history should identify treatable, potentially reversible comorbid conditions, functional and cognitive impairment, and current medications that can cause or exacerbate UI in frail older people (grade B). The mnemonic DIAPPERS has been commonly utilized to remember these conditions. The basic assessment must include an evaluation of the frequency and duration of symptoms, associated factors or events, precipitating and influential factors, and any measures of control that have already been used. During the history, account should be taken of the patient's medical and surgical history (i.e., bowel, menstrual, obstetric, and sexual history), and risk factors which help recognize possible influencing factors on symptoms. Furthermore, fluid/volume status, symptom severity, accessibility to toilets and social support, patients' and caregivers' expectations for UI care, should be explicitly explored (grade B). It is also essential to consider the patient's likely level of cooperation, overall prognosis and life expectancy (grade C).

In frail elderly people with bothersome nocturia, the treating physician should focus on detecting any potential triggering factors, including sleep apnea, nocturnal polyuria, and conditions associated with elevated post-void residual (PVR). A complete and precise bladder diary (frequency-volume chart) of a minimum 3 days' duration can be a useful tool in the assessment of individuals with nocturia (grade C). However, this may not always be feasible for all patients and caregivers.

Physical Examination

The initial step is to perform a relevant pelvic or genital and rectal examination to evaluate for vaginal/genital atrophy, pelvic organ prolapse, prostate nodules or masses, sphincter tone, fecal impaction and the presence of a distended bladder or a pelvic mass. The initial physical examination should also include cognitive and functional assessments as well as examination for relevant neurological conditions (e.g., Parkinson's disease, stroke, spinal stenosis, and cauda equina syndrome) to rule out potential comorbid illnesses, which can directly influence continence status.

Table 32.2 Recommendation for Initial Evaluation of Older Adults with Urinary Incontinence*

Recommendations

Assess, treat, and re-assess potentially treatable conditions (DIAPPERS)

Medical history

Evaluate treatment expectations regarding the continence paradigm

Physical examination including cognition, functional assessment, neurological and rectal examinations

Urine analysis

* Modified from 2012 update: guidelines for adult urinary incontinence collaborative consensus document for the Canadian Urological Association. Can Urol Assoc J. 2012;6(5):354–363.

Useful Tools for the Diagnosis of UI

Basic investigations

- Dipstick urinalysis is recommended as an initial UI assessment; it helps to identify urinary tract infections as well as other abnormalities such as hematuria, pyuria, and/or bacteriuria. All patients should be screened for hematuria (grade C), while persistent pattern should prompt further evaluation, including upper tract imaging and cystoscopy.

- Measurement of the post-void residual volume is considered fundamental to an initial UI assessment to investigate for incomplete bladder emptying in frail older patients with long-standing diabetes mellitus, previous history of urinary retention, recurrent urinary tract infections, medications known to decrease detrusor contractility (e.g., anticholinergics), severe constipation, complex neurologic disease, as well as persistent or deteriorating UI despite treatment (grade C).

- Bladder diaries recording details of fluid intake, voiding times, and volumes are an appropriate assessment tool which help determine UI type, severity, and circumstances. A minimum of three days' diary is recommended.

- Serum electrolytes, creatinine, and glucose maybe required if there is concern for renal impairment or in older adults with polyuria.

Specialist investigation

- Routine multichannel urodynamics testing is not necessary, but possibly warranted when diagnostic uncertainty may impact treatment decisions, in patients who have not experienced significant improvement in symptoms despite prior therapy, and for patients considering invasive treatment. Urodynamic evaluation in frail older persons is safe, feasible, and reproducible.

- More invasive investigation such as cystourethroscopy is a potential diagnostic tool used in outpatient urology settings, indicated in the presence of hematuria or otherwise unexplained pelvic pain.

WHAT ARE THE INTERVENTIONS TO REVERSE UI?

Before recommending a therapeutic intervention, it is crucial to determine the factors contributing to UI in the specific case presentation (review the mnemonic DIAPPERS). In the frail elderly patient, initial management is based first on the precise diagnosis of the type of UI experienced by the patient, severity of symptoms and bother, expectations and concerns of the patient and their caregiver(s). Treatment preferences, the level of cooperation, and the overall prognosis and life expectancy should also be considered. Figure 32.1 is an algorithm with an approach to treatment of UI.

Conservative and behavioral treatment strategies are useful in the broad management of UI (grade C). lifestyle modifications and behavioral interventions that may be helpful include:

- Avoiding excess fluid intake, caffeinated drinks, and alcohol.

- Weight loss has been shown to be beneficial in reducing UI in morbidly obese women.

- Bladder training for capable patients and prompt voiding for frail and cognitively impaired individuals (grade B).

- Pelvic muscle exercises may be considered, but evidence on their effectiveness is deficient (grade C).

- Adjunctive management considerations for the geriatric population involve appropriate continence products and devices, along with proper skin hygiene and breakdown prevention of the external genitalia, and perineum.

Pharmacotherapy does not cure UI, but is often considered for symptomatic relief particularly in UUI. In the elderly population, any drug treatment should be started very carefully due to several factors, which include polypharmacy, drug-drug interactions, impact on cognitive function, high potential for adverse events in this patient population. Additionally, it should be started with a low-dose regimen and titrated gradually with regular assessment of clinical benefits and side effects. Table 32.3 summarizes recommendations for pharmacologic therapy in the geriatric population with urinary incontinence.

Figure 32.1 Active screening of urinary incontinence in frail/older adults.

Source: Modified from 2012 update: guidelines for adult urinary incontinence collaborative consensus document for the Canadian Urological Association. *Can Urol Assoc J*. 2012;6(5):354–363.

Abbreviations: UI: urinary incontinence; BOO: bladder outlet obstruction; DHIC: detrusor hyperactivity with impaired contractility; UTI: urinary tract infection; CIC: clean intermittent catheterization.

These interventions should be individually tailored; and in certain patients a combination of these approaches may be utilized. However, compliance may be a concern with some forms of therapy. Ultimately, consideration of specialist referral is recommended for older adults with hematuria, pelvic pain, complex neurologic disease, prior pelvic surgery, and a response to initial management that is insufficient. Identifying incontinence is the most important step. Nowadays, various therapeutic interventions are available for this prevalent geriatric problem, but the first priority should be directed to encourage elderly people to discuss their urinary symptoms with their healthcare provider(s).

Many older people will require continence products (pads and protective garments). However, these products should be offered following a proper assessment and management plan or as a short-term relief until definitive diagnosis is explored. Indwelling urethral catheters or intermittent catheterization may be necessary for older adults with a significant PVR [Post Void Residual] and impaired bladder

Table 32.3 Summary of Age-Related Pharmacokinetics Changes, and Their Potential Effect on Urinary Incontinence Drugs

Parameter	Age-Related Changes	Potentially Affected UI Medications
Absorption	Minimal quantitative change despite delayed gastric emptying	Extended-release formulations
	Decrease subcutaneous fat	Topical preparations
Distribution	Decrease in lean body mass leads to: -Longer half-life of lipophilic agents -Higher serum concentration of hydrophilic agents	Tricyclic antidepressants
	Low protein binding in older adults with low albumin level gives rise to greater concentration of free drug molecules	Tolterodine
Metabolism (hepatic)	Decreased oxidation/reduction reactions	Tricyclic antidepressants
	No change in hepatic glycosylation	
	Decreased hepatic blood flow and hepatic mass: less first-pass effect and increased serum level of un-metabolized drug	Oxybutynin, tolterodine, solifenacin, darifenacin
	Stereoselective selectivity in metabolism (hypothetical)	Enantiomers
	Cytochrome P450	Oxybutynin, tolterodine, solifenacin, darifenacin, mirabegron, 5-hydroxymethyl tolterodine
Excretion (renal)	Decrease in renal clearance (–GFR)	Tolterodine, fesoterodine

Source: Modified from CUA guideline on adult overactive bladder. *Canadian Urological Association Journal* 11.5 (2017): E142.
Abbreviation: GFR = glomerular filtration rate.

emptying. It should be reserved when medical or surgical treatment is not possible and should not be considered as a replacement approach for nursing care of older adults with incontinence.

SUMMARY

UI is a highly prevalent condition in the geriatric population and is associated with considerable patient, caregiver, and healthcare system burden. It represents a geriatric condition with multiple risk factors and modifiers that include age-related changes, potentially comorbid conditions, medications, and functional impairments. Active screening for UI among frail older people is strongly recommended. A comprehensive initial evaluation requires assessment of potentially reversible conditions and impairments, as well as detailed history, physical exam, and urinalysis.

UI management in this population involves a multidisciplinary and stepwise approach progressing from lifestyle and behavioral modifications, pharmacotherapy to more invasive treatment strategies, as needed.

Appendix A: Grade of recommendation*

Grade	Nature of Recommendations
A	Based on clinical studies of good quality and consistency addressing the specific recommendations and including at least one randomized trial
B	Based on well-conducted clinical studies but without randomized clinical trials
C	Made despite the absence of directly applicable clinical studies of good quality
D	Evidence inconsistent/inconclusive (no recommendation possible) or the evidence indicates that the drug should not be recommended

* Modified from 2012 update: guidelines for adult urinary incontinence collaborative consensus document for the Canadian Urological Association. Can Urol Assoc J. 2012;6(5):354–363.

REFERENCES

1. Bettez M, Tu le M, Carlson K, et al. Update: guidelines for adult urinary incontinence collaborative consensus document for the Canadian urological association. *Can Urol Assoc J.* 2012; 6 (5): 354–363.

2. Thuroff JW, Abrams P, Andersson KE, et al. EAU guidelines on urinary incontinence. *Eur Urol.* 2011; 59 (3): 387–400.

3. Shaw C, Wagg A. Urinary incontinence in older adults. *Medicine.* 2017; 45 (1): 23–27.

4. Searcy JAR. Geriatric urinary incontinence. *Nurs Clin North Am.* 2017; 52 (3): 447–455.

5. Weiss BD. Diagnostic evaluation of urinary incontinence in geriatric patients. *Am Fam Phys.* 1998; 57: 2675–2694.

6. Corcos J, Przydacz M, Campeau L, et al. CUA guideline on adult overactive bladder. *Can Urologic Assoc J.* 2017; 11 (5): E142.

33 Sleep Disorders in Older Persons

Shachi Tyagi, MD, MS

CONTENTS

Poor sleep is one of the most prevalent health concerns encountered in clinical practice, especially among older adults. Over 50% of community-dwelling older adults complain of some form of sleep difficulty. Aging does not cause sleep problems; however, it is associated with increased sleep complaints and chronic sleep disturbances. This chapter will review sleep disorders in older adults, including information on presentation, etiology, evaluation, and management of sleep-related issues.

CLINICAL VIGNETTE

Ms. F is a 78-year-old woman who came to the geriatric clinic for care. She states her chief complaint as, "I have tried everything for my sleep, and nothing works!" Her sleep complaints started a couple of years ago. She denies any prior sleep-related difficulties. Currently, she can fall asleep but is unable to stay asleep. She has multiple awakenings throughout the night within an hour of falling asleep with difficulty returning to sleep. She spends up to 12–13 hours in bed to "catch up" on lost sleep and still struggles with daytime lethargy and difficulty concentrating. She notes that her sleep complaints started almost concurrently with her gastric complaints of daily nausea, repetitive burping, and acid reflux. This affected her appetite and she lost almost 25 lbs in a year. She underwent a detailed work-up, and now her reflux symptoms are controlled on esomeprazole. She has gained some of her weight back, though she remains over 10 lbs below her pre-illness baseline. Yet, her sleep complaints persist. Ms. F tried several medications for sleep with variable success and adverse effects including zolpidem, trazodone, lorazepam, alprazolam, temazepam, gabapentin, mirtazapine, and melatonin. She is not taking any prescription or over-the-counter sleep aids at this time.

Ms. F's medical issues include hypertension, hyperlipidemia, a remote history of myocardial infarction with percutaneous coronary intervention and a stent to the left anterior descending artery, heart failure with preserved ejection fraction, and degenerative joint disease with chronic low back and bilateral knee pain. She also noted increased stress and anxiety since her husband was diagnosed with cancer a couple of years ago. He is in remission but continues to struggle with chemo-related side effects. She lives with her husband; her two adult children live out of state. She does not use tobacco and drinks socially, half a glass of wine 1–2 times a month. Current medications include Lisinopril 40 mg/d, carvedilol 12.5 mg bid, atorvastatin 40 mg/d, aspirin 81 mg/d, esomeprazole 40 mg bid, acetaminophen 1000 mg bid. Ms. F has no drug allergies. She is healthy and independent, uses a cane for outdoor mobility. Her exam is remarkable for BMI of 28.12, blood pressure 158/85, and pulse 69/min. She has bilateral lower extremity edema up to mid-calf, worse around ankles. Cardiovascular examination otherwise is unremarkable.

DOI: 10.1201/9781003344476-38

Changes in Sleep with Aging

There is a change in circadian tendency with age displayed as an earlier bedtime and an earlier wake-up time. Also noted are changes in sleep architecture, including spending an increased proportion of time in stages N1 and N2 sleep (i.e., the lighter stages of sleep), a decreased proportion of time in stage N3 sleep (i.e., a deeper stage of sleep), and in rapid eye movement (REM) sleep. These changes reflect a decrease in deep, restorative sleep and an increase in light, transitory sleep. In addition, older adults tend to spend slightly less time asleep than younger adults. These "age-related" sleep changes begin in the early- and mid-adult years and become relatively constant in healthy adults over the age of 60. Many older adults have good sleep quality until the end of their lives. Therefore, it is critical that sleep problems in the elderly are not attributed to and disregarded as physiological changes but are identified and addressed appropriately.

Common Sleep Complaints in Older Adults

Older adults often complain of poor sleep. Specific issues include insomnia (difficulty initiating and/or maintaining sleep), early morning awakenings, nonrestorative sleep, daytime sleepiness, restless legs, periodic limb movements, snoring, and apneas (more apparent to the sleep partner than the patient). Of these, insomnia is most prevalent.

Insomnia

Insomnia is a patient-reported problem characterized by difficulty falling asleep or difficulty maintaining sleep (i.e., frequent awakenings, difficulty returning to sleep after awakenings, or awakening too early with the inability to return to sleep). Although nonrestorative sleep is often a symptom of insomnia, it has different functional correlates than other insomnia symptoms, including a greater degree of daytime impairments like sleepiness and fatigue. Additionally, the sleep complaints must persist with adequate opportunity and circumstances for sleep and cause significant daytime consequences, including difficulty concentrating, mood disorders, fatigue, and memory changes.

Insomnia is often subtyped by the predominant symptoms (i.e., sleep onset vs sleep maintenance). In epidemiological studies, sleep maintenance symptoms are more prevalent among individuals with insomnia (approximately 50%–70%), followed by difficulty initiating sleep (35%–60%), and nonrestorative sleep (20%–25%). However, multiple sleep symptoms are more common than any single symptom.

Insomnia in late life often (60% or more) occurs in association with other medical or psychiatric disorders (comorbid insomnia) and leads to decreased quality of life, the risk for falls, psychological and physical disabilities, economic and social costs, the risk for nursing home placement, and even mortality.

Factors That Contribute to Insomnia

Many factors contribute to insomnia and sleep disturbances in older adults. These factors include medical and psychiatric illnesses, medications and the problems of polypharmacy in this population, changes in circadian rhythms, and a higher prevalence of specific primary sleep disorders.

Comorbid Medical and Psychiatric Illnesses

Medical disorders can cause comorbid insomnia. These include pain disorders, such as arthritis and fibromyalgia; neurologic disorders, such as restless leg syndrome, dementia, and Parkinson's disease; psychiatric disorders, such as depression, anxiety, and substance use disorders; cardiopulmonary diseases, such as angina, congestive heart failure, asthma, and chronic obstructive pulmonary disease; and other fluid overload conditions like poorly controlled diabetes, heart failure, and lower extremity edema.

One of the most common causes of sleep maintenance insomnia in older adults is nocturia or nighttime awakenings to void. Three-quarters of participants in a survey of US residents 18 years or older cited the need to void as the most frequent reason for nocturnal awakenings. The proportion of participants reporting nocturia as the primary reason for nighttime awakening increased with age: 39.9% in those aged 18–44 years, 57.6% in those aged 45–64 years, and 77.1% in those aged 65 or above.

Diagnosis and Work-Up

The evaluation and diagnosis of insomnia is based on a careful clinical history of the sleep problem and relevant comorbidities. The 3-P model (predisposing, precipitating, and perpetuating) is a helpful heuristic framework for assessment. *Predisposing factors* include risk factors that increase older adults' likelihood of experiencing poor sleep, such as poor health, lifelong propensity for

Table 33.1 Commonly Used Medications That Affect Sleep

Medications	Examples	Sleep
β-blockers	Atenolol, metoprolol, propranolol	Affect sleep maintenance, nightmares
α1-agonist	Prazosin, terazosin	Sedation
α2-agonist	Clonidine	Daytime sleepiness, disrupted rapid eye movement sleep, early morning awakening
Corticosteroids	Prednisone	Daytime restlessness, insomnia
Diuretics	Chlorthalidone, furosemide	Diuresis, electrolyte abnormality/hypokalemia, sleep interruption secondary to increased awakening to void if taken close to bedtime
SSRI	Fluoxetine, sertraline, paroxetine	Decreased rapid eye movement sleep
Bronchodilators	Theophylline	Wakefulness (like caffeine)
Thyroid	Levothyroxine	Insomnia (at higher doses)

stress-related poor sleep, family history of insomnia, or low socioeconomic status. *Precipitating factors* include medical, environmental, or psychosocial stressors that can acutely disrupt sleep, such as depressive episodes, exacerbation of chronic medical issues like heart failure, chronic obstructive pulmonary disease, hospitalization, loss of a loved one, etc. *Perpetuating factors* are the aspects of their daily behavior that lead to a vicious circle of continued sleep disturbance. For instance, many individuals with poor sleep spend more time in bed to "catch up" on sleep, but this increased time in bed and attention to sleep fuel hyperarousal and perpetuate insomnia.

Key elements of assessment include the patient's sleep characteristics, daytime behaviors, medical-psychiatric history, symptoms of other sleep disorders, and medications (Table 33.1). Some self-report questionnaires such as Insomnia Severity Index have been validated in older adults. However, the retrospective recall of sleep quality necessary for these questionnaires may be difficult for older adults. Prospective sleep-wake diaries, which evaluate the timing and variability of sleep, capture useful information regarding sleep timing, quantity, and quality across consecutive days and may identify targets for behavioral interventions.

Treatment

The goals of insomnia treatment are to improve quantitative and qualitative aspects of sleep, reduce the distress and anxiety associated with poor sleep, and improve daytime function. Treatment of late-life insomnia includes psychological strategies, pharmacologic agents, or both. Psychological treatment approaches are highly effective in reducing insomnia, producing short-term and long-term positive changes in sleep habits and the subjective perception of better sleep.

Psychological Interventions

Psychological interventions for insomnia encompass various techniques, including sleep hygiene, stimulus control, sleep restriction, and cognitive-behavioral treatments (CBT). These treatments address the maladaptive behaviors, thoughts, and beliefs regarding sleep that perpetuate insomnia.

BOX 33.1   SLEEP HYGIENE RULES FOR OLDER ADULTS

- Do not "try to" sleep.
- Avoid stimulants after lunch (caffeine, nicotine).
- Limit alcohol intake.
- Limit liquids in the evening.
- Keep a regular bedtime–wake time schedule.
- Avoid naps or limit to 1 nap a day, no longer than 30 minutes at least 8 hours before the regular bedtime.
- Get regular exercise at least 6 hours prior to sleep.
- Spend time outdoors, particularly in the late afternoon or early evening.

BOX 33.2   STIMULUS CONTROL TECHNIQUES FOR OLDER ADULTS

- Go to bed only when sleepy.
- Use the bed and bedroom for sleep only.
- Do not read, watch TV, worry, or plan activities in the bedroom.
- If unable to fall asleep within 20 minutes, leave the bedroom. While out of bed, do something quiet and relaxing.
- Return to bed only when feeling sleepy again.
- If unable to fall asleep within 20 minutes, again get out of bed.
- Set the alarm and wake up at a regular time every day.
- Do not nap during the day.

BOX 33.3   SLEEP RESTRICTION THERAPY FOR OLDER ADULTS

- Restrict time awake in bed by setting strict bedtime and rising schedule.
- Keep a fixed wake-up time, regardless of actual sleep duration.
- Calculate the average amount of time in bed per night as reported by patient.
- If after 10 d sleep efficiency is lower than 85%, further restrict bedtime by 15–30 minutes.
- When sleep efficiency has reached 85%, increase time in bed by 15 minutes.
- Repeat this procedure until patient can sleep for 8 hours.

Sleep hygiene is an educational approach designed to guide older adults with insomnia to maintain a healthy sleep-wake routine. Box 33.1 summarizes sleep hygiene rules adapted explicitly for older adults.

Stimulus control therapy aims to address psychophysiological insomnia. Patients with insomnia often have negative associations with the bedroom environment, and stimulus control therapy is designed to break any preexisting associations between the bed (and bedroom) and wakefulness, which are often the result of maladaptive classical conditioning. Box 33.2 summarizes instructions for stimulus control therapy.

Sleep restriction is a behavioral strategy designed to increase the homeostatic sleep drive by reducing time in bed and maintaining a consistent wake time in the morning to strengthen the circadian signal through more closely aligning time spent in bed with time spent asleep. To increase compliance, clinicians should help patients understand the underlying theory behind this method and educate them on initial difficulties they may experience, such as initial sleep loss and daytime sleepiness. Box 33.3 summarizes the instructions for sleep restriction therapy.

Cognitive-behavioral therapy of insomnia (CBT) involves multimodal treatment combining elements of these techniques. The educational component involves encouraging the patient to determine which factors might predispose, precipitate, and perpetuate insomnia. The therapist helps the patient identify and eliminate the perpetuating factors with behavioral and cognitive strategies. The cognitive component deals with maladaptive thoughts or dysfunctional beliefs that the patient has about insomnia. CBT is typically delivered in 6–8 individual sessions, each lasting between 30 and 60 minutes, but the efficacy of brief versions and internet delivery have also been demonstrated.

Pharmacotherapy

Medication treatment of late-life insomnia should be used in a minority of patients; however, sedative-hypnotic medications are the most commonly prescribed treatment approach for insomnia in older patients. Hypnotic agents approved by the US Food and Drug Administration (FDA) include benzodiazepine receptor agonists (BzRAs), antihistamine drugs (e.g., hydroxyzine, diphenhydramine), a tricyclic drug (doxepin), melatonin receptor agonist (ramelteon), and orexin antagonists (suvorexant). Physicians also prescribe several medications without an FDA indication for insomnia, including anxiolytic benzodiazepines, sedating antidepressants, sedating antipsychotics, and anticonvulsants.

BzRAs are the most widely used drugs for the treatment of insomnia. These drugs include benzodiazepines (e.g., temazepam, triazolam), and "non-benzodiazepine" drugs (e.g., zolpidem, zaleplon, eszopiclone). The short-term efficacy of the BzRA drugs is well established, with improvement in sleep quality, sleep latency, and sleep efficiency depending on the drug's duration of action, with efficacy for up to 6 months of nightly or intermittent use. However, it is essential to consider their adverse effects among older adults, who are more susceptible to experience these. The adverse effects include morning sedation, anterograde amnesia, anxiety, impaired balance, increased falls and hip fractures, and complex sleep-related behaviors such as sleepwalking. Additional concerns include rebound insomnia, withdrawal, and dependence.

Other medications commonly used as hypnotics are listed in Table 33.2. Ramelteon is a melatonin 1 and melatonin 2 receptor agonist with properties similar to melatonin. It helps with sleep latency and sleep duration but has inconsistent effects on wakefulness after sleep onset. Doxepin, a tricyclic compound, is FDA approved for depression at doses of 100 to 200 mg and for insomnia at doses 3 mg to 6 mg. Doxepin affects wakefulness after sleep onset and sleep efficiency across the entire night. Suvorexant, a newer hypnotic, is an orexin antagonist, the first drug in this class approved by the FDA for insomnia treatment. It improves sleep latency and sleep efficiency. Long-term efficacy data at 1 year is remarkable for subjective sleep improvement in total sleep time and time to sleep onset.

Other prescription medications are also used to treat insomnia, but none have been systematically evaluated for their efficacy and safety. Trazodone is commonly used for insomnia. It improves sleep latency and sleep efficiency. Although trazodone has a relatively short half-life, morning sedation is a common adverse event. Mirtazapine is FDA approved for the treatment of depression and anxiety but is used off-label for sleep. It decreases sleep latency and helps with sleep maintenance too. In addition to causing sedation, mirtazapine is associated with increased appetite, weight gain, and dry mouth, probably related to its antihistaminic properties. Clinical observations suggest that mirtazapine may be less sedating at doses 30 mg per day or more than at lower doses. This counterintuitive weaker effect on sleep at a higher dose is hypothesized to be related to greater noradrenergic effects at higher doses relative to antihistaminic and serotonergic effects at lower doses.

Table 33.2 Pharmacotherapy for Insomnia

Drug Class	Generics	Elimination Half Life (h)	Tmax (h)	Indication
Benzodiazepines	Estrazolam	10–24	1.5–2	Sleep maintenance
	Flurazepam	48–120	1.5–2	Sleep maintenance
	Quazepam	48–120	2–3	Sleep maintenance
	Temazepam	8–22	1–2	Sleep maintenance
	Triazolam	2–4	2–6	Sleep onset
Benzodiazepine receptor agonists (BzRA)	Zaleplon	1	1	Sleep onset
	Zolpidem	2.5	1.6	Sleep onset
	Eszopiclone	6	1	Sleep maintenance
Melatonin agonist	Ramelteon	1–2.6	0.75	Sleep onset
H antagonist	Doxepin	15	3.5	Sleep maintenance
Orexin antagonist	Suvorexant	12	2	Sleep onset and maintenance
Sedating antidepressant	Trazodone	9–15	1–2	Sleep maintenance
	Mirtazapine	20–40	2–5	Sleep onset and maintenance
Sedating antipsychotics	Quetiapine	6	1–2	Sleep onset
Anticonvulsant	Gabapentin	5–9	1–3	Sleep onset
	Pregabalin	6	1.5	Sleep onset

Gabapentin and pregabalin are often used to treat common pain conditions with comorbid insomnia, including fibromyalgia. Sedating antipsychotics, such as olanzapine, quetiapine, and risperidone, are also used off label for insomnia, but because of their potential for serious side effects, including weight gain and cardiometabolic effects, clinicians should limit their use to those with serious psychiatric disorders.

Sleep-Disordered Breathing

Sleep-disordered breathing (SDB) is commonly encountered in older adults. SDB is characterized by respiratory events during sleep, including hypopneas (partial respiration) and/or apneas (complete cessation of respiration), during sleep. These respiratory events occur repeatedly throughout the night, with each event lasting at least 10 seconds or more. Clinical diagnosis of SDB is made when a patient has 10 to 15 apnea-hypopnea episodes per hour of sleep (called apnea-hypopnea index or AHI).

There are three types of apneic events: central, obstructive, and mixed. Central events are a result of a dysfunction of the respiratory neurons. Obstructive events are far more common and caused by anatomic obstruction of the upper airways despite the respiratory effort. Mixed events are a combination of central and obstructive components.

Patients usually complain of excessive daytime sleepiness, and bed partners may report snoring. Snoring is reflective of the airway collapse and is a component of breathing cessation during an apneic event; however, not all snoring is associated with sleep apnea. Excessive daytime sleepiness seen in SDB is associated with sleep fragmentation or repeated nighttime awakenings that frequently follow apneic events. Patients also report cognitive deficits with difficulty in concentration as a common complaint. SDB is often associated with other serious medical issues, including hypertension and cardiac and pulmonary disease, leading to increased morbidity and mortality.

Upon initial evaluation of an older adult with sleep-related issues, complaints such as snoring and excessive daytime sleepiness may suggest SDB. However, many older adults may not have a bed partner to relay the history of snoring or overnight apneic events. Therefore, it is imperative to collect information on daytime behaviors and contributory risk factors, including recent weight gain or obesity (excessive fatty tissue may contribute to airway obstruction), smoking history, alcohol intake, and use of sedative-hypnotics (may result in airway relaxation, thus facilitating obstruction).

Diagnosis

If SDB is suspected, clinicians should refer the patient to a pulmonary sleep specialist for overnight polysomnography (PSG) or ambulatory monitoring of sleep and respiration in the patient's home. PSG is the gold standard for SDB testing. Based on the results of the objective recording, treatment recommendations are made.

Treatment

In general, treatment of SDB in the elderly depends upon 1) the disease severity, 2) the extent of morbidity (i.e., daytime symptoms), and 3) the presence of comorbid illnesses. The dietary and lifestyle habits affecting or exacerbating SDB should be assessed and addressed first, including obesity, alcohol use, smoking, and prescription or over-the-counter sedatives or anticholinergics.

Positive airway pressure (PAP) remains the standard treatment for SDB. There are several types of devices that provide positive airway pressure, including continuous positive airway pressure (CPAP), bilevel positive airway pressure (BiPAP), and auto-CPAP. CPAP includes a nose mask connected via a hose to a machine that provides continuous air pressure. The air pressure acts as a splint to maintain the upper airway opening, thereby preventing the obstruction. The degree of air pressure is individually set for each patient at the sleep laboratory and depends on the underlying disease severity.

BiPAP acts similar to the CPAP but allows variation in positive airway pressure during expiration and inspiration: with reduced positive airway pressure during expiration compared to inspiration. The auto-CPAP allows the overnight variability in airway pressure to be adjusted automatically depending on the extent of airway obstruction, which may fluctuate with specific sleep stages and body position. There is no data to suggest BiPAP or auto-CPAP is better than CPAP, although better compliance is noted with BiPAP.

For patients who cannot tolerate PAP treatment and for those with mild disease, an oral appliance to maintain airway patency may provide good outcomes. These devices are dispensed by dentists and customized for each patient. These oral appliances are anchored on the patient's teeth or gums and work by moving the tongue or the mandible forward thereby preventing the obstruction at the hypopharyngeal level.

Patients with severe disease or those with poor response to PAP or oral appliance may be referred for surgical evaluation. Current procedures include maxomandibular advancement (MMA), laser-assisted uvulopalatoplasty (LAUP), uvulopalatopharyngoplasty (UPPP), pharyngeal implants, implanted hypoglossal nerve stimulators, etc. Clinicians should approach surgical methods with caution in elderly patients as the effectiveness of treatment may be lower, and the recovery may be prolonged and difficult.

Sleep-Related Movement Disorders

Periodic limb movements in sleep (PLMS) and restless legs syndrome (RLS) are sleep-related movement disturbances that become more severe with age. Repetitive limb movements that occur during sleep and cause sleep interruptions and awakenings characterize PLMS. Uncomfortable sensations in legs with urge to move the legs, which begin or worsen during periods of rest or inactivity and are partially or totally resolved by movement or stretching are indicative of RLS. If PLMS or RLS cause insomnia, treatment with ropinirole or with the off-label use of other dopamine agonists such as pramipexole should be considered. Ropinirole and pramipexole reduce both the number of kicks and awakenings. Levodopa/carbidopa have a similar effect on limb movements and awakenings but may increase daytime restlessness. Adverse events with these drugs should be monitored.

Parasomnia

REM sleep behavior disorder (RSBD) is a parasomnia; a catchall term for unusual behaviors that people experience before falling asleep, while asleep, or during the arousal period between sleep and wakefulness. During normal REM sleep, the body experiences atonia of skeletal muscles, while the brain shows activity similar to wakefulness, blood pressure rises, and breathing becomes irregular.

In REM sleep behavior disorder, normal muscle paralysis does not occur, enabling the person to act out their dreams physically. REM sleep behavior disorder can manifest as small muscle twitches and quiet sleep talking to loud shouting, punching, kicking, grabbing their bed partner, and jumping out of bed. The dreams associated with REM sleep behavior disorder are often intense and frightening. RSBD is associated with a neurodegenerative disorder in 48%–73% of cases, including Parkinson's disease, multiple system atrophy, or dementia with Lewy bodies.

CASE DISCUSSION

Ms. F's sleep complaints highlight the multifactorial etiology of sleep-related issues among older adults. Ms. F had no bothersome sleep complaints until two years ago when she faced significant social stressors related to her husband's illness and increased caregiving responsibilities, which, perhaps in addition to change in her appetite and diet, precipitated her gastric issues leading to acid reflux and weight loss. These factors together *precipitated* her sleep complaints, but her insomnia persisted even after the precipitating factors resolved. The factors *perpetuating* her sleep issues include increased time in bed to "catch up" on lost sleep, underlying anxiety, ongoing arthritic pain issues, heart failure exacerbation with poor blood pressure control, and increased lower extremity edema causing an increase in nighttime urine output and contributing to frequent awakenings to void.

Before considering pharmacologic treatment for Ms. F, detailed sleep information should be gathered, including symptoms of other sleep disorders and additional history regarding sleep timing and duration. A sleep diary would more accurately portray day-to-day variability and time in bed. This information could reveal different targets for specific behavioral and cognitive interventions, such as reducing time in bed to increase homeostatic sleep drive or cognitive techniques to address arousal. Treating heart failure, blood pressure, ongoing pain disorder, and underlying anxiety disorder may be valuable adjuncts to address Ms. F's sleep complaints.

KEY REFERENCES

1. Ohayon MM, Carskadon MA, Guilleminault C, Vitiello MV. Meta-analysis of quantitative sleep parameters from childhood to old age in healthy individuals: developing normative sleep values across the human lifespan. Sleep. 2004 Nov 1;27(7):1255–1273. doi: 10.1093/sleep/27.7.1255. PMID: 15586779.
2. Ancoli-Israel S. Sleep and aging: prevalence of disturbed sleep and treatment considerations in older adults. J Clin Psychiatry. 2005;66 Suppl 9:24–30; quiz 42–3. PMID: 16336039.

3. Ohayon MM. Nocturnal awakenings and comorbid disorders in the American general population. J Psychiatr Res. 2008 Nov;43(1):48–54. doi: 10.1016/j.jpsychires.2008.02.001. Epub 2008 Mar 28. PMID: 18374943.

4. Rodriguez JC, Dzierzewski JM, Alessi CA. Sleep problems in the elderly. Med Clin North Am. 2015 Mar;99(2):431–439. doi: 10.1016/j.mcna.2014.11.013. Epub 2014 Dec 30. PMID: 25700593; PMCID: PMC4406253.

5. Bloom HG, Ahmed I, Alessi CA, Ancoli-Israel S, Buysse DJ, Kryger MH, Phillips BA, Thorpy MJ, Vitiello MV, Zee PC. Evidence-based recommendations for the assessment and management of sleep disorders in older persons. J Am Geriatr Soc. 2009 May; 57(5):761–789. doi: 10.1111/j.1532-5415.2009.02220.x. PMID: 19484833; PMCID: PMC2748127.

6. Morin CM, Mimeault V, Gagné A. Nonpharmacological treatment of late-life insomnia. J Psychosom Res. 1999 Feb;46(2):103–116. doi: 10.1016/s0022-3999(98)00077-4. PMID: 10098820.

7. Morin CM, Kowatch RA, Barry T, Walton E. Cognitive-behavior therapy for late-life insomnia. J Consult Clin Psychol. 1993 Feb;61(1):137–146. doi: 10.1037//0022-006x.61.1.137. PMID: 8450099.

8. Buysse DJ, Rush AJ, Reynolds CF 3rd. Clinical management of insomnia disorder. JAMA. 2017 Nov 28;318(20):1973–1974. doi: 10.1001/jama.2017.15683. PMID: 29059360.

9. Chowdhuri S, Patel P, Badr MS. Apnea in older adults. Sleep Med Clin. 2018 Mar;13(1):21–37. doi: 10.1016/j.jsmc.2017.09.003. Epub 2017 Nov 10. PMID: 29412981.

34 Polypharmacy and Deprescribing in the Elderly

Louise Mallet, B.Sc.Pharm., Pharm.D., BCGP, FESCP, FOPQ

CONTENTS

CLINICAL VIGNETTE

Mrs. D is a 92-year-old woman who lives alone in an upper duplex. She sustained a fall last week. She has two daughters who are involved in her care and visit their mother at least twice a week. Mrs. D needs help with ADLs (Activities of Daily Living) such as washing. She receives private help once a week for bathing. She also has a cleaning person who comes once a week. She still cooks but her daughters bring her meals that can be heated in the microwave. She dresses by herself and goes out with friends twice a month. It is mentioned by the daughters that Mrs. D does not always take her medications as prescribed. They often find pills on the floor when they visit. There are no known allergies.

Past medical history is significant for hypertension, diabetes type 2, hypothyroidism, dyslipidemia, insomnia, constipation and a history of falls.

Weight: 50 kg. Height: 165 cm. Patient says she lost 5 kg in past 3 months.

Laboratory results from a week ago disclose (normal values in parenthesis):

- Na: 129 mmol/L (133–143).
- K: 4.4 mmol/L (3.5–5.0).
- Mg: 0.60 mmol/L (0.75–1.25).
- Creatinine: 85 μmol/L (40–85; stable).
- Albumin: 39 g/L (8–50).
- TSH: 9 μU/mL (04–4.4).
- Vitamin B12: 176 pmol/L (> 133).
- Hb A1c 6.5% (4.3–6).
- Calculated Cr Cl using Cockcroft/Gault formula: 30 mL/min (> 60).
- Blood glucose reported by daughter: between 4 and 7 mmol/L (3.9–11; done once a week at different times during the week).

Her current medication list is as follows:

- Amlodipine 5 mg po daily.
- Pantoprazole 40 mg po daily.
- Furosemide 40 mg po daily.
- Levothyroxine 88 mcg po daily.
- Metformin 850 mg po bid.
- Atorvastatin 40 mg po daily.

DOI: 10.1201/9781003344476-39

- Glyburide 5 mg po bid.

- Docusate sodium 100 mg po bid.

- Citalopram 20 mg po daily for the past 10 years.

- Lorazepam 1 mg po at bedtime, prn.

- Acetaminophen (Tylenol PM^MD) 1 tablet po at bedtime, prn.

Her medications are delivered in vials. She has her own system to organize her medications. She prepares her medications for one week at a time using vials.

This case illustrates the problems with polypharmacy in older patients. This chapter will present a systematic process to optimize the medications prescribed for Mrs. D.

When an elderly patient presents with a status change, unless proven otherwise, it should be assumed to be a medication related problem.

Jerry Gurwitz, M.D.

WHAT IS POLYPHARMACY?

Polypharmacy is common in the elderly. However, there is no standard definition for polypharmacy. The World Health Organization (WHO) defines polypharmacy as multiple medicines for chronic use at the same time, usually more than 4 medications. Some authors have defined polypharmacy as the prescription of more medications than clinically indicated, use of unnecessary drug, use of ineffective medication, the presence of therapeutic duplications or the concurrent use of 2 to 9 different therapeutic agents. Excessive polypharmacy is defined as the concurrent use of at least 10 medications in older adults.

Polypharmacy has been associated with decreased physical and social functioning, increased risk of falls, delirium, decreased adherence to medication, higher costs, emergency room visits, hospital admissions, nursing home placement and death.

In Canada, 20% of older adults aged 65 to 74 take 10 medications or more per day. This percentage increases to 32% for those aged 75 to 84 and to 40% for those ≥ 85 years of age. It is reported that 30% of hospitalizations in older adults 75 years of age and over are related to medications (Canadian Institute for Health Information 2014).

WHAT IS DEPRESCRIBING?

Deprescribing is the process of stopping an inappropriate medication, supervised by a health care professional with the goal of managing polypharmacy and improving outcomes. Inappropriate medications are defined as medications in which risks outweigh benefits. Patient's goals, life expectancy, values, preferences and level of care should be discussed in the context of deprescribing. The activity of deprescribing should be part of the continuum of prescribing. It is a patient-centered intervention which includes patient consent and close monitoring. Deprescribing encompasses the process of deciding with the patient which medications can be discontinued, planning a cessation protocol when needed and monitoring the plan and follow-up.

Which factors should be considered when evaluating medications in the elderly?

Is the Patient Really Taking the Medication?

- Ask the patient to bring medications (prescribed, over the counter, vitamins, eye drops, natural products, essential oils, etc.). Mrs. D has a bottle of Tylenol PM^MD which contains Acetaminophen 500 mg and diphenhydramine 25 mg. Diphenhydramine is an anticholinergic medication which can have an impact on her cognition and also cause falls. She has a history of falls and sustained a fall last week. She says that she recently bought this product as suggested by a friend. She took it once and did not like the feeling of it.

- TSH is elevated. Is Mrs. D taking her levothyroxine correctly? Daughter says that pills are found on the floor on a regular basis when she visits. It is suggested to continue the same dose of levothyroxine for now and repeat TSH in one month.

- Verify which system is used to help take her medication; Dispill, Dosett or a self-created system. Ask Mrs. D what she does when she forgets to take her medications. Verify with the community pharmacist whether she renews her medication on a regular basis. For example, Mrs. D has a prescription for lorazepam, a benzodiazepine, prescribed "prn" or as needed for sleep. It is important to verify if she takes it every night on a regular basis or say, once a week to avoid the risk of precipitating withdrawal symptoms. Benzodiazepines have been shown to increase the risk of falls, hip fractures, cognitive impairment, delirium, dementia and traffic accidents.

■ Ask Mrs. D if she knows the indication for each her medications; is she taking all her prescribed medications on a regular basis and if not, the reasons why (side effects, too many medications or forgetting to take them).

What Are the Current Indications for Each Drug?

■ Verify the indication for each medication.

■ Verify the presence of a medication cascade. A prescribing cascade is observed when an adverse drug reaction is misinterpreted as a new medical problem. A second medication is prescribed which places the patient at risk of adverse drug reaction or potential drug-drug interactions. This domino effect can go on if not recognized by the health care provider. Some examples of prescribing cascades can be found in Table 34.1.

■ Consider discontinuation or tapering the medication if no valid indication.

■ Match each medication with a medical problem.

Medications	Medical Problems
Amlodipine	Hypertension
Furosemide	Lower leg edema from use of amlodipine? Medication cascade?
Atorvastatin	Hypercholesterolemia?
Metformin	Diabetes
Glyburide	Diabetes
Pantoprazole	GI problems?
Levothyroxine	Hypothyroidism
Docusate Sodium	Constipation
Insomnia	Lorazepam, Tylenol PM
Citalopram	Depression?

What Is Mrs. D's Life Expectancy and What Are Her Expectations and Preferences?

■ Discuss with Mrs. D her expectations and preferences in terms of her medications.

■ Estimate Mrs. D's life expectancy and objectives of treatment. She has a limited life expectancy between 1.9 and 3.9 years based on published literature.

■ Define the therapeutic objective for the use of atorvastatin for Mrs. D. Suggest to discontinue considering her age.

■ If a new medication is added, verify the time for benefit before prescribing considering her limited life expectancy.

■ Identify medications which may cause harm. For example, use the American Geriatrics Society (AGS) Beers Criteria for potentially inappropriate medication (PIM) use in older adults, to verify which medications are potentially inappropriate (Table 34.2).

Table 34.1 Prescribing Cascade

Examples of Prescribing Cascade

Furosemide → urinary incontinence → oxybutynin
Amlodipine → peripheral edema → furosemide
Risperidone → rigidity → levodopa + carbidopa
Ciprofloxacin → hallucination → risperidone
Atorvastatin → leg pains → quinine
Digoxin → nausea/vomiting → metoclopramide
Venlafaxine → hyponatremia → salt supplements

Table 34.2 Potentially Inappropriate Medication

AGS Beers Criteria for PIM	Reasons
Glyburide	Severe hypoglycemia
Citalopram	Hyponatremia, falls
Lorazepam	Slowness, confusion, falls
Pantoprazole	Use > 8 weeks causes hypomagnesemia, risk of *Clostridium difficile* infection

Considering Pharmacokinetic Modifications with Aging, Which Factors Should Be Taken into Consideration When Evaluating Mrs. D's Medication?

Pharmacokinetic changes should be considered when evaluating Mrs. D's medications. With aging, a decrease in renal function is reported. Mrs. D's creatinine clearance calculated using the Cockcroft and Gault formula is 30 mL/min. Medications that are renally excreted should be adjusted. Metformin in this case is contraindicated with a creatinine clearance of less than 30 ml/min. Metabolites of glyburide are also renally excreted and not indicated with a CrCl of less than 50 ml/min due to their accumulation and increased risk of hypoglycemia. Age-related changes with absorption, distribution, metabolism and elimination of medications with normal aging and in the frail elderly are described in Table 34.3.

What Are the Therapeutic Objectives for Her Diabetes and Hypertension?

Considering her life expectancy and level of autonomy, therapeutic objectives for Hb A1c of < 8.5% and glucose level between 5 and 10 mmol/L would be appropriate for this patient to avoid hypoglycemia (cause of falls). Metformin and glyburide can be discontinued with close monitoring of blood glucose. Her daughter can be involved in documenting blood glucose for the next few weeks. If needed, another antidiabetic agent such as an inhibitor of the dipeptidyl peptidase-4 (DPP-4) can be prescribed.

For her hypertension, blood pressure goals should be less than 150/90 without orthostatic hypotension. Evaluation of orthostatic hypotension should therefore be done. If Mrs. D has peripheral edema due to her amlodipine and was prescribed furosemide for this problem (medication cascade), these drugs should be discontinued. An angiotensin-converting-enzyme inhibitor should be considered.

Why Should Drugs with Anticholinergic Properties Be Avoided in the Elderly?

Studies have shown that medications with anticholinergic properties have been associated with falls, and a decline in functional and cognitive capacity. A withdrawal plan should be implemented when stopping these medications. As discussed, Mrs. D is taking Tylenol PM which has acetaminophen and diphenhydramine as active ingredients. This should be stopped and discussion of the treatment of her "insomnia" initiated.

As per Beers Criteria for PIM, Table 34.4 illustrates a list of medications with strong anticholinergic drugs that should be avoided in the elderly. The table illustrates the most common anticholinergic drugs used in clinical practice.

WHICH DRUGS CAN BE DISCONTINUED IN MRS. D'S CASE?

When the decision is made to implement a drug deprescribing plan, thus discontinuing medications, a plan should be put in place for monitoring and follow-up. This is an on-going re-evaluation. Table 34.5 illustrates the problems, drugs, therapeutic objectives and other considerations to evaluate if needed.

- For example, are the treatment goals achieved?
- Can a non-pharmacological approach be implemented?
- Determine if you need to taper a medication.
- Supervision of drug discontinuation should be made by one physician. Collaboration can be made with a community pharmacist, for example to taper a benzodiazepine.

Table 34.3 Age-Related Changes in Pharmacokinetics with Normal Aging and in the Frail Elderly

	Age-Related Changes	Normal Aging	Frail Elderly
Absorption	No changes	No clinical impact	↓
Distribution	Body fat	↑ volume of distribution for liposoluble drugs. Adjust dosage for fat-soluble drugs such as antipsychotics, antidepressants, benzodiazepines	↑↑
Distribution	Total water	↓ Volume of distribution for water-soluble drugs. Adjust dosage for water-soluble drugs such as diuretics, digoxin, oral hypoglycemic	↓↓
	Albumin	↓ Free fraction for drugs that are more than 90% bound to albumin such as phenytoin, valproic acid, warfarin	↓↓
Metabolism	Hepatic blood flow	↓ First-pass extraction by the liver for drugs such as verapamil, propranolol.	↓↓
	Esterase enzymes	↓ Metabolism of drugs metabolized by esterase enzymes. For ex: decreased metabolism of prodrug-enalapril to enalaprilat	↓↓
	Phase I metabolism	↓ Metabolism of drugs metabolized by oxidation reaction	↓↓
	Phase II metabolism	No changes with normal aging	↓Changes in glucuronidation of acetaminophen and clearance of metoclopramide
Elimination	Glomerular filtration rate	↓ Elimination of drugs renally excreted	↓↓
	Tubular secretion	↓ Elimination of drugs excreted by tubular secretion such as cimetidine, trimethroprim	↓↓
	Serum creatinine	No changes with normal aging	↓↓For low-weight patient with decreased muscle mass, decrease in serum creatinine level
	Creatinine clearance	↓ With normal aging	↓

Table 34.4 Common Drugs with Anticholinergic Properties as Listed in AGS Updated Beers Criteria 2015

Antiemetic	Dimenhydrinate, promethazine
Antihistamines	Chlorpheniramine, cyproheptadine, diphenhydramine, hydroxyzine, meclizine
Antidepressants	Amitriptyline, desipramine, doxepin (> 6 mg), nortriptyline, paroxetine
Antimuscarinics	Darifenacin, fesoterodine, oxytubynin, solifenacin, tolterodine, trospium
Antiparkinsonian	Benztropine, trihexyphenidyl
Antipsychotics	Cloxapine, loxapine, olanzapine
Antispasmodics	Atropine (excludes opthalmic), clidinium-chlordiazepoxide, dicyclomine, scopolamine
Skeletal muscle relaxants	Cyclobenzaprine, Methocarbamol, orphenadrine

Table 34.5 Match Problems, Drugs and Therapeutic Objectives

Problems	Current Drugs	Therapeutic Objectives	Others
Falls	Acetaminophen/ diphenhydramine (Tylenol PM)	Pain control with acetaminophen alone	Gait evaluation and rehabilitation
Diabetes	Metformin 850 mg po bid Glyburide 5 mg po bid	Hb A1c < 8.5% Glucose between 5 and 10 mmol/L	
Hypertension	Amlodipine 5 mg daily Furosemide 40 mg daily	SBP < 150 without orthostatic hypotension	Moderate salt intake
Hypothyroidism	Levothyroxine 88 mcg po daily	TSH 0.4 and 4.4	Verify compliance
GI	Pantoprazole 40 mg po daily	Clarify indication	Discontinue. Suggest looking at www. Deprescribing.org
Cholesterol	Atorvastatin 40 mg po daily	Discontinue	
Depression	Citalopram 20 mg po daily	No clear indication	Geriatric Depression Scale
Insomnia	Lorazepam 1 mg po at bedtime	Better sleep	Sleep hygiene
Constipation	Docusate sodium 100 mg po bid	Regular bowel movement as per patient	Docusate sodium not effective long term. Change for Lax-a-day 17 g po daily

CONCLUSION

Evaluating medications in the elderly should be done on a regular basis, in order to modify risk factors to avoid geriatric syndromes such as falls, delirium, etc. When prescribing a new medication to an elderly patient, the patient's expectations and preferences, and the objective of treatment according to life expectancy, should be included in the discussion.
It takes one minute to prescribe a medication but years to discontinue it.

SUGGESTED READING

American Geriatrics Society, Beers Criteria Update Expert Panel. American Geriatrics Society 2015 updated Beers criteria for potentially inappropriate medication use in older adults. J Am Geriatr Soc 2015; 63: 2227–2246.

Bowles S. Polypharmacy. In: Huang A, Mallet L. ed. Medication-Related Falls in Older People: Causative Factors and Management Strategies. Springer Nature, Switzerland, 2016, p. 41–54.

Holmes HM et al. Life expectancies predictions for women and men on the basis of US life tables. Arch Intern Med 2006; 166: 605–609.

Mallet L. Pharmacology of drugs in aging. In: Huang A, Mallet L. ed. Medication-Related Falls in Older People: Causative Factors and Management Strategies. Springer Nature, Switzerland, 2016, p. 55–66.

Reeve E, Shakib S, Hendrix I et al. Review of deprescribing processes and development of an evidence-based, patient-centred deprescribing process. Br J Clin Pharmcol 2014; 78: 738–747.

Rochon P, Gurwitz JH. The prescribing cascade revisited. Lancet 2016; 389: 1778–1780.

Scott IA, Hilmer SN, Reeve E et al. Reducing inappropriate polypharmacy. The process of deprescribing. JAMA Intern Med 2015; 175: 827–834.

35 After Menopause

Ronald M. Caplan, MD, CM, FACS, FACOG, FRCS(C)

CONTENTS

CLINICAL VIGNETTE

An independent 96-year-old woman, living alone with daytime cleaning help, visits her gynecologist for a routine checkup. She has no specific complaints. She never smoked, and rarely drinks a glass of wine.

She stopped menstruating at age 52 and has not bled vaginally since. She does visit her gynecologist once yearly, before her annual trip to her childhood home, Switzerland. She travels alone.

She is well oriented, rational, and aware of her surroundings. She is mobile without the use of any support. Her body habitus is normal, and she stands erect. She sees adequately with corrective lenses.

She does see a cardiologist for a longstanding, right bundle branch block but is not currently on any medication for this. Her only regular medication is atorvastatin, prescribed by the cardiologist, which keeps her low density lipoprotein (LDL) within normal limits.

Physical examination, including breast and pelvic examination, is normal. Her vital signs are normal.

A complete blood count and blood chemistries are reported as normal. Urinalysis is normal.

MENOPAUSE

Menopause means the stopping of the menstrual flow, at an average age of approximately 50. Women do not normally menstruate beyond the age of 55.

The normal function of the ovaries is lost. There is a high density of nerve fibers in postmenopausal ovaries, implying altered communication. There is diminished output of estrogen and progesterone by the postmenopausal ovary. The pituitary gland puts out increased amounts of follicle stimulating hormone (FSH) and luteinizing hormone (LH). The pituitary gland itself is controlled by the hypothalamus situated at the base of the brain. Gonadotropin-releasing hormones (GNRH) from the hypothalamus act on the pituitary gland to release FSH and LH in rhythmic fashion.

Increasing wealth of societies, better nutrition, and implementation of public health measures are factors that contribute to the lengthening of the reproductive years. These factors help women to stay healthy longer.

Abnormal bleeding in a woman in the menopausal age group and beyond must always be investigated because of the possibility of abnormal growth, notably of the lining of the uterus.

DOI: 10.1201/9781003344476-40

The symptoms of menopause vary widely in intensity, type and duration from woman to woman.

Hot flushes, the sudden onset of a feeling of heat and flushing of short duration, are a classic symptom.

There may be night sweats. Other symptoms may include sleeplessness, irritability, lack of concentration, changes in appetite and headache.

There may be a change in libido, or sexual desire and satisfaction.

Hair may be less lustrous. The skin can lose some of its smoothness and glow.

OSTEOPOROSIS AND HORMONAL REPLACEMENT THERAPY (HRT)

A big concern for women in the postmenopausal years is osteoporosis, which involves demineralization of the bones. There is a reduction in bone quantity. The supporting fibers of the interior of the bone, the trabeculae, become scanty and thin, leading to a propensity for fractures, and postural abnormalities, including "hump" formation at the level of the thoracic spine, an outward curvature indicative of osteoporotic change with anterior compression of thoracic vertebrae (kyphosis). The process in the spinal column can result in compression fractures of the vertebrae. A woman can end up being shorter as she ages.

Of course, menopause is not the only precursor of osteoporosis, and a lesser, but significant, proportion of older men have to deal with osteoporosis as well.

It is important for a woman's longevity and wellbeing that postmenopausal osteoporosis be minimized. As a woman ages, it is increasingly important for her to remain mobile. A hip fracture in an older woman can be particularly devastating. She is temporarily immobilized. The fracture may not heal well at least partially because of the osteoporosis. As well, she is subject to blood clots that can travel through her circulatory system to her heart and lungs: a life-threatening pulmonary embolism.

In normal bone, the activity of osteoblasts, cells that form bone, and osteoclasts, which absorb and remove bone, are in balance. Bone resorption can be inhibited by drugs, causing bone density to increase, resulting in stronger bones.

Fair, slim women tend to be more at risk for osteoporosis, although all women should be on guard against it. A healthy lifestyle, including regular aerobic and weight bearing exercise, as well as sports activities, are important. Lean muscle mass is important in itself, and for its impact on bone density. These active skeletal muscles are attached to bone. When the muscle contracts, the bone moves.

More information on exercise can be found in Chapter 4, "Physical Activity as a Countermeasure to Frailty", by Guy Hajj Boutros and Dr. Antony D. Karelis.

Cigarette smoking should be avoided. Alcoholism is a risk factor for osteoporosis. The diet should be healthful and rich in calcium, which is notably present in milk and milk products. The use of skim milk and skim milk products cuts down on caloric intake. Ideally, three glasses of skim milk a day or the equivalent should be included in the diet. A calcium pill is roughly equivalent to the calcium in one glass of milk. If there is no milk in the diet, three 500 mg calcium tablets may be needed each day. However, too much calcium intake can be associated with kidney stone development.

Vitamin D is important in bone metabolism. An adequate diet should generally supply enough vitamin D, but especially in older persons when the diet might be deficient, daily supplementation with 800 International Units (IU) of vitamin D can be helpful.

More information on diet can be found in Chapter 10, "Could My Patient Be Malnourished?" by Dr. Jose Morais.

A variety of treatment options are available for prevention of osteoporosis, which may also have the beneficial effect of lessening menopausal symptoms, notably "hot flushes".

Watchful waiting can be employed if symptoms are not bothersome, if the diet is nutrient rich including adequate calcium intake, if regular aerobic exercise is enjoyed, and if bone density testing remains normal. However, intake of calcium and vitamin D alone is usually not sufficient to stop bone loss.

Osteoporosis occurs along with decreased estrogen production by the ovaries. Estrogen replacement therapy by itself, however, can lead to cancer, notably cancer of the endometrium, the lining of the uterus. This undesirable effect is largely obviated by the addition of progesterone, another naturally occurring female sex hormone, to the regimen. Estrogen with progesterone is classic hormonal replacement therapy.

HORMONAL REPLACEMENT THERAPY (HRT)

Estrogen can be taken orally or by skin patch. There are vaginal preparations as well. Oral estrogen is processed in the liver, which can lead to problems in women with liver disease. Conversely, because of passage of oral estrogen through the liver, there can be beneficial effects on cholesterol levels, with low density lipoprotein (LDL) cholesterol being lowered and high density lipoprotein (HDL) being raised. However, levels of C-reactive protein are raised. C-reactive protein is associated with inflammation, and inflammation can be a contributing factor in heart disease.

With estrogen, with or without progesterone replacement, postmenopausal bleeding can occur, sporadically or cyclically. When postmenopausal bleeding occurs, whether in the presence of HRT or not, it should not be assumed that the bleeding is simply due to HRT or some other benign factor. Postmenopausal bleeding is a classic warning sign of gynecologic malignancy, and that possibility has to be ruled out with appropriate investigation by a gynecologist.

HRT should be individualized, after careful examination, and after the risks and benefits have been explained, as well as the possibility of using other therapy, such as denosumab, bisphosphonates or specific estrogen receptor modulators (SERMS).

Benefits of HRT can include lowering of LDL as explained earlier, and improvement of vaginal lining atrophy (thinning).

In most women, after four years of use soon after menopause, the risk of hormonal replacement therapy with estrogen and progesterone outweighs any possible benefits. However, in some women, symptoms are persistent, even after the age of 65. Risks include cardiovascular disease, heart disease, thrombosis (blood clot) and stroke, and possibly an increased risk of ovarian cancer, with prolonged HRT. HRT can increase the eventual risk of getting breast cancer. There may be an increased risk of cognition impairment and dementia.

The diagnosis of osteoporosis is confirmed by bone density studies. These painless tests are performed with the use of DXA machines (dual energy X-ray absorptiometry) and reported as T-scores.

Osteoporosis can be counteracted by aerobic exercise, calcium and vitamin D intake, HRT, denosumab, bisphosphonates or SERMs. Although statins, other drugs or "natural" alternatives (which could contain varying amounts of unopposed estrogenic substances) may be helpful in some cases, it is important that these are not taken without proper consultation, and with regard to risks as well as benefits.

DENOSUMAB

Denosumab is a human monoclonal IgG2 antibody. "Monoclonal" refers to the fact that the antibody protein is derived from one clone of cells, all of which are identical. The antibody goes to a specific receptor site. The receptor site is a distinctively shaped area on a cell surface, designed to receive a specific substance. In this case, denosumab binds to the receptor activator of nuclear factor-kB ligand (RANKL). It inhibits bone resorption by impairing the development, activation and survival of osteoclasts. Denosumab has become, along with bisphosphonates, a widely used osteoporosis treatment. Its effect on bone turnover is quickly reversible. However, stoppage may result in an increased propensity to fracture, and usage may impact response to infection.

Denosumab has been shown to improve bone mineral density (BMD) more than bisphosphonate treatment at the lumbar spine, total hip and femoral neck.

BISPHOSPHONATES

These nonhormonal drugs specifically combat osteoporosis. Bisphosphonates selectively adhere to and remain within bone. They act at the level of bone resorbing cells known as osteoclasts, inhibiting their activity by inactivation or by promoting apoptosis (programmed cell death). Less bone is absorbed, so bone remains dense and strong. Bisphosphonates provide persistent antiresorptive effect after discontinuation.

The risk of hip and vertebral fractures in older women is reduced significantly with the use of bisphosphonates.

SPECIFIC ESTROGEN RECEPTOR MODULATORS (SERMS)

These drugs that bind to estrogen receptors are an alternative to HRT in preventing osteoporosis. However, SERMs do not take away symptoms of menopause, including hot flushes. Specific SERMs may actually decrease the incidence of breast cancer.

Benign tumors of the uterus (fibroids) may shrink. However, the incidence of endometrial cancer is increased with certain of these drugs. There can be an increased risk of thromboembolism.

CALCITONIN

This hormone that inhibits bone resorption tends to be ineffective in early menopause. However, it can have some effect more than ten years after menopause in increasing bone mineral density.

PARATHYROID HORMONE

The tiny parathyroid glands are situated very close to the thyroid gland in the neck. Parathyroid hormone can be genetically engineered. The hormone promotes bone growth.

GROWTH HORMONE

Growth hormone output decreases as a woman ages. Theoretically, giving growth hormone to women approximately 70 years of age could lessen the decline in their bone mass, as well as the decline in their muscular strength, while gaining less abdominal fat.

STATINS

Statins influence the metabolism of cholesterol by inhibiting cholesterol production in liver cells. This prompts liver cell receptors to remove LDL from the bloodstream so that liver cells get the cholesterol they need for cell function. The primary use for this class of drugs is to reduce the risk of cardiovascular disease. Statins can reduce the risk of thrombosis in veins. Additionally, statins can reduce the risk of bone fracture. They increase bone formation and bone density and may inhibit bone resorption.

PHYTOESTROGENS

Some natural supplements contain phytoestrogens which are derived from plants. The problem with taking such supplements is that the dosage ingested into the human body is often unregulated and unknown. There is no progesterone to counteract the increased incidence of endometrial cancer.

Phytoestrogens may not improve menopausal symptoms, and do not alleviate hot flashes.

OSTEOPOROSIS GENES

An international research team led by Dr. Brent Richards (McGill University) reported in 2018 on genes associated with low bone mineral density (BMD) and fracture risk. It was found that a gene called DAAM2 influences bone density, mineralization, porosity and strength. Five other genes were found to probably be important for BMD and fracture as well.

CARDIOVASCULAR EVENT RISK AFTER MENOPAUSE

Cardiovascular disease risk is greater after menopause. Much of this increase simply goes along with general aging. However, it was noted as far back as the classic Framingham Study that menopause itself did seem to increase cardiovascular disease risk.

BREAST CANCER SCREENING

In the average-risk woman after menopause, breast examination and mammography may be done yearly, with the possibility of decreasing the frequency to every second year at approximately age 55, if agreed upon by the woman and her physician. The decision to continue mammography past age 75 should be made by each woman in consultation with her physician.

CERVICAL CANCER SCREENING

Women should be tested with cytology (Papanicolaou or Pap smear) and tested for human Papillomavirus (HPV) until age 65. If testing has been negative to that point, it may be stopped by her physician. Women who are now menopausal did not have the benefit of being vaccinated against the HPV virus when they were young: the vaccine was not then available.

LIBIDO AND SEXUAL FUNCTION

The frequency of sexual intercourse and sexual satisfaction does not necessarily correlate to the cessation of menses. There is, however, a possible diminution in libido and sexual desire.

This is often compounded by the fact that a male partner may be losing sex drive, having erectile problems (erectile dysfunction: ED), and may be incapable of having intercourse or achieving orgasm. Urological examination may detect problems including prostatic enlargement that may require intervention. Sex coaching by a professional counselor may be necessary. Drugs such as tadalafil and sildenafil promote erection. Tadalafil use can counteract benign prostatic hyperplasia.

After menopause, there is a decrease in androgen production from the ovaries and from the adrenal glands. Dehydroepiandrosterone (DHEA), DHEA sulphate (DHEAS), androstenedione, and testosterone are all decreased. Estrogen replacement therapy (HRT) further decreases bioavailable free testosterone because of an increase in sex hormone–binding globulin (SHBG). Decreased testosterone can possibly lead to muscle wasting, depression, loss of energy and decreased libido, as well as osteoporosis.

A recently FDA-approved injectable drug for the treatment of hypoactive sexual desire disorder (HSDD) in premenopausal women is bremelanotide (Vileesi) which activates melanocortin receptors.

This is in addition to the previously FDA approved, for premenopausal women, oral flibanserin (Addyi) which is a serotonin 1A receptor agonist and a serotonin 2A receptor antagonist.

Libido can possibly be enhanced by small amounts of testosterone. Giving testosterone to women is not without hazard. Acne, irreversible changes in the voice and male pattern hair growth are possible. The clitoris may enlarge. Oral methyltestosterone can be toxic to the liver. If a preparation that combines estrogen with testosterone is prescribed, there can be an increased incidence of endometrial cancer.

VAGINAL DIFFICULTIES

After menopause, the vagina may gradually tighten. This effect can be more pronounced if sexual intercourse is infrequent or absent. The vagina loses elasticity, and much of its lubrication. If intercourse is resumed, it may be painful or even impossible. The lower end of the vulva (area of the vaginal opening) called the fourchette, can tear and bleed. There may also be tears with penile penetration further up the vagina. With regular intercourse and the use of vaginal lubrication when needed, these problems generally do not occur.

In severe cases of vaginal tightening, the gynecologist may prescribe the use of vaginal dilators in graduated sizes.

Hormonal replacement therapy (HRT) with estrogen and progesterone cyclically, or in combination orally, or by skin patch, can keep the vagina supple and lubricated.

DISCUSSION

With our burgeoning population of seniors, the majority of whom are women, the postmenopausal years have become an increasingly significant proportion of life. If the average age of menopause today is approximately 50, and a woman can reasonably now expect to live well into her eighties or even beyond, then this span can easily represent more than a third, even up to half, her life. The implications for the individual, her family, and society at large are vast. If the individual is fortunate enough to be free of major debilitating disease and keeps herself properly nourished and mentally, physically and socially active, and finds the work she may be doing to be rewarding, her opportunities for a long and fulfilling life lie before her.

RESOLUTION OF THE CLINICAL VIGNETTE

This autonomous, independent woman with intact faculties in her mid-nineties represents a growing cohort of the older old. She is traveling to a place that she knows well, where competent medical care is available if needed: *Bon voyage!*

REFERENCES

1. Ronald M Caplan. Long Life: Prolonging the Productive, Fulfilling Lives of Women. A Survival Strategy, Morgan James Publishing. 2008. 183–227.
2. ACOG Practice Bulletin: Cervical Cancer Screening and Prevention: Number 168, October 2016 (reaffirmed 2018).
3. ACOG Practice Bulletin: Breast Cancer Risk Assessment and Screening in Average-Risk Women: Number 179, July 2017 (Reaffirmed 2019).
4. ACOG Practice Bulletin: Management of Menopausal Symptoms: Number 141, January 2014 (Corrected January 2016, March 2018).

5. Bone Density Exam/Testing https://www.nof.org/patients/diagnosis-information/

6. https://www.health.harvard.edu/heart-health/ask_the_doctor_is_bundle_branch_block_serious (Published January 2009, updated April 3, 2019).

7. https://www.nih.gov/news-events/nih-research-matters/genes-linked-abnormal-bone-density-fracture (Published January 15, 2019).

8. Lyu H, Jundi B et al., Comparison of denosumab and bisphosphonates in patients with osteoporosis. J Clin Endocrinol Metab. 2019; 104(5): 1753–1765.

9. Morris John A, Kemp John P, Richards J Brent et al., An atlas of genetic influences on osteoporosis in humans and mice. Nature Genetics. 2019; 51, 258–266.

10. Kannell WB, Hortland MC et al., Menopause and risk of cardiovascular disease: The Framingham study. Ann Intern Med. Oct 1, 1976; 85 (4): 447–452.

11. US Cardiology. 2008: 5 (1): 12–14.

12. https://www.uscjournal.com/articles/Menopause-cholesterol-cardiovascular-disease

13. Ouyang, Pamela MD. Menopause and the Cardiovascular System.https://www.hopkinsmedicine.org/heart_vascular_institute/clinical_services/centers_excellence/womens_cardiovascular_health_center/patient_information/health_topics/menopause_cardiovascular_system.ht

14. https://en.wikipedia.org/wiki/RANKL

15. https://www.nature.com/articles/s41413-018-0040-9

16. Perelman, Michael, Sex Coaching for non-sexologist physicians: how to use the sexual tipping point model. J Sex Med 2018; 15: 1667–16672.

17. https://www.fda.gov/news-events/press-announcements/fda-approves-new-treatment-hypoactive-sexual-desire-disorder-premenstrual-women

18. http://www.addyi.com

36 The Senior Adult Eye

Peter M. Odell, MD, FACS

CONTENTS

Older adult eyes have the same problems as eyes of younger people, but these problems tend to be more frequent, requiring closer observation as people age. The three most common senior eye care ocular issues are cataracts, macular degeneration and glaucoma. There are, of course, other important considerations with senior eyes, some of which are the red eye, the painful eye and sudden loss of vision.

CATARACT

The natural clear lens of the eye is located immediately behind the pupil. A cataract is a cloudiness/opaqueness of the natural lens. The cloudiness usually is progressive at varied unpredictable rates and results in increasingly blurred vision. In the initial stages, often simply changing the spectacle prescription minimizes the blurring.

As of this writing there are no proactive measures to prevent the progression of cataracts. Changing diet, activity, or medications will in fact have no influence on the rate of progression and decreasing vision. Sometimes, cataracts do not progress at all! Please remember that the diagnosis of a cataract itself does not mandate surgery. Surgery should only be performed when the patient feels the need to improve his/her visual function.

If cataracts reduce vision to an unacceptable level, surgery can be considered. The interpretation of visual impairment can vary considerably from patient to patient, even with the same objective degree of visual loss. Patient #1 may barely notice the visual loss and surgery should then be deferred while patient #2 with the identical visual impairment may feel incapacitated and surgery would then be considered.

Cataract surgery is usually done under local anesthesia in an outpatient setting. Patients are typically home within two hours of the surgery. Preexisting medical problems do not necessarily contraindicate surgery. Each case, of course, is different, requiring coordination between the ophthalmologist and the primary care physician.

Twenty-five percent of patients who have cataract surgery will, at some point, need a subsequent in-office laser treatment.

GLAUCOMA

The most common type of glaucoma is chronic open angle glaucoma, COAG. COAG occurs randomly in 2% of the population (with a family history the incidence is much higher). In the early stages of glaucoma there are no symptoms; however, if untreated the symptoms can become quite devastating.

Diagnosis is made by your eye care professional. The most basic part of a glaucoma evaluation consists of intraocular pressure measurement with inspection of the optic nerves. Measurement of corneal thickness, visual field examination, and measurement of retinal nerve fiber layer thickness may become indicated.

In the vast majority of COAG cases, eye drops alone will successfully lower eye pressure to an acceptable level, therefore preventing ocular damage. Sometimes two or three different types of drops will be used simultaneously. Beta blockers such as timolol maleate (Betimol, Istalol) function to decrease aqueous production. Carbonic anhydrase inhibitors such as dorzolamide hydrochloride ophthalmic (Trusopt) and brinzolamide ophthalmic suspension (Azopt) likewise inhibit aqueous production (sometimes used in oral form, acetazolamide (Diamox), for very short term). Brimonidine tartrate ophthalmic solution (Alphagan) and apraclonidine (Lopidine), alpha agonists, function to decrease aqueous production and also to increase the rate of drainage. There also are combination drops such as dorzolamide/timolol (Cosopt) and brimonidine/timolol (Combigan) which often are easier for the patient to manage.

DOI: 10.1201/9781003344476-41

Irritation/allergic reactions can occur from these topical medications. Often, the preservative in the bottle is the issue as opposed to the active ingredient. Some of these medications are available in a preservative-free unit dose format: tafluprost (Zioptan), timolol PF, dorzolamide/timolol (Cosopt PF).

In more difficult cases, office-based laser treatments become indicated. These are easy for the patient and effective in lowering intraocular pressure. In a very small percentage of COAG cases, surgery will become indicated.

The other glaucoma variants are managed in a similar manner. The exception, however, is acute narrow angle glaucoma. This can be a true medical emergency manifested by sudden loss of vision, severe pain, nausea, and vomiting necessitating immediate care.

Routine yearly ophthalmic examination can usually detect COAG and enable early treatment and can also detect narrow angles. In this situation an office-based laser treatment can be performed to prevent an acute episode.

Yearly preventive eye examinations are important to diagnose glaucoma at early stages and thereby prevent its secondary effects.

MACULAR DEGENERATION

The older adult population is also very susceptible to macular degeneration, a disease which affects reading vision disproportionately to distance vision. Although measuring only 1.5 mm in diameter, the macula is the most sensitive part of the retina and is integral to good functional vision.

Macular degeneration can not only cause blurry vision but also can cause distorted vision. Straight lines can look curved and letters can appear to have missing segments.

There are two types of macular degeneration, dry and wet (leakage of blood and fluid into the usually dry macula). Differentiating between the two types is very important in deciding the appropriate treatment. The less severe dry type usually progresses very slowly over long periods of time and is currently treated with over-the-counter antioxidants with lutein based on the AREDS study. The wet/exudative type is currently being treated with periodic intraocular injections of anti-VEGF (vascular endothelial growth factor) medications. (See Glossary.)

Once again, a yearly evaluation with your eye care professional will usually enable early diagnosis and treatment.

Common ocular disorders

1. Conjunctivitis, redness of the white part of the eye and/or inside of eyelids with or without discharge. Conjunctivitis can have varied etiologies: infection both viral and bacterial, less commonly fungal, allergic reactions, environmental factors, and chemical irritants. If wearing contact lenses, possible allergy to the lenses or lens solution or ulcers of the cornea should be considered. Bacterial conjunctivitis is treated with topical antibiotics in drop or ointment format. Tobramycin, gentamicin, ciprofloxacin, neomycin/polymyxin B/bacitracin (Neosporin), and bacitracin (ophthalmic) are a few of the commonly used antibiotics. Steroid/cortisone drops should never be used without an eye examination.

2. Floaters are very common, appearing as "bugs" moving inside the eye. Most people will develop floaters in their lifetime and the floaters are usually harmless. However, if the floaters suddenly increase in number or are accompanied by flashing lights, an urgent ocular exam is necessary as these symptoms can also herald an impending retinal detachment (although in the majority of cases the retina is normal).

3. Ocular migraine manifests itself with blurred vision lasting 1–2 minutes up to an hour associated with shimmering lights in the peripheral vision. As the vision improves, a pressure sensation behind the eye or mild headache often ensues. If this has happened early in life there is no concern. However, if ocular migraine occurs for the first time after age 65, a medical evaluation is indicated.

4. Dry eyes present with a sandy scratching sensation, usually worsening as the day progresses. Sometimes, paradoxically, dry eyes can cause increased tearing! Dry eye etiologies can be random, related to eyelid disease, systemic disease, or even prior refractive surgery. Treatment varies with severity of symptoms. Topical lubricants with or without preservatives are the entry level treatment. Omega 3/6 supplements, cyclosporine drops, heat therapy, daily lid cleansing

and/or punctal plugs, which block tear drainage, are other available treatment modalities determined by the severity the symptoms.

5. Acute pain with sudden loss of vision with nausea and vomiting can be acute glaucoma, requiring immediate medical attention.

6. Sudden loss of vision can be related to acute retinal detachment, retinal vascular occlusions, acute inflammation of the optic nerve or other parts of the eye as well as intraocular blood or inflammation. This also demands immediate medical attention.

7. A red blotch on the eye can be a superficial hemorrhage from the spontaneous rupture of a surface capillary. While often dramatic in appearance, it usually is not serious. It can be related to inadvertent trauma, bleeding disorders, or hypertension, and often the precise etiology cannot be determined. This needs to be evaluated by a medical professional.

8. Double vision can be both vertical or horizontal and requires examination, as neurologic causes are a possibility.

9. If pupils become unequal in diameter (anisocoria), the causes are varied, from OTC (over the counter) eye drops to neurologic conditions. Medical attention is required.

10. Light sensitivity has many causes and requires an examination.

11. Chalazions are one of the most common causes of eyelid swelling and discomfort. Chalazions usually manifest themselves with a localized swelling of one lid with tenderness to touch. This reaction most commonly is inflammatory (not infectious) and is treated with warm compresses four times a day. Drops are not indicated. In selected situations oral antibiotics can become indicated. If the chalazion is large and not responsive to medical measures, in-office drainage sometimes becomes indicated.

12. Redness of eyelid skin (one lid only) with groups of small cysts that also involves the skin of both the brow and scalp is strongly suggestive of shingles (Herpes Zoster). Often, discomfort precedes the skin eruption by weeks or days.

13. Redness of all four eyelids can represent an allergic dermatitis, infection, systemic disease and should be evaluated if lasting more than 48 hours.

14. Eyelids can roll inwards (entropion) rubbing on the surface of the eye causing varying degrees of discomfort and tearing. In these cases, the eyelashes are usually not visible. Entropion typically requires surgical correction.

15. Eyelids can also pull away from the eye (ectropion) causing deformity, tearing and irritation. Surgical repair is usually elective.

16. Upper eyelids can develop lowered elevation levels above the pupil (ptosis). If the eyelid level obstructs the pupil, surgery becomes indicated on a functional/elective basis. If lids are above the pupil and not affecting vision, surgical repair is cosmetic in nature.

17. Eyelid growths are most commonly benign; however, eyelid cancers account for 25% of all facial skin cancers. Therefore, any persistent or enlarging eyelid growth needs to be evaluated.

18. Facial asymmetry of sudden onset with inability to close one eye is suggestive of Bell's palsy, again requiring immediate attention.

19. Baggy eyelids, both upper and lower with or without puffiness, can evolve with age and time. Surgical correction can be elective and most commonly is cosmetic.

20. Sudden changes in peripheral vision can result from neurologic issues, retinal issues, and many of the already mentioned ocular conditions. Again, examination is imperative.

21. Diabetes mellitus both Type I and Type II can cause eye issues and requires at least yearly monitoring.

22. Oral medications can have significant ocular side effects that necessitate periodic eye examination. Ethambutol, hydoxychloroquine (Plaquenil), tamoxifen, and amiodarone are just a few of the more common drugs with negative effects on the eye. Primary care physicians should, of course, be alerting their patients.

23. Many systemic diseases can have ocular involvement. The following are just a partial list: kidney disease, hematologic diseases, hypertension, thyroid disease, various cancers, arteriosclerosis, autoimmune disease, neurologic disease. All of these systemic complications can be detected by routine periodic examination.

24. Sinus and nasal disease can extend through the bony tissue surrounding the eye (orbit) with many negative effects. These are usually managed jointly with ENT consultants.

25. Tearing can result from blockage of the tear drain or from other diseases already discussed.

All of the conditions listed will require examination/evaluation by an eye care professional and treatments can vary dependent upon individual circumstance. The listed conditions are some of the more common ocular problems and concerns. The list is certainly not intended to be all encompassing; rather it is to be used as a reference guide for the more commonly encountered ocular disorders.

SOURCES

1. AREDS: https://www.nei.nih.gov/research/clinical-trials/age-related-eye-disease-studies-aredsareds2
2. https://www.nei.nih.gov/learn-about-eye-health/eye-conditions-and-diseases/age-related-macular-degeneration/wet-amd-type-late-age-related-macular-degeneration-read-about-treatments-wet-amd-anti-vegf

37 Hearing Loss and Aging

Joseph J. Montano, Ed.D.

CONTENTS

SCENARIO A

Janice looked at her father, Richard Abrams, during her baby's 6th birthday party. He was smiling, he seemed to be attentive, but something just didn't feel right. He seemed to be present in the room but not participating in the festivities. She was worried. Janice had noticed her father beginning to disengage. She was worried perhaps he was beginning to have increased cognitive issues. Could this be the beginning of dementia? She had lived through the difficulty with memory loss and confusion with her mother a few years ago and was afraid she might have to relive it again with her dad. She called to him, but he did not reply. When anyone engaged him in conversation, he sat and smiled nodding his head in agreement. Finally, a friend at the party asked her if her father was able to hear. Hearing? Could this be the problem? She was so fearful of cognitive decline she never even considered the possibility of hearing loss. But it made sense. He struggled during their phone conversations. He asked for repetitions all the time. The television was always so loud. And now, he just seemed to be withdrawing. She became very concerned about her father's hearing.

This scenario highlights a frequent reality of hearing loss: it is an invisible condition. There are no obvious signs of hearing loss. People look normal, ears look fine. There is no pain, discomfort or outward indications that a hearing loss exists. The most common identifiers are changes in behavior. In this story, it wasn't until Janice started worrying about cognitive decline that the possibility of her father's hearing loss was considered. Many of these changes are subtle and may not be identified at first. Hearing loss is a complex problem because it does not merely impact a person's ability to hear, it is much worse than that; it impacts their ability to communicate. This chapter will focus on issues related to hearing loss and some options available to help a person you suspect may have diminished hearing ability.

It is no surprise to anyone that as people age, the incidence of hearing loss increases. What however may be surprising is that it probably started decades before anyone even noticed. Hearing loss as a result of aging is referred to as presbycusis, or age-related hearing loss. It is a process that can begin in the third or fourth decade and progress through a lifetime; typically, a loss of hearing occurs gradually over the years at such a slow rate that people do not even realize their hearing is changing. It is perceived as normal. People learn to live with this hearing loss and frequently develop strategies to overcome the barriers presented, such as hearing at parties, in restaurants, at business meetings or even during religious services. It may become more apparent as the hearing loss increases and the person begins to ask for repetitions all the time, and the strategies they developed over the years begin to fail. The worst scenario is that the adult with hearing loss begins to withdraw, isolate and disengage from their normal behaviors.

Hearing loss is a common characteristic of aging. As we age, the ear functioning begins to lessen and the brain's ability to process the information we hear begins to decrease. According to the NIH (2016) approximately one-third of adults over the age of 65 have hearing loss. That number increases significantly as we reach our 80s and 90s. Age-related hearing loss is

DOI: 10.1201/9781003344476-42

often a difficult condition to identify when in its early stages. Since hearing decreases over time, most have significant hearing loss for ten or more years before they begin to seek treatment, and even then, it can take several years before they actually agree to pursue hearing aids or amplification (2018). Whether they self-identify the presence of a hearing loss or are urged by family and friends to have their hearing tested, many people delay or even reject the notion of getting a hearing aid. Some report they are too expensive or don't like the cosmetic appearance of the instruments, but most resist because of stigma. Cohen and Williams (2018) report that stigma is a leading cause of the lack of hearing aid uptake, because of the fear of aging and being perceived as imperfect. While the number may vary, most researchers report that only about 25 to 30% of those who need hearing aids actually pursue amplification. This statistic has been consistent for many years and is also seen in many other countries around the world (2017). This combination of factors, stigma, cost and self-perception contribute to a dramatically underserved population of older adults with hearing loss.

Hearing Loss and Cognition

Research has been pointing to a relationship between hearing loss and cognitive functioning. Many older adults with cognitive disorders also experience hearing loss; the more significant the degree of hearing loss, the more severe the cognitive decline (2013). There has been a concern for many years about this relationship and the questions being currently researched concern whether there is indeed a cause-and-effect relation between the two or if early adoption of hearing aids or amplification can slow the rate of cognitive decline. Certainly, the presence of hearing loss puts an individual at risk for inadequate communication function and may indeed contribute to possible cognitive decline. As research in this area is underway, future findings may have an impact on hearing aid uptake for people with hearing loss and may be the necessary means for overcoming the obstacles presented by stigma.

As a result of these issues (cognitive decline, cost of hearing aids, stigma, etc.), government officials have been meeting over the past few years and have recommended the introduction of over-the-counter (OTC) hearing aids. Currently, the FDA is in the process of preparing the guidelines for the safety and efficacy of OTC instruments and they have just released the preliminary recommendation. At the time of this writing, the guidelines are out for review. Once formulated, OTC hearing aids will be available for adults with mild to moderate hearing loss and should be provided at a reduced cost compared to the traditional methods of hearing aid acquisition. The outcome of this is yet to be determined but the prospect of more people with hearing loss having access to hearing aid devices seems like a positive move for all concerned.

Early Signs of Hearing Loss

Since the onset of age-related hearing loss is so slow over so many years, the symptoms can be subtle and often missed. Most people begin exhibiting hearing issues when they are in the presence of background noise. This is often easily explained away because of the environment. For example, many restaurants and family gatherings take place in noisy rooms, so even if a person is having difficulty, they blame the problem on the background sound rather than on a change of hearing. While it is true that even people with normal hearing may experience difficulty in some situations, a person with hearing loss will have a reduced ability to compensate for the environment condition and experience significantly more difficulty. To add complexity to the situation, as we age, not only is hearing beginning to suffer, but our ability to interpret speech in noise also decreases as a result of brain changes in auditory processing. So, even in the case of an older adult with mild hearing loss, understanding speech in noise can be very difficult.

Another frequent complaint made by those with age-related hearing loss is difficulty experienced in listening to grandchildren or groups of people. In order to maximize communication ability of older adults, it is recommended that conversation take place in quiet environments and include the ability to take advantage of the visual cues of speech. This refers to what people commonly refer to as lipreading. While most people are not actually lipreading speech, the movement of the mouth, facial expressions, environmental cues all contribute to understanding speech. When we are talking to children or in groups, we are often denied these resources and must rely on our hearing ability alone. Most people do not realize the importance of visual cues when engaged in a conversation and clear conversation is compromised. Our daily communication behaviors make hearing difficult especially with hearing loss because frequently we are guilty of not facing the person when speaking, having a conversation with the television or radio playing in the background, talking from other rooms and speaking at a fast rate. Suggestions for improved communication strategies will be reviewed later in this chapter.

SCENARIO B

Janice decided to call her family physician about her dad's hearing, and he gave her the name of a local otolaryngologist (ear, nose and throat [ENT] doctor). The doctor examined her father's ears and there was no ear wax noted. He ordered a hearing test and her father was seen by an audiologist. The results indicated the presence of a moderate to severe degree of sensorineural hearing loss, enough that participation in daily conversation would be compromised and difficult. After a discussion with Mr. Abrams and Janice, it was decided they would consider options to help improve his ability to hear and engage with family and friends. With many options available, they decided on a set of hearing aids. Soon after, Mr. Abrams became noticeably more engaged in discussions, the television volume was lower, and Janice relaxed as her fear the possibility of her father's decreasing cognitive functioning was alleviated.

Types of Hearing Loss

Certainly, aging is not the only cause of a loss of hearing, but it is the most prevalent. Hearing is a complex function. Sound is directed into the ear and travels into the ear canal. At the end of the ear canal, the ear drum, or tympanic membrane, begins to vibrate and send a signal across the small bones, the ossicles of the middle ear. This causes movement within the cochlear part of the inner ear. As a result, small hair cells in the cochlea send a signal along the auditory nerve to the brain where the sound is then interpreted. Any disruption along this pathway can result in a hearing loss. The location of the problem will determine the classification of the hearing loss, either conductive, sensorineural or mixed. Table 37.1 identifies the types of hearing loss and their location in the ear.

Conductive hearing loss occurs as a result of problems occurring with the outer ear, ear drum or middle ear. Frequent causes of conductive hearing loss include impacted ear wax, ear infections with fluid in the middle ear cavity, ear drum perforations or problems with the ossicles. Frequently, there are medical treatments available for many of these causes of conductive hearing loss.

Sensorineural hearing loss occurs when there is a problem within the inner ear system including the cochlea or the auditory nerve. Hearing loss that is sensorineural in nature is frequently not responsive to medications and medical treatment and requires the use of amplification devices to help improve communication ability. Within this category, loss as result of aging, loud noise

Table 37.1 Types of Hearing Loss

Ear	Type of Hearing Loss	Common Causes	Functioning
Outer Ear	Conductive	Ear wax, foreign object in the ear	Decrease in hearing but able to understand speech when it is loud enough
Tympanic Membrane (Ear Drum)	Conductive	Perforation, scarring from old perforations, ear drum infection	Decrease in hearing but able to understand speech when it is loud enough
Middle Ear	Conductive, sometimes mixed	Fluid in the ear, middle ear infections, damage to the bones of the middle ear	Decrease in hearing but able to understand speech when it is loud enough
Inner Ear	Sensorineural	Aging, noise exposure, genetics, side effect of some drugs	Varying degrees of hearing loss sometimes with poor understanding of speech. Sometimes can be accompanied by balance issues.
Auditory Nerve	Sensorineural	Tumor-like growth on the 8th nerve	Varying degrees of hearing loss, very poor understanding of speech, tinnitus and vertigo

exposure or drug toxicity may be evident. Within the inner ear is also the balance mechanism and therefore some people with sensorineural conditions also suffer from dizziness and vertigo. This type of hearing loss is the most commonly seen in adults.

The final type of hearing loss is referred to as a mixed hearing loss because its origins are located within the outer/middle and inner ears. An example of this type of condition could be a person who has had lifelong middle ear infections resulting in a conductive hearing loss and then develops a sensorineural hearing loss as she/he ages. Thereby the loss affects both areas of the ear.

Regardless of the type of hearing loss, if medical and surgical treatment options cannot restore hearing to normal limits, amplification may need to be considered. There are many different types of amplification devices including hearing aids, hearing assistive technology systems (HATS), personal sound amplifiers and OTC devices. Choosing the right device for an individual takes the skill and knowledge of an audiologist or hearing healthcare provider as the options can at times be overwhelming.

Types of Amplification Devices

With the higher risk of social isolation, psychosocial effects and even cognitive decline, managing hearing loss is an important part of aging health and care. Luckily, there are many non-invasive options available to help modify the risks associated with hearing loss. Hearing aids are perhaps the most effective way to improve communication ability and are readily available through hearing healthcare providers, online, at big box stores and soon, over the counter. While there will be a difference in the types of hearing aids, certainly the consumer has a variety of amplification options to consider. For many families, the challenge is not the hearing aid, it is the ability to motivate the family member to pursue hearing aids in the first place. As mentioned earlier, hearing aids are considered by many to be a symbol of the stigma of aging. In this next session, I will discuss styles and functions of hearing aids as well as some alternatives to them called hearing assistive devices.

Hearing Aids

Hearing aids are electronic devices that that bring amplified sound to a person's ears. There are some hearing aids that can be extremely sophisticated with robust programming capabilities such as Bluetooth streaming possibilities, multiple listening programs for various environments, rechargeability and cosmetically appealing designs. These devices require a visit to a hearing care professional. Audiologists are doctoral-level professionals trained to provide the rehabilitation services to help a family manage the presence of hearing loss. Not only can they expertly program these devices, but they provide the therapeutic interventions necessary for adjustment to hearing loss. Hearing instrument specialists are experts in hearing aids and are able to dispense and program devices. Ear, nose and throat doctors are responsible for the medical management of hearing loss but typically refer patients to audiologists for hearing aid fittings.

Hearing aids come in various styles and price ranges. The most common style is an instrument that is referred to as a behind the ear model. This style has the capability of meeting the needs of most individuals with hearing loss. Because of its position, located physically behind the ear, and the device housing, these hearing aids are the most flexible and can add improved hearing in various listening conditions. They contain two microphones: one that is useful in quiet rooms and another that is directional, meaning the microphone picks up sound best in front of the person. These devices are now often rechargeable, relieving the patient and or family of the burden of changing batteries. They can easily be connected to cell phones for telephone use, streaming music or television and can be paired with other devices like external microphones that can be used to enhance direct speech input. Accessories can be added to these hearing aids that can be paired to televisions and personal computers which would allow families to watch television together without complaints about the volume being too loud, or participate in video conference calls and family FaceTime, Skype or Zoom.

Many of these hearing aids are equipped with a telecoil or T switch. This component allows the hearing aid to be compatible with an induction listening system. This technology requires the installation of a special wire loop within the listening environment. For example, many theaters and places of worship have begun installing these loops. This would allow any attendee or parishioner to simply put their hearing aid in the T coil program to access the audible signals. It is a cost-effective way for venues to make sound available for people with hearing aids and it opens up endless possibilities for those with hearing loss. Loops allow hearing aids to improve their functions in spaces that frequently pose communication difficulties.

The style referred to as in the ear hearing aids has all the components built into the body of the instrument and fits directly inside the ear canal. It comes in various styles from very small (depending on the size of the ear and hearing loss) to devices that fit the entire opening of the ear. Smaller instruments may not have all the features of the behind the ear devices but can certainly provide good functional hearing for many with varying degrees of hearing loss. Some people believe this style has improved cosmetic appeal and, while for some that could be true, there can be a sacrifice in performance.

As mentioned earlier, OTC hearing aids are soon to be available at many retail outlets without the need of seeing a hearing professional. They are meant for people with only a mild to moderate hearing loss and will be self-fitted. Standards for these devices are currently under review. The devices are expected to appear in stores sometime in the next few years. The availability of OTC hearing aids can help make the cost of hearing help less expensive and more accessible. Given how few individuals who can benefit from hearing aids actually wear them, increased availability may be able to close that gap.

Once a person has hearing aids, care and maintenance of the devices is extremely important. Caregivers are frequently required to manage the day-to-day hearing aid performance and should be comfortable with hearing aid devices. If a family member has a home health aide, that person must be included in hearing aid maintenance training.

Certainly, one of the most important components of hearing aid maintenance is to ensure that the power is on and the hearing aids are operating properly. This would require that batteries are fresh, or the devices have been charged. Battery life in a hearing aid can range from a few days to perhaps up to a week depending on the use and features. For this reason, batteries should be assessed daily, and hearing aid function verified. Most devices provide the user with a signal to warn that the hearing aid battery is about to expire and needs to be changed or recharged. If the person is an independent user of the hearing aid, they would change the battery or replace it in the charger. If the person requires assistance, the caregiver must be competent with this task.

Since all hearing aids are placed in the ear canal, they are prone to being clogged by ear wax. All hearing aids should be wiped after use and any debris removed from the instrument. Sometime wax actually clogs the hearing aid and needs to be removed. Hearing aids come with a small wax filter that can easily be changed if occluded. When occluded, however, the hearing aid will not work even if the battery is good.

Hearing Assistive Technology Systems (HATS)

While not a hearing aid, hearing assistive technology systems (HATS) have been available for many years and can help provide improved hearing access for specific listening conditions. Perhaps the most common devices in this category are amplifiers used in theaters, places of worship and large group amplification. HATS take sound from one source and send it directly to another. How the sound is transmitted distinguishes the type of device. For example, infra-red is a common transmission signal for the devices worn by people attending theaters and watching television. FM systems are commonly used for one-to-one communication or small group gatherings. An FM system requires the speaker to use a microphone and, through FM waves, the speech is transmitted to the listener with hearing loss either through a receiver attached to hearing aids or headphones. Some FM microphones can be placed on a dinner table to allow improved access to dinner conversation. Many hearing aids have an accessory known as a partner or external microphone. The following is an example of how this technology can be used.

SCENARIO C

Janice took her father to an audiologist where he was evaluated for a hearing aid. A variety of instruments were discussed. They decided to purchase a set of behind the ear hearing aids. The hearing aids were able to stream information from Mr. Abrams's smart phone and he was better able to communicate with Janice. He was thrilled to learn he was now able to hear music that he played on the phone directly in his hearing aids. There was an immediate improvement in her father's ability to follow conversation and hear the television. His interaction with the grandchildren improved and he no longer disengaged during family gatherings. She did notice however, when she went to a restaurant with her dad, that he appeared to struggle because of the background noise. Even though the hearing aids improved conversations over all, some noisy environments were very challenging. She obtained a partner mic and decided to wear it during their next lunch restaurant visit. She turned the microphone on and placed it on the lapel of her jacket close to her mouth. Immediately her dad was able to hear and respond appropriately to the conversation and the voice was clear and louder than the background noise in the restaurant. Following this positive experience, she decided to use the microphone every time she visited her dad.

Some types of personal amplification can be very inexpensive and simple to use. A hardwire device is a microphone used by the speaker, connected to an amplifier then to a set of headphones worn by the person with hearing loss. This is a wonderful device for one-on-one communication and has a variety of uses. It is especially useful when trying to communicate with a family member who may be sick and unable to manage hearing aids. It can be used for with someone who may be bedridden, or even on palliative care. Some families use hardwired systems for family members who may already have hearing aids but fear they may be lost if a hospitalization occurs. There are many people who, perhaps because of stigma, reject the notion of wearing a hearing aid even in the presence of hearing loss. For those people, family can use a simple hardwired system when involved in conversation to help improve communication attempts. There are a number of creative uses for this type of technology with the ultimate goal of improving an individual's communication ability when hearing aids are rejected or unavailable.

Other types of HATS include a category of devices known as alerting technology. Alerting systems are used to identify important signals and sounds that people with hearing loss need to be aware of in their environments. These might include things like the doorbell ringing, a smoke detector screaming or an alarm clock buzzing. These devices would provide a visual, vibratory or amplified signal as the means to increase awareness of important sounds. Telephones can also include alerting signals such as a light or loud ring. Since telephones are often important communication aids for many families caring for older adults, it is also possible to obtain captioned telephones. These phones transcribe the telephone conversation in real time and are often provided free of charge as a function of the Americans with Disabilities Act. They can be ordered through any hearing health care provider with documentation of the presence of hearing loss.

Communication Strategies

Table 37.2 highlights suggestions for improving communication when speaking with individuals with hearing loss. While hearing aids are valuable and will enhance the sound of speech, best communication is achieved when strategies are used to enhance the listening situation. It is important to remember that people with hearing loss will frequently still have difficulty hearing some speech and conversation. Understanding is affected by many variables with the most significant being the lack of visual cues, presence of noise and ability to attend to conversation.

The availability of visual cues is extremely important for people with hearing loss. While most are not consciously aware that they are lipreading, performance increases when the speakers face each other and lips are visible. The use of face masks during Covid has been extremely difficult since they not only distort speech but deny the available of visual cues. Whenever possible, conversations should take place in areas that are well lit, and individuals are seated in such a way as to allow access to these important cues.

One of the biggest complaints people make about hearing loss is the difficulty they experience when they are trying to have a conversation in noisy environments. Restaurants are perhaps some of the most difficult places for people with hearing loss. Everyone is affected by the presence of noise during conversation, even those with normal hearing. However, individuals with hearing loss are at a significant loss since they do not have the capability to effectively compensate for the noise. While most hearing aids have programs available to enhance speech in noise, they do not remove all the interference from a conversation. It is important to chose quieter restaurants when visiting with a person with a hearing loss. Hearing aids attempt to raise the speech signal above the level of the background noise, but these environments can still be challenging for many. The use of assistive technologies like the external microphone mentioned earlier may be a better solution to enhance speech in noise, but most people do not have this technology and need to maximize their situation with hearing aids. Some advance planning is suggested in order to locate the quieter restaurants in the area to maximize hearing ability for all.

Regardless of the environment, successful communication for people with hearing loss requires a great deal of effort. The luxury of being a passive listener, that is, the ability to not pay full attention during a communication event, is impossible. Listening must always be an active behavior. They must be listening attentively, watching faces, asking for repetitions and seeking assurance that they heard the conversation successfully. This can be exhausting. As a result, many people

Table 37.2 Communication Strategies for People with Hearing Loss

- Directly face your communication partner. Try and be on the same level, in good lighting. People with hearing loss rely on visual cues for communication. Even when they are not aware of it, they might be lipreading.
- People tend to raise their voice when they are speaking with a person who has hearing loss. It is preferable to speak slowly and clearly.
- Avoid exaggerating speech. If the person is using visual cues, over-emphasizing speech will make the visual cues unnatural and perhaps even take away from successful communication.
- Do not speak from other rooms. This is a very common trait among couples and families and may be difficult to overcome. Even if a person is wearing a hearing aid, this communication attempt will likely be unsuccessful.
- Get the person's attention before beginning a conversation. This will help the person cue into the speaker and take advantage of the cues available.
- Inform the person that the topic is changing. It is best that the person with hearing loss is aware of the topic, especially when with a group of people talking about many different issues.
- Try and arrange seating with a group so the person with hearing loss has visual access to the speakers.
- Keep noise at a minimum. If entertaining guests in your home, avoid playing music or having the television on in the background.
- If in a restaurant or noisy area, try and find the quietest section of the restaurant, preferably in a corner. Many hearing aids have directional microphones, so facing a wall will help reduce some background noise and enhance speech.
- Try to avoid noisy restaurants if possible. These environments are difficult for even people with normal hearing.
- If a word or phrase is misunderstood, repeat or rephrase to allow for an improved chance of understanding.
- Have the person repeat important information such as meeting times, phone numbers, directions, etc. Do not assume all the information has been heard and understood.
- Look for signs that the person with hearing loss might not have understood what was said. They may be afraid to ask someone to repeat something. Often, they may nod their head to make the speaker believe they heard the conversation.
- Always remember that a person with hearing loss may miss some information when in a conversation. Have patience and provide additional cues whenever possible.

with hearing loss complain they are tired because of the effort they need to use in order to have a conversation. Using the strategies described can help them reduce effort and increase communication success.

SCENARIO D

To celebrate her dad's 80th birthday, Janice arranged for a family gathering at a restaurant near his home. She visited the restaurant to check the amount of noise and availability of light for good communication. She spoke to the owner and explained that her father had a hearing loss and they needed to arrange for a round table that would seat 12 in the quietest section of the facility. They chose the space, and she made the reservation. The night of his party, he was seated in the center of the table facing Janice who was directly across the table in the corner of the restaurant. She knew her father's hearing aids would be facing forward so she did not want them in the direction of the most noise in the restaurant. They were facing the quieter side of the room in the corner. She placed a special microphone in the center of the table and informed everyone to speak slowly and clearly, one person at a time. Mr. Abrams participated in the party, blew out his candles and had a successful evening with his family—something he had not done in a very long time.

Care and Management of an Older Adult with Hearing Loss

Hearing loss can impact every aspect of a person's life. Not only will it interrupt conversation and make communication difficult and even impossible at times, but it can lead to severe psychosocial issues such as depression and isolation. Cognitive decline been associated with hearing loss and it is vital that one provide optimal listening conditions when possible. If hearing loss is suspected, make arrangements for a hearing evaluation and obtain some type of hearing assistance, whether it is prescribed hearing aids, OTC devices or assistive technology. Create a comfortable listening environment by providing the necessary technology and using the appropriate communication strategies.

If you suspect a loved one of having some hearing loss, look into it immediately. There are many options available to help improve communication, interpersonal relationships, engagement and perhaps even delay the onset of cognitive decline. There is nothing greater than our ability to communicate. While there may be many obstacles preventing a person to seek hearing aids or amplification, once this challenge has been overcome, quality of life can begin to improve for many. There are many resources available for people trying to find local hearing professionals, information on hearing loss or even peer support. For additional information, contact the American Speech-Language-Hearing Association, American Academy of Audiology, Academy of Otolaryngology–Head and Neck Surgery and the Hearing Loss Association of America.

REFERENCES

1. Cohen H, Williams H. (2018 September). Incorporating stigma counseling into audiology practice. *The Hearing Journal*, 71(9): 18, 19, 22.
2. Lin FR, Yaffe K, Xia J, Xue Q, Harris TB, Purchase-Helzner E, Satterfield S, Ayonayon HN, Ferrucci L, Simonsick EM, Health ABC Study Group. (2013). Hearing loss and cognitive decline in older adults. *JAMA Internal Medicine*, 173(4): 293–299.
3. NIH. (2016). Age-related hearing loss. NIH Pub No 97–4235. Age-Related Hearing Loss (Presbycusis)—Causes and Treatment (nih.gov) accessed October 27, 2021.
4. Simpson A, Matthews L, Cassarly C, Dubno J. (2019). Time from hearing aid candidacy to hearing aid adoption: a longitudinal cohort study. *Ear and Hearing*, 40(3): 468–476.
5. Valenti M, Amlani A. (2017). Cost as a barrier for hearing aid adoption. *JAMA Otolaryngology–Head & Neck*, 143(7): 647–648.

38 Skin Care of the Older Person

The Skin and Its Associated Changes

Aziz Khan, MD and Hao Feng, MD, MHS

CONTENTS

CASE SCENARIO

Mr. X, an 80-year-old male, was referred from the primary care physician's office for evaluation of a growth on the scalp. He was otherwise healthy with no significant past medical or surgical history. He took over-the-counter multivitamin and vitamin D tablets. He had noticed multiple growths on the face, scalp, and hands. One of the lesions that had been slowly growing in size over the prior six months was particularly concerning for him and his physician. He had significant sun exposure in the past, including blistering sunburns. On physical examination, he had a firm hyperkeratotic, indurated papulonodule with ulceration. In addition, there were multiple rough, scaly papules on the scalp, ears, face, and hands.

What is the likely diagnosis?

How should you proceed further?

AGING SKIN

The skin is the largest organ in the body and acts as a barrier between the body and the external world. As a barrier, the skin protects the body against harmful environmental stimuli, including physical, chemical, and infectious agents. Also, the skin is a dynamic, complex organ with a variety of other functions beyond barrier function and a sensory organ. These functions include temperature, fluid and electrolyte regulation, as well as biosynthesis and metabolism of different substances.

The skin additionally functions as a social organ and is in constant communication with the outside world. In the current society that we are living in, aesthetic appearance is given high importance. Throughout history, people have often been judged based on their appearance and the color of their skin. The visible signs of aging (i.e., wrinkling, gray hair, age spots) mostly involve the skin. The cosmetic industry has invested heavily in improving this aesthetic problem and prevention of signs of aging. However, of late focus has been shifting towards dermatological issues associated with advancing age.

Skin aging involves two processes. Intrinsic aging is genetically encoded and is an inevitable part of the normal aging process. The epidermis becomes thinner, resulting in skin atrophy and increased fragility. Other changes include decreased elasticity, impaired wound healing, loss of thermoregulation, and impaired metabolic functions. Changes in the skin appendages result

DOI: 10.1201/9781003344476-43

in other visible signs of aging, including hair loss and gray hair. Extrinsic aging, also known as photo-aging, is skin damage caused by external harmful agents, mainly ultraviolet (UV) radiations from sun exposure. It is often challenging to differentiate changes associated with intrinsic aging from extrinsic aging. Some of the characteristic changes associated with photo-aging include a more pronounced wrinkling, telangiectasia, variation in skin pigmentation, and cellular atypia/dysplasia. Skin growths like actinic keratosis and skin cancers are usually features of sun-damaged skin as UV exposure is a major risk factor for their development.

COMMON BENIGN SKIN CONDITIONS IN THE ELDERLY

Pruritus and Eczematous Dermatoses

Pruritus, or itch, is a common dermatological complaint in the elderly and can be caused by both primarily dermatological and systemic conditions. Dermatological conditions often cause pruritus with associated rash, while systemic diseases can cause pruritus without rash. Common dermatological conditions associated with pruritus in the elderly include skin dryness (xerosis), seborrheic dermatitis, incontinence-associated dermatitis, venous stasis dermatitis, allergic contact dermatitis, lichen simplex chronicus, and urticaria.

Xerosis is one of the common conditions associated with aging skin. Decreased production of lipids and sebum contributes to diminished natural skin moisturizing. Xerosis is the most common cause of pruritus in the elderly. Xerosis typically causes pruritus without a rash. However, in severe cases, it can lead to an eczematous reaction, called asteatotic dermatitis. Extremities are the most commonly involved sites in asteatotic dermatitis. Aggravating factors for xerosis include low humidity (cold, dry weather, central heating), frequent bathing, and exposure to harsh detergents or irritants.

A variety of systemic conditions can also cause pruritus without rash in the elderly. These conditions include renal disease, liver disease, iron deficiency anemia, thyroid disease, and malignancy. Drug eruptions cause pruritus with associated rash, depending on the type of drug eruption.

Depression and anxiety can further contribute to pruritus. Chronic pruritus in itself can lead to insomnia and depression. A psychological evaluation should be considered in patients with chronic pruritus, and underlying depression/anxiety should be treated accordingly as appropriate.

Treatment of pruritus involves both topical and systemic agents. Work-up for underlying systemic disease, review of medications, and assessment of skin should be performed before initiating therapy. Nutritional status should be assessed as malnutrition can worsen xerosis. Aggravating factors should be avoided. Topical moisturizers (emollients) should be used liberally every day and should be continued to prevent recurrence after treatment. Topical anti-pruritic agents like menthol can be added to the emollients to decrease pruritus in the short term. Other agents for short-term relief of pruritus include topical steroids, systemic steroids, and systemic antihistamines.

Seborrheic dermatitis is another common pruritic skin condition affecting the elderly. Dandruff is a mild form of seborrheic dermatitis characterized by scales with minimal inflammation. Seborrheic dermatitis characterized by erythematous patches with overlying scales, distributed mainly in areas with a high density of sebaceous glands (nasolabial folds, eyebrows, retro-auricular folds, etc.), is more common and severe in patients with HIV infection and neurological disease (particularly Parkinson's disease). Treatment options include topical antifungal and/or topical anti-inflammatory agents.

Contact dermatitis is also a frequently seen inflammatory dermatosis in the elderly. Contact dermatitis can be divided into allergic contact dermatitis (a delayed-type hypersensitivity response to a particular substance) and irritant contact dermatitis (direct damage to the skin from a specific material). Irritant contact dermatitis is more common. Treatment involves avoidance of the causative agents and the use of topical anti-inflammatory agents.

Stasis dermatitis is a common inflammatory skin condition in the elderly. Stasis dermatitis mainly involves the lower extremities and is associated with chronic venous insufficiency. Risk factors for chronic venous insufficiency include old age, family history, obesity, standing occupation, deep venous thrombosis, diabetes mellitus, hypertension, certain medications, and heart failure. Stasis dermatitis presents as an ill-defined erythematous patch or plaque in chronically edematous legs. Ulceration may occur in severe cases. Chronic changes include thickening of the skin and hyperpigmentation. Management of stasis dermatitis includes treatment of underlying venous insufficiency, frequent emollients use, and topical anti-inflammatory agents for pruritus.

Bacterial superinfection is common and should be treated with systematic antibiotics when indicated.

Pressure-Induced Skin and Soft Tissue Injury

Pressure-induced skin and soft tissue injuries, commonly known as pressure ulcers or bedsores, are common in the elderly. These are caused by sustained, unrelieved pressure resulting in ischemia and tissue damage. Immobility, sensory impairment, reduced perfusion, and malnutrition are major risk factors. Pressure ulcers commonly develop in areas of bony prominence. The deeper tissue is more susceptible to damage than superficial skin. Hence, a small external ulcer may turn out to be a more significant, extensive ulcer after debridement. Pressure ulcers are classified according to the extent of skin/tissue injury. Management of pressure ulcers requires multidisciplinary care and coordination. Relief of pressure, local wound care, adequate nutrition, pain control, and treatment of underlying medical conditions are the primary treatment measures. Bacterial superinfection is common. Common local signs and symptoms of infection include tenderness, erythema, purulent discharge, and foul odor. However, these are not universally present, and impaired wound healing may be the only sign of infection. Daily monitoring and documentation are essential for wound healing and to prevent a recurrence.

Skin Infections

Common skin infections in the elderly include fungal, bacterial, and viral infections.

Superficial fungal infections (dermatomycoses) are common in the elderly and may go unnoticed for a prolonged period due to their benign nature. Dermatophyte infections can affect any part of the body and are classified according to anatomic involvement. Tinea pedis (infection of feet) and tinea unguium (infection of nails, also known as Onychomycosis) are the most common dermatophyte infections in the elderly. Cutaneous candidiasis often develops in body folds like groins. Obesity and immobility are major risk factors. Diagnosis is usually made from the clinical appearance and can be confirmed with direct microscopy. Topical antifungal therapy is often sufficient; however, in severe or refractory cases, oral antifungals can be used.

Bacterial infections include cellulitis, folliculitis, erysipelas, impetigo, skin abscesses, and erythrasma. Cellulitis often involves the lower extremities. Interdigital fungal infection of the feet is a major risk factor. Cellulitis should be differentiated from stasis dermatitis and contact dermatitis. Deep venous thrombosis should be considered if there is a unilateral swelling with other risk factors for venous thrombosis, including immobility. These conditions can be treated with appropriate topical or systemic antibiotics.

Herpes Zoster/shingles is a painful, viral skin infection affecting the elderly. Immune suppression and old age are the major risk factors for the development of shingles. Treatment involves the systemic administration of anti-viral agents and pain medications use. Other viral infections in the elderly include viral warts and molluscum contagiosum.

Scabies is another pruritic skin infection which should be considered in nursing home residents. Scabies mostly involves inter-digital spaces. Visualization of the organism on direct microscopy from skin scraping of burrows confirms the diagnosis. Treatment options include topical permethrin or oral ivermectin.

Benign Skin Tumors

Benign skin growths and neoplasms are common in the elderly. Acrochordons (also known as skin tags) are outgrowths of healthy skin. Skin tags are more common in the elderly and are frequently seen in patients with obesity and diabetes mellitus. They appear as pedunculated lesions and commonly occur on the neck and intertriginous areas. They are diagnosed clinically, and treatment options include removal with forceps and fine-grade scissors, cryotherapy, or electrodesiccation.

Seborrheic keratosis is the most common epidermal tumor in the elderly, with a prevalence of up to 60%. Genetic predisposition, old age, and sun exposure are major risk factors. They appear as well-demarcated, round to oval, pigmented papules or plaques with stuck-on appearance. Face, trunk, and upper extremities are the most commonly affected sites. They are diagnosed clinically, and treatment options, if desired, include cryotherapy, curettage/shave excision, or electrodesiccation.

Cherry angiomas are mature capillary proliferations commonly seen in the elderly. They manifest as bright red, blanchable, dome-shaped papules on the trunk. These are asymptomatic but may bleed profusely with traumatic rupture. Treatment options, if desired for cosmetic regions, include electro-cauterization, laser therapy, or cryotherapy.

Solar lentigo, also known as "old age," "liver" spots, occur as a result of the proliferation of normal melanocytes due to chronic sun exposure. These manifest as uniformly pigmented macules in areas of actinic skin damage. These are asymptomatic. However, lesions with a change in color, border irregularity, or raised lesions should be biopsied to rule out lentigo maligna or melanoma.

Other common benign skin growths in the elderly include lipomas, venous lake, calluses, cutaneous horns, benign nevi, and dermatofibromas.

Pre-Malignant Growths

Actinic keratoses (AKs) occur as a result of the proliferation of atypical keratinocytes in sun-exposed areas. AKs have the potential to progress to squamous cell carcinoma (SCC) of the skin. They manifest as an erythematous, gritty, scaly papules which are more easily felt than seen. Chronic sun exposure is the leading risk factor. Diagnosis is often made clinically; however, a biopsy should be obtained if there is a concern for underlying SCC. Treatment options for AKs include cryotherapy, topical therapies (5-fluorouracil (5-FU) 5% cream, imiquimod 5% cream), and photodynamic therapy. Protection from the sun is important for prevention. Patients with AKs require ongoing monitoring for lesion recurrence and progression to SCC.

COMMON MALIGNANT TUMORS IN THE ELDERLY

Epidemiology of Skin Cancer

Skin cancer is the most common cancer in the United States. It is estimated that one in five Americans will develop skin cancer in their lifetime. The worldwide incidence of skin cancer has increased considerably over recent decades, reaching an "epidemic" proportion. This is attributed mainly to increased cumulative sun exposure in a progressively aging population. However, skin cancer is preventable in most cases. Skin cancer greatly affects the quality of life, contributes to the overall burden of skin conditions in the elderly, and can be fatal if not diagnosed early.

There are two main types of skin cancers, cutaneous melanoma (CM) and non-melanoma skin cancers (NMSC). Basal cell carcinoma (BCC) and cutaneous squamous cell carcinomas (SCC) are the two most common forms of NMSC. NMSC accounts for the majority of skin cancers (80%), the most common being BCC (70%). The majority of the deaths from skin cancer are attributed to CM. BCC and SCCs are highly curable if diagnosed early and treated appropriately.

Exposure to ultraviolet (UV) light is the major risk factor for all types of skin cancer. Cumulative UV light exposure during one's lifetime is associated with an increased risk of CM and NMSCs. Hence, the incidence of skin cancers increases with age. One blistering sunburn in childhood can nearly double the risk of developing melanoma. Skin cancers arise mostly in areas of chronic actinic skin damage. Other risk factors for the development of all types of skin cancers include exposure to tanning beds, skin that burns easily, blond or red hair, immunocompromised conditions (including immunosuppressive medication use), and a history of skin cancer. The presence of multiple moles (more than 50), atypical moles, large moles, family or personal history of CM increases the risk of developing CM. Patients with a history of melanoma are nine times more likely to develop a second melanoma as compared to the general population.

Caucasians are at increased risk of developing skin cancer; however, skin cancer can develop in anyone, regardless of skin color. In individuals with darker skin types, skin cancer is often diagnosed at a later stage and develops in areas that are not commonly exposed to the sun. Patients with a skin of color are less likely to survive melanoma as compared to Caucasians.

Clinical Features

Cutaneous Melanoma

There are four main types of invasive cutaneous melanoma. These include superficial spreading melanoma, lentigo maligna melanoma, nodular melanoma, and acral lentiginous melanoma. Superficial spreading melanoma is the most common form of melanoma (accounting for 70% of cases) and presents as a slowly enlarging macule/patch with variable pigmentation. Nodular melanoma is the second most common form and presents as a rapidly enlarging pigmented papule or nodule. Lentigo maligna melanoma (LM) and acral lentiginous melanoma are less common. Acral lentiginous melanoma is not related to sun exposure and occurs on the palms, soles, and beneath the nails.

The "ABCDEs" rule and the "Ugly Duckling" sign help clinicians in identifying skin lesions concerning for melanoma. ABCDE is an acronym which stands for A: asymmetry, B: border irregularity, C: color variation, D: diameter > 6 mm, and E: evolving or changing with time. "Ugly Duckling" refers to a skin lesion/mole which looks different from the rest and sticks out. Most normal moles on one's skin should look similar. In contrast, a lesion concerning for melanoma stands out like an "ugly duckling." These signs help in the identification of potential melanoma; however, these are not specific for melanoma, and not all melanomas will display these characteristics.

Non-Melanoma Skin Cancers

Both BCC and SCC develop in areas of chronic actinic damage. The most common variants of BCC include the nodular, superficial, morpheaform subtypes. Nodular BCC typically presents as a pearly, pink, or flesh-colored papule or nodule on the sun-exposed areas of the head and neck. Superficial BCC usually presents as a shiny, erythematous macule, patch, or thin plaque on the trunk. Morpheaform BCC might resemble a scar.

The presentation of invasive SCC varies with the degree of tumor differentiation. Well-differentiated tumors present as firm hyperkeratotic, indurated papules or plaques while poorly differentiated tumors present as flesh-colored papules/nodules with frequent ulceration and bleeding.

REVISITING THE CASE

Mr. X was evaluated in the dermatology clinic and underwent a full-body skin examination with dermatoscopy. He was found to have multiple actinic keratoses (AKs) on the scalp, ears, nose, and dorsum of hands. Biopsy of the scalp lesion showed a moderately differentiated squamous cell carcinoma with positive margins on biopsy. He was scheduled for Mohs micrographic surgery for definitive removal of the tumor. For the AKs, he was given the option of freezing with liquid nitrogen therapy vs. application of 5-fluorouracil (5-FU) 5% cream. Due to an increased number of lesions, the patient opted for 5-FU therapy.

Management Options

The prognosis of melanoma depends on the stage at the time of diagnosis. The thickness of the tumor (measured in millimeters) is most strongly associated with the probability of metastasis. Patients with stage 0 (in situ melanoma) and stage 1 (localized invasive) have a better prognosis and are curable with surgical treatment. Those with more advanced disease (stage a 2–4) are likely to develop metastatic disease. Surgical excision remains the mainstay of treatment. Surgical management of CM is complex and is beyond the scope of this writing. However, wide local excision with regional lymph node sampling is the preferred surgical option. Resection margins depend on the stage of the disease. Immunotherapy can be used as an adjunct to surgery and as primary therapy for metastatic disease.

BCC generally carries a very favorable prognosis, and a complete cure can be achieved with timely intervention. SCC has a higher potential to metastasize as compared to BCC; however, a complete cure can be achieved with early recognition and treatment. Treatment selections depend on patient demographics and patient preference. Mohs micrographic surgery (MMS) provides the best long-term cure rates and cosmetic outcomes. It is the first-line therapy for high-risk BCCs and SCCs. Also, in low-risk patients, MMS can be used as an alternative therapy if the patient desires an improved cosmetic outcome. Standard excision can be used for lower-risk tumors. Non-surgical treatment options including cryosurgery, topical therapies (5-fluorouracil (5-FU) 5% cream, imiquimod 5% cream), are reserved for patients with BCC who refuse surgery, are poor surgical candidates, and those with multiple superficial BCCs. Topical therapies, however, are not approved by the Food and Drug Administration (FDA) for the treatment of SCCs.

REVISITING THE CASE

Mr. X successfully underwent MMS. On follow-up visit, the wound was healing well with no evidence of local recurrence. There was no regional lymphadenopathy. He was counseled that he will need regular follow-up every 3–6 months for 2 years, followed by every 6–12 months for 3 years, and then annually for life. He was also counseled about skin cancer preventive measures.

Prevention of Skin Cancer

Chronic sun exposure is the most important and preventable risk factor for the development of both melanoma and non-melanoma skin cancers. Regular sunscreen use has been associated with a decreased CM risk. Increased incidence of CM in men might be partly due to reduced rates of sun protection. Protection from the sun (sunscreen use, avoidance of sun, protective clothes is the most critical defense against the development of skin cancers.

Sun protection is recommended for all age groups as damaging effects of sun exposure are cumulative over time. A broad-spectrum sunscreen with a sun protection factor (SPF) of at least 30 should be liberally used while out in the sun. Reapplication every two hours is recommended, even on cloudy days. The shade should be sought when possible, especially between 10 am and 4 pm, when UV radiation is the strongest. Shade decreases the amount of UV radiation by 50 to 90%. In contrast, snow, water, metallic surfaces, and concrete can reflect up to 90% of the UV rays. In addition, sun-protective clothing, including hats and sunglasses, provides adequate protection against UV radiation. Tanning beds should be avoided. Strict sun avoidance may increase the risk of vitamin D deficiency; however, oral vitamin D supplementation is an effective, safe, and well-tolerated alternative for achieving adequate vitamin D levels.

REFERENCES

1. Apalla Z, Nashan D, Weller RB, Castellsagué X. Skin Cancer: Epidemiology, Disease Burden, Pathophysiology, Diagnosis, and Therapeutic Approaches. Dermatology and Therapy. Springer Healthcare; 2017. Vol. 7, pp. 5–19.
2. Garcovich S, Colloca G, Sollena P, Bellieni A, Balducci L, Cho WC, et al. Skin cancer epidemics in the elderly as an emerging issue in geriatric oncology. Aging and Disease. International Society on Aging and Disease; 2017. Vol. 8, pp. 643–661.
3. Norman RA. Geriatric dermatology. Dermatol Ther [Internet]. 2003 Sep [cited 2020 Jun 28];16(3):260–268. Available from: http://doi.wiley.com/10.1046/j.1529-8019.2003.01636.x
4. Wey SJ, Chen DY. Common cutaneous disorders in the elderly. Journal of Clinical Gerontology and Geriatrics. Elsevier B.V.; 2010. Vol. 1, p. 36–41.
5. Blume-Peytavi U, Kottner J, Sterry W, et al. Age-Associated Skin Conditions and Diseases: Current Perspectives and Future Options. Gerontologist. 2016. Vol. 56(Suppl 2), pp. S230–S242. doi:10.1093/geront/gnw003

39 Caring for the Older Person Undergoing Plastic Surgery

Subhas Gupta, MD, CM, PhD, FRCSC, FACS and Erin O'Rorke, MD

CONTENTS

PROLOGUE

"Doctor, I would really like you to make me look younger as all of this loose skin in my neck makes me appear much older than I feel." This patient presented for an aesthetic surgery evaluation hoping to have a facelift. Her story is much more complex.

We first met this patient six months earlier following her aortic valve replacement surgery that was complicated by mediastinitis and sternal dehiscence. Her first plastic surgery procedure was a chest wall reconstruction using both of her pectoralis muscles and her right rectus abdominis muscle while she was still a patient in the surgical intensive care unit on both inotropic agents and pressors. Fortunately, her reconstruction was successful, and she was discharged home in much improved condition a week later. But was this "improved condition" good enough for her to undergo a facelift?

PLASTIC SURGERY IN THE OLDER PATIENT

The U.S. population has steadily become older, in large part due to progressive medical and surgical advances. While just over 15% of the North American population is 65 years of age or older, this group accounts for over 40% of surgical cases. With higher rates of comorbid conditions compared to younger patients, the older population requires specialized preoperative workup, risk assessment, and preparation before undergoing surgery, as well as attentive postoperative care.

Within the field of plastic and reconstructive surgery, elderly individuals make up a large percentage of the patient population, particularly for a subset of commonly performed procedures. This chapter will identify some of the most common plastic surgery procedures requested by elderly patients, discuss special techniques in preoperative preparation for surgery, and outline crucial perioperative and postoperative recommendations to maximize both functional and aesthetic outcomes in the older patient population.

COMMON PLASTIC SURGERY PROCEDURES AMONGST OLDER PATIENTS

While the field of plastic surgery is incredibly diverse in its range of surgical and non-surgical procedures, there is a well-defined subset of procedures that have remained amongst the most commonly performed on older patients over the past two decades. Physicians caring for elderly patients should have an understanding of the purpose and potential outcomes of these procedures, as they will undoubtedly frequently encounter patients considering and actually undergoing them. Tables 39.1–39.4 include the most common plastic surgery procedures performed on elderly patients, along with their indications and potential complications, divided into the categories of Hand; Breast and Trunk; Head and Neck Skin Cancers; and Facial Aesthetic operations.

"PREHABILITATION"—OPTIMAL PRIMING OF THE OLDER PATIENT FOR PLASTIC SURGERY

While the plastic surgery procedures performed in older patients vary in their associated morbidity, optimizing these patients for surgery reduces their risk of complication and enhances their recovery. Prehabilitation is defined as a process of improving the functional capability of a patient prior to a surgical procedure so the patient can better withstand the stress of a surgical procedure. This is most important in the elderly patient. In our plastic surgery practice, we have been using prehabilitation protocols for the past two decades. A whole person optimization view of the

DOI: 10.1201/9781003344476-44

Table 39.1 Common Hand Pathology Requiring Surgical Procedures in the Elderly Patient

Pathology	Non-Surgical Management Options	Surgical Management	Complications
Carpal tunnel syndrome	Nighttime splinting Corticosteroid injections	Surgical division of the transverse carpal ligament (TCL) • Palmar fascia and TCL incised longitudinally to expose median nerve. • Appropriate for patients with prolonged symptoms or advanced disease.	Pillar pain Scar tenderness Persistent symptoms
Trigger finger (stenosing tenosynovitis)	Hand therapy NSAIDs Corticosteroid injections into the flexor sheath at the A1 pulley	Release of the A1 pulley via pulley division	Stiffness Tenderness Incomplete release Tendon bowstringing Digital nerve injury
1st carpometacarpal arthritis (basal joint arthritis)	Activity modification Joint protection Thenar muscle strengthening/physical therapy NSAIDs Corticosteroid injections into CMC joint (use with caution—potential to accelerate arthritic degeneration)	Arthroplasty • Trapeziectomy. • Removal of surrounding osteophytes. Ligament reconstruction with tendon interposition (LRTI) • Flexor carpi radialis tendon used to reconstruct the volar beak ligament and fill the space created from removal of trapezium bone from wrist.	Reduction of pinch strength Loss of joint height Stiffness Persistent pain

Table 39.2 Common Breast and Trunk Malignancy Reconstructions

Sternal Wound Reconstruction

Reconstructive Option	Procedure Considerations
Pectoralis major flap	Close proximity to sternum Limited ability to cover lower third of sternum unless anastomosed to internal mammary artery (IMA) perforators, which may not be available after certain thoracic surgeries such as coronary artery bypass grafts
Rectus abdominis flap	Can provide coverage of the lower sternum Can still be used in cases where the IMA has been harvested by relying on musculophrenic perforators
Omentum flap	Large, versatile flap that can cover the length of the sternum Easily contoured and can fill small wound cavities Limited use in patients with previous abdominal surgery due to adhesions or in patients not stable enough to undergo laparotomy Possible complications include epigastric hernia, bowel obstruction, and bowel adhesions
Latissimus dorsi flap	Best for coverage of lateral chest wall defects Harvested in prone/lateral position; necessitates intraoperative patient position change Significant distance from sternum Distal flap blood supply may be tenuous

Breast Reconstruction

Reconstructive Option	Procedure Considerations
Implant-based reconstruction	*Indications* Unilateral or bilateral breast reconstruction May be one-stage or two-stage (tissue expander to implant) May be immediate or delayed *Benefits* Often shorter operative time compared to autologous tissue reconstruction Prosthetic implants do not affect rate of detection of locoregional breast cancer recurrence *Challenges* Symmetry can be challenging to achieve, particularly in unilateral reconstructions May require contralateral symmetry procedures (mastopexy, reduction mammaplasty) May require revisions over time
Autologous reconstruction	*Indications* Unilateral or bilateral breast reconstruction in patients desiring more natural-appearing reconstruction and/or avoidance of prosthetic devices Common techniques include deep inferior epigastric artery perforator (DIEP) flap and transversus abdominis myocutaneous (TRAM) flap, amongst others *Benefits* Uses patient's native tissue without need for prosthetic device Improvement in reconstructed breast softness and symmetry *Challenges* Additional donor site with potential for donor site complications (seroma, hematoma, infection, abdominal weakness, hernia formation) Longer operative time and hospital stay compared to implant-based reconstruction

Table 39.3 Surgical Reconstruction after Excision of Dermatologic Malignancies of the Face and Scalp

Reconstructive Option	Indications	Procedure Notes	Complications
Primary closure	Scalp lesions up to 3 cm in diameter Forehead lesions up to 2.5 cm in diameter Facial defects with sufficient surrounding skin laxity	Devitalized or fibrotic wound edges sharply debrided prior to wound closure	Wound dehiscence Delayed healing Wide scar in cases of high-tension closure
Closure by secondary intention	Forehead defects in which wound edges cannot be approximated	Granulation tissue matrix fills in wound defect with eventual epithelial covering of wound	Relatively slow wound healing option Discouraged in scalp defects due to lengthy process, and formation of hairless scar
Skin grafts	Allografts (from other human) or xenografts (from different species) may provide temporary closure while awaiting pathology results and execution of final reconstructive plan Split-thickness autografts (from same individual) indicated for closure of superficial wounds of face and scalp with well-vascularized tissue bed at base of defect	Skin grafts for facial defects should not be meshed for optimal aesthetic outcome	Seroma Hematoma Graft loss Variable color and texture match (may result in shiny/patch-like appearance of healed graft)

(Continued)

Table 39.3 (Continued)

Reconstructive Option	Indications	Procedure Notes	Complications
Local flaps	Allow for closure of most scalp defects 3–6 cm in diameter Larger scalp defects (6–9 cm in diameter) may be closed with a local skin flap with skin grafting of flap donor site (secondary defect)	Superior functional and aesthetic results compared to skin grafts, particularly in patients who require postoperative local radiation therapy Wide undermining of scalp should be performed to maximize scalp mobilization and cover secondary defect as much as possible	Follicular damage/ incisional alopecia Need for skin graft coverage of secondary defect
Free tissue transfer	Useful for scalp defects larger than 9 cm in diameter Useful for defects with exposed bone without pericranium	Superficial temporal vessels commonly used as recipient vessels Frequently used options include latissimus dorsi and rectus abdominis muscle flaps, serratus anterior muscle flap and anterolateral thigh fasciocutaneous flap	Skin graft closure of secondary defect may be necessary in larger free flaps Infection Hematoma Flap necrosis

Table 39.4 Aesthetic Surgery of the Face

Procedure	Indications	Procedure Notes	Complications
Forehead and brow lift	Forehead and brow ptosis Horizontal forehead skin wrinkles Vertical glabellar furrows	Goal is to soften transverse forehead lines and glabellar creases without creation of a "surprised" look This may be achieved by elevating the lateral brow with minimal to no elevation of the central and medial brow	Scalp paresthesias Frontalis muscle weakness Incisional alopecia Hematoma
Blepharoplasty	Brow ptosis Eyelid ptosis Tarsoligamentous laxity	Excises excess eyelid skin, muscle and/or orbital fat	Corneal irritation Ectropion Lid malposition Swelling of conjunctiva Need for reoperation
Facelift	Ptosis and atrophy of facial tissues Generalized facial and neck skin laxity Jowls Platysmal bands Loss of neck definition	Does not address quality of facial skin Is not a treatment for sun damage, or irregular pigmentation	Hematoma Skin necrosis Facial nerve injury Hypertrophic scarring

patient prior to a plastic surgery procedure has many facets and addresses physical, psychological, nutritional and lifestyle parameters.

Over the past several years, there have been several studies performed to demonstrate the value of prehabilitation. These studies have generally included all age groups of patients undergoing a specific procedure. An increase in functional capacity before surgery as measured by the 6-minute walk test (6MWT) is strongly correlated with improved outcomes from specific procedures. The 6MWT assesses distance walked over 6 minutes as a sub-maximal test of aerobic capacity or endurance. Studies geared at a broader multimodal prehabilitation program have included nutritional guidance and anxiety reduction through education. These studies have also shown reduced morbidity from surgical procedures.

In our practice, we have developed a prehabilitation pathway that aims to empower patients, modify key behaviors, and improve outcomes with reduced complications along with lowered costs. There are several goals for prehabilitation:

- Improve cardiovascular, pulmonary, and/or musculoskeletal function.
- Improve balance and reduce the risk of falls.
- Reduce anxiety and improve coping with specific cognitive behavioral strategies.
- Improve quality of sleep with sleep hygiene education.
- Optimize surgical outcomes with smoking cessation interventions.
- Optimize diet with nutrition counseling.
- Implement home safety strategies to avoid falls.
- Facilitate return to work with adaptive equipment.

The general postoperative decline in physical and psychological function creates the most significant risk for morbidity. Additionally, this decline has an important impact on functional disability during the recovery from plastic surgery specifically impairing the following:

- Return to work.
- Caring for others.
- Mobility due to safety concerns (walking, driving).
- Ability to travel and take vacations.
- Activities of daily living, including feeding, dressing, bathing and walking.
- Instrumental activities of daily living that allow an individual to live independently in the community.

The four parts of Plastic Surgery Prehabilitation are functional and nutritional optimization, lifestyle choices, and stress management. This is summarized in Figure 39.1.

The Prehabilitation L-A-N-E

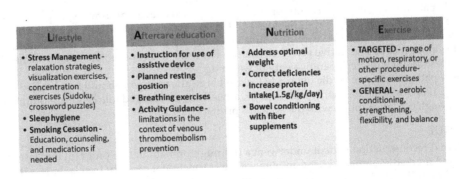

Lifestyle	Aftercare education	Nutrition	Exercise
• Stress Management - relaxation strategies, visualization exercises, concentration exercises (Sudoku, crossword puzzles) • Sleep hygiene • Smoking Cessation - Education, counseling, and medications if needed	• Instruction for use of assistive device • Planned resting position • Breathing exercises • Activity Guidance - limitations in the context of venous thromboembolism prevention	• Address optimal weight • Correct deficiencies • Increase protein intake (1.5g/kg/day) • Bowel conditioning with fiber supplements	• TARGETED - range of motion, respiratory, or other procedure-specific exercises • GENERAL - aerobic conditioning, strengthening, flexibility, and balance

Figure 39.1 The Prehabilitation L-A-N-E.

Medical Optimization

Figure 39.2 Medical optimization of the elderly plastic surgery patient.

The program has a duration range of 4 to 10 weeks for elective procedures and serves to increase functional reserve as it physically and mentally optimizes patients for surgery. The categories of assessment and intervention are summarized in Figure 39.2.

ENHANCED PERIOPERATIVE AND POSTOPERATIVE CARE OF THE OLDER PATIENT UNDERGOING PLASTIC SURGERY

Prehabilitation is not yet widely adopted in surgical practices. Efforts focused on improving patient outcomes have been centered on the intraoperative and postoperative periods. During any surgery, including plastic surgery, special care should be taken both intraoperatively and postoperatively to minimize complications and optimize outcomes in older patients. Intraoperatively, this begins with proper patient positioning. Elderly patients benefit from careful padding and positioning to avoid skin breakdown and pressure injuries, a complication older skin is particularly prone to.

To decrease the risk of postoperative disorientation and delirium, a multimodal nonnarcotic pain regimen should be employed in the operating room. This can include a combination of regional pain blocks, acetaminophen and gabapentin, among other nonnarcotic medications. Physicians should also avoid prescribing medications associated with an increased risk of adverse events in elderly patients, such as anticholinergic nausea medications, benzodiazepines and sedatives such as zolpidem.

In the postoperative period, elderly patients can benefit from a multidisciplinary care team including input from specialists in geriatrics, hospital medicine, physical and occupational therapy, nutrition and social work. Physical therapy focused on improving postoperative strength, mobility and balance decreases length of hospital stay and reduces the need for nursing home disposition in elderly patients.

Strategies to reduce the risk of delirium, in addition to minimizing the use of the aforementioned medications, include early mobilization after surgery and diligent monitoring and timely management of early signs of delirium.

Elderly patients who experience intraoperative dysglycemia have significantly longer length of ICU and length of hospital stays. Diabetes and longer surgery duration have been shown to increase the risk of intraoperative dysglycemia, and elderly patients with these risk factors may benefit from tighter perioperative glycemic control. The same improvement results from maintaining normothermia with perioperative patient warming.

Elderly patients who are medically ready for discharge after surgery should be provided with clear verbal and written discharge instructions, as well as prearranged follow-up appointments and thorough communication with the patient's primary care physician.

EPILOGUE

Our sternal reconstruction patient underwent a thorough prehabilitation program that lasted 10 weeks and markedly improved her 6-minute walk test functional capacity from a far less than ideal 250 m to 550 m. Her nutrition and glycemic control were optimized, and she underwent her facelift under monitored anesthetic care without incident.

REFERENCES

1. Bettelli G, Neuner B (2017) Postoperative Delirium: A Preventable Complication in the Elderly Surgical Patient. *Monaldi Archives for Chest Disease*, 87(2), 842.
2. Cameron AM, Cameron JL (2020) *Current Surgical Therapy*, 13th Edition. Philadelphia, Pennsylvania. Elsevier, Inc.
3. Gupta S (2021) Surgical Site Infections: Preventing and Managing Complications. *WoundSource Practice Accelerator*. October 2021.
4. Knaak C, Wollersheim T, Morgeli R, Spies C, Vorderwulbecke G, Windmann V, Kuenz S, Kurpanik M, Lachmann G (2019) Risk Factors of Intraoperative Dysglycemia in Elderly Surgical Patients. *International Journal of Medical Sciences*, 16(5), 665–674.
5. Matullo E (2007) CMC Arthroplasty of the Thumb: A Review. *Hand*, 2(4), 232–239.
6. Thorne CH, Chung KC, Gosain AK, Gurtner GC, Mehrara BJ, Rubin JP, Spear SL (2014) *Grabb and Smith's Plastic Surgery*, 7th Edition. Philadelphia, Pennsylvania. Lippincott Williams & Wilkins (Wolters Kluwer).
7. Townsend CM, Beauchamp D, Evers M, Mattox KL (2022) *Sabiston Textbook of Surgery*. St. Louis, Missouri. Elsevier, Inc.

PART VI
UNDERSTANDING, PROTECTING

40 Elder Abuse

Mark J. Yaffe, MDCM, MCISc, CCFP, FCFP

CONTENTS

CLINICAL VIGNETTE

Mrs. L. is an 88-year-old widow with stable ischemic heart disease and diet-controlled Type 2 diabetes mellitus. She has shown gradual deterioration in short-term memory and in judgment. She downplays deficits suggested by her MMSE score of 24, and is angry at her family doctor for notifying the license bureau about concerns about her ability to drive safely. Mrs. L. lives alone, with the exception of a housekeeper who comes to her apartment three half days per week to prepare some meals, do laundry, and to assist with bathing/hygiene. Mrs. L. downplays the need for the latter. The housekeeper had tried a number of times to attend to these issues, but in response to Mrs. L.'s lack of cooperation the housekeeper became physically rough with the bathing. As well she has gradually ignored skin sores on the upper legs and buttocks.

Social contact with friends decreased over the preceding few years, aggravated by hearing loss. Following audiology testing Mrs. L. was advised that she would benefit from a particular hearing aid that would be easily useable, despite severe osteoarthritis in her hands. Mrs. L. stated that she could not afford the co-payment cost of the apparatus. The housekeeper frequently yells at her that she is too tight with her money, but Mrs. L. gives into frequent pleas from the housekeeper for extra money to help with troubled members of her family.

The family doctor has suggested a home visit by a community nurse or social worker, but this has been turned down by Mrs. L. She does, however, reluctantly give the physician permission to telephone her only child, a daughter who lives 2000 miles away. The latter is hard to reach and voice messages that are left are not returned. When contact is eventually made, the daughter indicates that she talks to her mother about once every three to four weeks, and that, while her mother might be a little eccentric, she was a "normal 88-year-old who requires no new interventions." The family physician learns that the daughter has power of attorney for mother's affairs, that she hasn't made much attempt to keep track of her mother's finances, and that she was unaware of money regularly being given to the homemaker independent of her usual pay.

DOI: 10.1201/9781003344476-46

WHAT IS ELDER ABUSE?

Elder abuse encompasses mistreatment and neglect of an older adult (in some communities the use of the word "elder" would be inappropriate as it might be a designation for a community leader of any age). Elder abuse represents single or multiple acts of commission or omission inflicted on an older adult (commonly viewed as aged 60 or 65, or older) within a relationship where there is an expectation of trust (1). While mistreatment may occur as a result of ignorance, it is usually considered non-accidental or intentional, though intent to harm may in some cases be difficult to substantiate.

Elder abuse is important to detect and respond to not only to address the overt and sometimes covert sequelae of the mistreatment, but also to prolong the lives of the victims: Seniors who have been abused have a significantly higher mortality rate (independent of the abuse) when compared to seniors who have not been abused (2).

Health care professionals may encounter older adults with signs and/or symptoms of abuse in varied settings: during home visits, in office settings, in emergency rooms, on acute care hospital wards, and in long-term care institutions. Within institutions a distinction is encouraged between acts that are uniquely aimed at an individual (elder abuse) and those that may be due to institutional or systemic failure. Both are important to address, but solutions may rest at different levels of care.

As described next elder abuse is commonly divided into four categories: physical, psychological/verbal, financial/material, and neglect (3):

PHYSICAL ABUSE

Acts Associated with Physical Abuse

- Individuals who are hit, slapped, kicked, tied, shaken, choked, grabbed, pushed, shoved, punched, slammed against a wall, pinched, scratched, bit, burned, scalded.
- Twisted limbs.
- Rough transfers.
- Unexplained or poorly explained falls and injuries.
- Multiple visits to emergency departments.
- Use of a weapon.
- Improper use of physical or chemical restraint.
- Sexual abuse: unwanted sexual contact, touching, or rubbing; masturbation that is forced, tricked, coerced, manipulated; use of physical threats (hitting, holding down, use of weapon) to give or receive oral, genital, or anal sex.

Manifestations of Physical Abuse: Unexplained or Unusual

- Bruises (especially those that are finger or knuckle shaped).
- Need for new dental work.
- Lacerations, abrasions, scars.
- Sprains, fractures, multiple trauma.
- Genital inflammation, pain, tenderness.
- Signs of anxiety, depression, withdrawal, low eye contact.

PSYCHOLOGICAL/VERBAL ABUSE

Acts Associated with Psychological Abuse

- Lying.
- Humiliating or infantilizing.

- Demeaning talk or jokes.
- Coercion.
- Inappropriate shouting/yelling.
- Controlling verbal or physical contact with family or friends.
- Threatening to hit or throw something.
- Disrespect for privacy.
- Insulting, swearing, name calling, putting down.
- Threats with weapons, deprivation, punishment, guardianship, abandonment, institutionalization.
- Sexual: verbal threats to give or receive oral, genital, or anal sex; individuals forced to view or participate in pornographic or sexually explicit pictures or videos; offensive sexual talk.

Manifestations of Psychological Abuse: Unexplained or Unusual

- Apprehensiveness.
- Physical avoidance.
- Reduced eye contact or continual eye darting.
- Quietness, passivity, withdrawal.
- Depression, anger.
- Weight loss.
- Missed appointments.
- Caregivers who try to answer in place of the senior.

FINANCIAL OR MATERIAL ABUSE

Acts Associated with Financial/Material Abuse Include

- Disrespect for property, including taking, misuse, concealment of resources, property, or assets, with or without coercion, enticement, intimidation, or deception.
- Misappropriation of funds, bank accounts, or credit/debit cards against the will of a senior or without his/her knowledge.
- Forced to give power of attorney.
- Forged signature.
- Use of power attorney or employment of service people by others for personal gain.

Manifestations of Financial/Material Abuse: Unexplained or Unusual

- Anxiety, apprehensiveness, avoidance.
- Social withdrawal.
- Depression, tearfulness, weight loss.
- Clothes not appropriate to the weather.
- Under-medicated.

NEGLECT

Acts Associated with Neglect

- Inappropriately left alone or unsupervised.
- Withholding of necessary aids: walker, wheelchair, glasses, hearing aid, telephone.
- Living environment too hot or too cold.
- Clothing inappropriate to weather.
- Unsanitary living conditions, bed linens or incontinence products not changed.
- Medications not or irregularly supervised.
- Inappropriate or poor food supplied.
- Delays in seeking treatment.
- Inconsistent treatment.
- Frequent change of physicians.

Manifestations of Neglect

- Poor mobility.
- Cachexia.
- Decubitus ulcers, pressure sores, bed sores.
- Poor hygiene, body odor.
- Frequent infections.
- Unexplained medical problems.
- Fearfulness, anxiety, depression.

SYSTEMIC OR INSTITUTIONAL FAILURE

Acts Associated with Institutional or Systemic Failure

- Inadequate custodial care or supervision.
- Low or unpredictable nursing/nursing aide care.
- Delays in response time to seniors' calls for help.
- Inadequate nutrition.
- Overcrowded or unsanitary living conditions.
- Poor staff communication skills.
- Limited staff language competency.
- Recurrent inappropriate staff-resident interactions.
- Misuse of physical or chemical restraints.

DETECTION OF ELDER ABUSE

Risk Factors

Since physicians of varied backgrounds and experience may be the first or enduring point of contact for an abused senior, a knowledge of elder abuse is promoted despite sometimes vague signs and symptoms. Guidelines are neither for or against whether physicians should routinely screen

Table 40.1   Detection of Elder Abuse

Weak Association	Moderate Association	Strong Association
Social isolation (CR)	Females (CR)	Poor physical health (CR)
Dementia (CR)	Blacks (CR)	Childhood violence (CG)
Mental illness (CG)	Passive/dependent (CR)	Stress (CG)
Hostility (CG)	CG dependent on CR	CR dependent on CG
Drugs/alcohol (CG)	CG related to CR	Institutional care (CG)

for elder abuse. Research into risk factors has generated some of this uncertainty because of a lack of clarity about their impact. Nonetheless it is useful to be aware of such factors and the roles they may play in relation to elder abuse when considered from the perspectives of caregivers (CG) and care receivers (CR); see Table 40.1. (4)

DETECTION INSTRUMENTS

There are a small number of validated detection tools for use by clinicians (5). The Elder Abuse Suspicion Index© (EASI) is a practical one because its six questions take only 2–5 minutes to complete (6). The self-administered version, the EASI-sa, comprises five questions and is completed in a similar brief time frame (7). These tools use words understandable by, and acceptable to, older adults (7), and is available in ten languages (8). A nine question tool derived from the EASI has been specifically designed for use in the long-term care setting (EASI-ltc), and is pending formal testing (9). Copies of the Elder Abuse Suspicion Index tools and practical aspects of their application are found on a website devoted to it: http://www.mcgill.ca/familymed/research/projects/elder.

OUTCOME OF SUSPECTED ABUSE

Since a positive response on the EASI can be a false positive arising from cognitive impairment (delirium, dementia), a MMSE (or equivalent tool) should be performed as part of a mental capacity assessment, the EASI being validated for cognition scores of ≥ 24 on the MMSE. If the senior is found by this process to be inapt, then a declaration of such should be made according to the reporting protocol of the jurisdiction in which one is practicing.

Does identification of elder abuse by a cognitively intact senior legally bind a physician to report the mistreatment? It depends on the geographical jurisdiction in which one is practicing. Some do not impose mandatory reporting; some require it for abuse that occurs within a public institution that cares for seniors; and others require reporting irrespective of where the abuse has occurred. A dilemma for practitioners is that some cognitively intact victims do not want the abuse disclosed. There may be reluctance to see the abuser punished; they may be embarrassed, humiliated, or shamed that a family member was abusive; they may fear retaliation from the abuser; or they may realistically worry that removing the abuser may leave their global living situations worse than it was with the abuse.

Such situations are legally and ethically challenging. It would therefore be advisable for clinicians to seek the advice and collaboration of regionally designated resources for elder abuse: Adult Protective Services, social services, or police officers. What can health professionals expect from these experts? Where feasible, social workers will do a complete evaluation of the psychosocial needs of the older person and the caregiver. If indicated, along with a doctor's help, they will begin procedures to have the person declared under a protective regime (public, private curatorship, or homologation of a mandate). They will access homecare services, respite programs, caregiver support groups and placement, if necessary. If the senior is competent, they will respect the right of self-determination, but support the person to have a life without abuse. If indicated, they will involve the police or get a Human Rights Commission (or equivalent) involved.

CLINICAL VIGNETTE CONTINUED

The case history described self-neglect; self-neglect, however, does not appear in the cited descriptors of elder abuse. It is considered a different problem, with causes and possible solutions that require a unique approach. The vignette does however suggest neglect on the part of the homemaker and the out-of-town daughter. It does provide evidence of verbal as well as physical abuse by the homemaker. Both daughter and homemaker appear to be abusing the trust the mother had in them in far as her finances were concerned.

In the vignette the family physician has not directly used a detection tool to gather data; however he has taken advantage of his knowledge of the content of the EASI to ask Mrs. L. and her daughter relevant questions. As a result he feels more urgency in the situation and a need to get help for Mrs. L. He reminds her that over his 22 years of care for her that he has tried to respect her best interests. Responding positively to this reminder she agrees to have a visit from a social worker, but reserves the right to keep open whatever options may be available to her.

REFERENCES

1. World Health Organization. *The Toronto Declaration on the Global Prevention of Elder Abuse.* Geneva, Switzerland: World Health Organization, 2002.
2. Lachs MS, Williams CS, O'Brien S, Pillemer KA, Chartlson ME. The Mortality of Elder Mistreatment. *JAMA* 1998; 280 (5): 428–432.
3. Yaffe MJ, Tazkarji B. Understanding Elder Abuse in Family Practice. *Canadian Family Physician* 2012; 58: 1336–1340.
4. Yaffe MJ. Elder Abuse. Chapter in Calhoun K, Eibling DE, Wax MK, Kost K, eds. Geriatric Otolaryngology. New York: Taylor and Francis, 2006, 639.
5. McMullen T, Schwartz K, Yaffe M, Beach S. *Elder Abuse and Its Prevention: Screening and detection*, IOM (Institute of Medicine) and NRC (National Research Council: Elder Abuse and Its Prevention: Workshop Summary, April 2014, 88–93, The National Academies Press Washington, DC.
6. Yaffe MJ, Wolfson C, Weiss D, Lithwick M. Development and Validation of a Tool to Assist Physicians' Identification of Elder Abuse: The Elder Abuse Suspicion Index (EASI ©). *Journal of Elder Abuse and Neglect*, 2008; 20 (3): 276–300.
7. Yaffe MJ, Weiss D, Lithwick M. Seniors' Self-Administration of the Elder Abuse Suspicion Index (EASI): A Feasibility Study. *Journal of Elder Abuse and Neglect* 2012; 24 (2): 277–292.
8. http://www.mcgill.ca/familymed/research/projects/elder
9. Ballard SA, Yaffe MJ, August L, Cetin-Sahin D, Wilchesky M. Adapting the Elder Abuse Suspicion Index © for Use in Long-Term Care: A Mixed Methods Approach. Journal of Applied Gerontology. In press, June 2017.

41 Late-Life Anxiety

Jess Friedland, MD, FRCPC, Paulina Bajsarowicz, MD, FRCPC and Philippe Desmarais, MD, FRCPC, MHSc

CONTENTS

CLINICAL VIGNETTE

A 75-year-old female presents to her family doctor complaining of increased fatigue and worry. She lives alone, has been widowed for five years and has a son who was a strong source of support after her husband's death and with whom she has a close relationship. After her spouse passed away, she was treated for a first major depressive episode and diagnosed with mild generalized anxiety disorder. She still takes her SSRI antidepressant. Her past medical history includes mild iron-deficiency anemia (untreated), hypertension and dyslipidemia.

For the past six weeks she has been increasingly concerned about her son, who recently became unemployed and is having financial difficulties; she often has insomnia. Two weeks ago, while going to the bathroom, she tripped over the carpet and fell on her right knee; she has fallen several times in the past few months. The pain from this most recent fall has been unrelenting and she has been taking an over-the-counter NSAID regularly.

She has been feeling dizzy, weak, fatigued, feels her heart is racing and is short of breath. She has been taking previously prescribed benzodiazepines for the past week.

Her medications include: lorazepam 0.5 mg PO BID PRN (which she takes regularly), sertraline 75 mg PO QD, ibuprofen 200 mg PO QID, atorvastatin 20 mg PO QHS, and valsartan 40 mg PO QD.

CLINICAL SIGNIFICANCE

Anxiety is a universal and potentially useful human emotion, with deep evolutionary roots. It is a complex neurobiological experience, encompassing mind and body and involving the prefrontal cortex, the limbic and autonomic systems. Its primary manifestations are:

- Cognitive: fear, worry, irritability, distress.

- Physical: fatigue, muscle tension, insomnia, autonomic hyperreactivity.

- Behavioural: avoidance and other safety behaviours.

When anxiety's utility is consistently outweighed by associated distress and dysfunction, anxiety is considered disordered. Older adults are typically less prone to anxiety disorders, depression and other negative emotional states than younger adults, and it is relatively rare to have a new onset of an anxiety disorder in late life. However, the potential consequences of anxiety disorders and even subthreshold anxiety are important: they correlate with loneliness and lower life satisfaction; decreased physical and psychosocial functioning; increased risk of depression, heart disease and dementia; increased use of health services and lower satisfaction with care received.

EPIDEMIOLOGY

A number of large epidemiological studies have investigated the prevalence of late-life anxiety, including notably the National Comorbidity Study Replication (NCS-R) and the Longitudinal Aging Study Amsterdam (LASA). Findings of these and other studies are quite variable, perhaps because older adults tend to under-endorse anxious feelings and excessive worry and rather

DOI: 10.1201/9781003344476-47

present more somatic symptoms such as fatigue and pain. For example, the 12-month prevalence of generalized anxiety disorder (GAD) is reported as 0.8–1.8% in the NCS-R, whereas the 6-month prevalence per LASA is reported as 6.9–11.5%. The results converge somewhat when looking at the prevalence of having any anxiety disorder in late life, with the NCS-R finding 6.0–8.9% and LASA finding 10.4–13.9% of people over age 65 to have any anxiety disorder.

Older people living in institutional settings have not been as well described, but small studies indicate that the prevalence of anxiety in these settings is higher than in the community.

For people with neurocognitive disorders, anxiety is a common symptom, occurring in up to one-third of patients with mild neurocognitive disorder (mild cognitive impairment) and up to two-thirds of patients with major neurocognitive disorder (dementia).

What is clear from epidemiologic studies is that anxiety is common in late life, usually has its onset in childhood to middle age and has a decreasing prevalence with age. GAD, specific phobias and social anxiety disorder remain common throughout the lifespan, while panic disorder, post-traumatic stress disorder (PTSD) and obsessive-compulsive disorder (OCD) become relatively rare in later life.

In terms of course and prognosis, anxiety disorders are typically chronic illnesses with a waxing and waning course. Six-year follow-up of 112 anxiety disorder patients in the LASA study showed persistence of the disorder in about a quarter, subclinical anxiety in about half, high use of benzodiazepines (43%) and low use of antidepressants (7%).

RISK AND PROTECTIVE FACTORS

A number of risk factors for the development of anxiety disorders have been elucidated:

- *Demographic:* female sex, being divorced/separated/widowed/never married and/or childless.

- *Personality:* neurotic personality (tendency to have negative reactions to events) and poor coping skills.

- *Clinical conditions:* fear of falling, urinary incontinence, sensory impairment, hypertension, poor sleep, chronic medical condition, functional limitations.

- *External stressors:* early life stress, chronic disability in self or spouse, war experiences.

Other potential predisposing factors include new stressors such as losses and the degeneration of adaptation-associated brain regions such as the dorsolateral prefrontal cortex.

To explain the decrease in prevalence of anxiety disorders with age, a number of potential protective factors have been observed or hypothesized. These include the decline in propensity for negative affect over time (though it rises again starting in the mid-70s), increased exposure to stressors over the lifespan ("stress inoculation"), opportunity to practice emotion regulation, degeneration of anxiety-associated brain regions such as the locus coeruleus, and social support, religiosity, physical activity and cognitive stimulation.

DIAGNOSIS OF ANXIETY DISORDERS

Recognition and diagnosis of anxiety disorders in late life can be complicated by under-reporting of anxious feelings and excessive worry by older adults, accumulation of medical and cognitive co-morbidities and the psychosocial losses and transitions that are more common in older adults. The Diagnostic and Statistical Manual of Mental Disorders, 5th Edition, 2013 (DSM-5) provides diagnostic criteria for numerous distinct anxiety disorders along with several other psychiatric disorders, categorized as obsessive-compulsive, stressor-related, somatic or adjustment disorders, that involve significant anxiety components:

- *Specific phobia:* in which immediate and disproportionate fear or anxiety provoked by a specific object or situation leads to persistent avoidance or endurance with intense distress (e.g. fear of falling).

- *Social anxiety disorder:* also known as social phobia, in which the phobic stimulus is a social situation where the individual feels exposed to possible scrutiny by others (about e.g. tremor or forgetfulness).

- *Panic disorder:* involving recurrent, unexpected panic attacks that lead to fear of further panic attacks and maladaptive avoidance of panicogenic situations.

- *Agoraphobia:* involving avoidance of various public situations due to fear of difficulty escaping or getting help in the event of panic or other incapacitating symptoms (e.g. incontinence).

- *GAD (Generalized anxiety disorder):* in which the individual experiences excessive and difficult-to-control anxiety and worry about everyday, routine life circumstances (e.g. well-being of family or physical health or safety). The worry leads to cognitive and/or somatic symptoms.

- *Substance/Medication-induced anxiety disorder:* in which anxiety symptoms are clearly temporally and etiologically linked to medication exposure or to substance intoxication or withdrawal (see the following examples).

- *Anxiety disorder due to another medical condition:* in which clinically significant anxiety is demonstrated through history, physical exam or lab findings to be the direct pathophysiological effect of another medical condition (see examples later).

- *Illness anxiety disorder:* previously known as hypochondriasis, in which the anxious preoccupation relates to having or acquiring a serious illness, clearly disproportionate to the individual's absent or mild somatic symptoms and other findings.

- *OCD (Obsessive-compulsive disorder):* involving obsessions and/or compulsions that are time-consuming or cause significant distress or dysfunction.

- *Hoarding disorder:* whose central feature is a persistent difficulty discarding possessions, leading to accumulation of clutter that compromises living areas.

- *PTSD (Post-traumatic stress disorder):* in which a number of characteristic symptoms—nightmares, flashbacks and other intrusive phenomena, avoidant behaviours, negative thinking patterns and mood, and hyperarousal—arise following exposure to one or more traumatic events.

- *Acute stress disorder:* similar to PTSD but lasting from three days to one month after the exposure.

- *Adjustment disorder with anxiety:* in which disproportionate anxiety develops in response to an identifiable stressor and resolves within six months of the resolution of the stressor.

In older adults, fear of falling and anxiety in the context of delirium or dementia are also important clinical entities.

Principles of evaluation include ruling out other primary causes, including medication side effects (e.g. prednisone), medical conditions (e.g. chronic obstructive pulmonary disease) and dementia. A thorough physical examination is essential given the many medical conditions that can cause anxiety. The Canadian Network for Mood and Anxiety Treatments (CANMAT) also recommends laboratory work-up including CBC, fasting glucose and lipids, electrolytes, liver enzymes, serum bilirubin, serum creatinine, urine toxicology and TSH. Depending on clinical suspicion, consider urinalysis, vitamin B12 level and ECG. Co-morbidity with depression and substance use are common and must be evaluated. Dangerosity, including suicide risk and pathological avoidance behaviours, must be assessed.

Medical conditions known to have anxiety as a symptom include:

- *Endocrine:* hypo- and hyperthyroidism, pheochromocytoma, hyperadrenocorticism and hypoglycemia.

- *Cardiovascular:* congestive heart failure, pulmonary embolus, arrhythmia, mitral valve prolapse and coronary artery disease.

- *Gastrointestinal:* ulcerative colitis, diverticulitis, irritable bowel syndrome.

- *Respiratory:* COPD, pneumonia, hyperventilation.

- *Hematologic:* vitamin B12 deficiency and anemia.

- *Neurologic:* Parkinson's disease, neoplasms, vestibular dysfunction, encephalitis and neurodegenerative neurocognitive disorders.

- *Other:* Postural disturbance, dizziness and falls.

Medications known to have anxiety as a side effect include anticholinergics, cholinesterase inhibitors, inhaled beta-agonists, insulin, levodopa, montelukast, phenytoin, psychostimulants, steroids, SSRIs, thyroid medications.

Substances that can cause anxiety through either intoxication or withdrawal include alcohol withdrawal, amphetamine/cocaine intoxication, benzodiazepine withdrawal, caffeine use/intoxication, cannabis use and nicotine use.

SCALES

Validated rating scales for anxiety symptoms can be useful for quantifying symptoms and following response to interventions. Some scales are specific to older people and others are for the general population. Among the numerous anxiety symptoms scales, the following self-rated scales have been sufficiently validated in the older population: seven-item Generalized Anxiety Disorder Scale (GAD-7); Beck Anxiety Inventory (BAI); Geriatric Anxiety Inventory (GAI); Penn State Worry Questionnaire; and Worry Scale.

For people with dementia, for whom caregiver observations need to be taken into account, there is a multimodal anxiety-specific scale and other scales that include an item or set of items on anxiety or anxiety-like symptoms: Reliable Anxiety Scale In Dementia (RAID); Neuropsychiatric Inventory (NPI); and Cohen-Mansfield Agitation Scale.

KEY CO-MORBIDITIES: DEPRESSION AND COGNITIVE DISORDERS

Depression: Clinical pearls to help distinguish pure anxiety from anxious depression include: content of anxiety is more present/future-oriented in pure anxiety vs. related to the past in depression, early morning awakening with worse morning anxiety is more indicative of depression, and anxiety in the context of depression is generally more debilitating than in pure anxiety. About half of older persons with major depressive disorder (MDD) had a co-morbid anxiety disorder with severe anxiety symptoms, while about a quarter of older persons with anxiety disorders had MDD. Co-morbidity correlates with delayed or diminished response to antidepressants, greater somatic symptoms and greater suicidal ideation and risk of suicide.

Cognitive disorders: A recent systematic review and meta-analysis of the interplay between anxiety and cognition (Gulpers et al. *Am J Geriatr Psychiatry* 2016) showed incident cognitive impairment in community samples with RR (Relative Risk) 1.77 and incident dementia in community samples RR 1.57 (1.23 for people under age 80 and 2.51 for people over age 80). However, anxiety as a risk factor for conversion to dementia in memory clinic samples was not significant and it is not clear whether anxiety is prodromal or causal. In patients with established dementia, subjective reports of anxiety symptoms in dementia patients were similar in vascular and Alzheimer's dementia (29%)—subjective anxiety and physical tension were the most common complaints. NPI (Neuropsychiatric Inventory) ratings by caregivers showed higher rates of anxiety in vascular (46%) and frontotemporal (39%) dementias vs. Alzheimer's (30%). Five percent of patients with Alzheimer's have GAD; psychiatric history is a predictor of this co-morbidity.

TREATMENTS

Psychotherapy: Research has focused on GAD and mixed anxiety symptoms. The best evidence is for cognitive-behaviour therapy (CBT) for GAD, relaxation training and mindfulness therapies such as Mindfulness-Based Stress Reduction. There is some evidence for supportive therapy. A number of helpful adaptations of CBT in late life have been established, and these adaptations could also be considered for other psychotherapies. The adaptations include: simplified/less abstract treatment rationale and therapeutic interventions, slower pace with increased repetition and review of previous sessions, audiotaping sessions for patient to review, between-session reminder phone calls, at-home assignments, more focus on behavioural change and health concerns, engagement of the family in the treatment and integration of religion. Some evidence supports the use of telephone or internet-based psychotherapy, and this may help to address access issues.

Pharmacotherapy: The pharmacological treatment of late-life anxiety disorders can be effective based on clinical observations, but is complicated by limited evidence and safety issues. CANMAT recommends that pharmacological choices be guided by the evidence along with prior treatment response, the nature of the targeted symptoms, medication interactions and other safety issues and side effect profiles of the medications. Combination treatment with psychotherapy is recommended.

The available evidence demonstrates efficacy and tolerability for:

- Selective serotonin reuptake inhibitors (SSRIs), including citalopram, escitalopram and sertraline.

- Serotonin-norepinephrine reuptake inhibitors (SNRIs), including venlafaxine and duloxetine.
- Pregabalin.

SSRIs and SNRIs, while generally safe, do increase the QTc (QT interval corrected for heart rate) interval (especially citalopram, which should be limited to a maximum dose of 20 mg QD), the risk of falls and fractures and the risk of upper GI bleeding.

Although there is no geriatric-specific evidence to guide their use, the tolerability of mirtazapine and buspirone make them reasonable treatment options. Furthermore, our clinical experience and the favourable side effects of quickly improved sleep and appetite support the use of mirtazapine.

Cholinesterase inhibitors may improve anxiety in the context of dementia, though they can in some cases increase anxiety.

Because of issues with their safety profiles, the following medications are not first-line options, and should be used only with caution:

- Benzodiazepines have demonstrated effectiveness for late-life anxiety. However, their safety profile, including sedation, fall and fracture risk, cognitive impairment and link with dementia risk, argues against their regular long-term use. They could be used with great caution in the initial phase of treatment with SSRIs or SNRIs, since those medications can initially increase agitation and insomnia and take several weeks to effectively decrease anxiety.

- Older antidepressants such as tricyclic antidepressants (TCAs) can be effective but are not first-line choices given their significant anticholinergic and cardiac effects. Among the TCAs, nortriptyline is favoured for use in the elderly because it is relatively less anticholinergic.

- Low-dose atypical antipsychotics, particularly quetiapine, olanzapine and aripiprazole, can be effective as augmenting agents in severe mixed anxio-depressive states. Since they have black-box warnings for use in geriatric populations due to a small but significant risk of increased mortality, these should be used only after a well-documented discussion of their pros and cons.

RESOLUTION OF THE CLINICAL VIGNETTE

1. How would you approach this patient's problems?

   - High index of suspicion for anxiety disorder given that older adults are less likely to report anxiety and worry.

   - Although anxiety in this patient is multifactorial, a medical cause or exacerbating factor for her symptoms needs to be investigated. She is already known for mild anemia and has been taking NSAID medication regularly and this may be a source of bleeding. Her physical complaints may be primarily somatic symptoms of her anxiety, but an underlying general medical condition needs to be ruled out. Furthermore, pain can exacerbate anxiety and insomnia.

   - After you have investigated the patient, she is found to have a bleeding peptic ulcer which exacerbated her anemia. X-ray showed moderate osteoarthritis. Throughout the assessment, she perseverates about her concerns for her son's financial situation and how she cannot stop thinking about it as she has no means to help him. She tells you she is constantly feeling on edge and keyed up, and she cannot concentrate or sleep.

2. How would you address the anxiety?

   - The symptoms of her generalized anxiety disorder have worsened due to the stressor of her son's unemployment. If not for the ulcer, we would titrate sertraline to 200 mg as tolerated. However, since her ulcer is a relative contraindication to an SSRI, we can consider a cross taper to mirtazapine which could also help with her insomnia. Supportive therapy, CBT and sleep hygiene instructions can be offered to the patient for both anxiety and insomnia.

3. What else to consider?

   - Falls may be due to the weakness from the anemia, but also due to benzodiazepine use. A slow taper may be warranted. Furthermore, since she has been tripping in her apartment, a thorough home safety evaluation can be requested. Adequate pain control should be implemented.

   - Orthopaedic consultation in view of the unrelenting right knee pain.

SUGGESTIONS FOR FURTHER READING

Alvadaro C and Modesto-Lowe V: Psychotherapeutic Treatment Approaches of Anxiety Disorders in the Elderly. Current Treatment Options in Psychiatry. 2017; 4:47–54.

American Psychiatric Publishing: Diagnostic and Statistical Manual of Mental Disorders, 5th Edition (DSM-5). 2013.

Crocco EA et al.: Pharmacological Management of Anxiety Disorders in the Elderly. Current Treatment Options in Psychiatry. 2017; 4:33–46.

Therrien and Hunsley: Assessment of Anxiety in Older Adults: A Reliability Generalization Meta-Analysis of Commonly Used Measures. Clinical Gerontologist. 2013; 36:171–194.

Wolitzky-Taylor KB et al.: Anxiety Disorders in Older Adults: A Comprehensive Review. Depression & Anxiety. 2010; 27:190–211.

42 An Overview of Late-Life Depression

Artin Mahdanian, MD, MSc and Silvia Monti De Flores, MD, FRCPC, DFAPA

CONTENTS

CLINICAL VIGNETTE

Mr. D is a 73-year-old divorced man who was brought to the emergency room by his daughter for suicidal ideation and depression. He described a few months' history of continuous excessive worry about his future, panic attacks and loss of interest in life. He self-isolated and avoided seeing family and friends. He had gradually stopped all of the physical exercise activities (swimming, jogging and yoga) that he used to do, because he did not have the physical energy and mental joy. He had difficulty sleeping, decreased appetite and had lost about 10 pounds in the past few months. Recently, he had been feeling very guilty about how he had treated his ex-wife who died of suicide by hanging 20 years ago, 10 years after their divorce. He thought he deserved to die and started to think about ending his life. He denied any delusions or hallucinations. He did not have any anxiety or other psychiatric symptoms prior to this episode except for few months of "psychotherapy" with a psychologist 30 years ago after his divorce.

His symptoms started a few months ago when his company went bankrupt following a few months of struggling with a tax audit and numerous financial problems. Then, he decided to retire. He used to be a very successful and high-achieving accountant who ran the company with his brother for more than 40 years. He suffers from diabetes mellitus type II, gout and a frozen shoulder. His medication list includes vitamin B12, metformin-sitagliptin 1000mg+50mg, valsartan-HCTZ 160mg+25mg, and allopurinol. The only important family history was chronic treatment-resistant depression in his mother.

WHAT IS DEPRESSION?

Depression is a general term which is used for Major Depressive Disorder (MDD). Diagnosis is always a clinical one and it is based on meeting the diagnostic criteria for either DSM-5 or ICD-10. For the diagnosis of MDD based on DSM-5, there must be 5 symptoms; one of them should be either depressed mood or lack of interest (anhedonia) and 4 other symptoms out of psychomotor slowness, decreased/increased appetite, weight changes, sleep disturbances, suicidal ideation, decreased energy, decreased concentration or feeling guilty. The symptoms must be persistent and present most of the time for a period of at least two weeks. Moreover, there should be a decline in baseline functioning of the patient.

WHY IS DEPRESSION AN IMPORTANT CLINICAL PROBLEM IN THE ELDERLY?

MDD is one of the most common causes of disability worldwide. It is a highly prevalent disorder characterized by episodes of persistent depressed mood or loss of interest/pleasure (affective symptoms) plus other vegetative and cognitive symptoms as already described.

Late-life depression (LLD), with an estimated prevalence of about 15%, is a common psychiatric disorder in people >65y. LLD is associated with increased morbidity and mortality. It is associated

DOI: 10.1201/9781003344476-48

with increased healthcare cost. LLD has also been shown to be highly recurrent with research reports varying between 30% and 65% over 3 to 20 years follow-up. The consequences of untreated LLD include poor quality of life as well as worse outcome and exacerbation of other chronic illnesses, and most importantly, suicide.

Predictors of poorer outcome may include adverse childhood events, age of onset, limited education and the number of previous recurrences and length of untreated episodes. Additionally, personality disorder diagnosis (avoidant, obsessive compulsive and introvert personality traits) may predict a further episode, while somatoform disorders may predict time to recurrence. Due to the atypical presentation, the diagnosis of LLD is often missed by primary care physicians, which leads to under-treatment of the disease. However, a timely diagnosis can be life-saving and, when treated, it has a good prognosis; up to 70% of treated older patients achieve full remission.

WHAT ARE THE CHALLENGES IN DIAGNOSIS OF DEPRESSION IN THE ELDERLY?

In the geriatric population, depressive symptoms may be masked by unexplained physical complaints (e.g., fatigue, diffuse pain or back pain, headache, chest pain, etc.) and, subsequently, the classical DSM-5 criteria may sometimes seem to fail in terms of diagnosing depression. Furthermore, the conditions mentioned next can exist concomitantly.

Therefore, the differential diagnosis of LLD in the elderly is broad, including, but not limited to, central nervous system disorders (dementia, Parkinson's disease and neoplastic lesions), other psychiatric disorders (dysthymia, bipolar and anxiety disorders), endocrine disorders (hypo-/hyperthyroidism and hyperparathyroidism), medication side effects (e.g., β-blockers, centrally active antihypertensive medications, steroids, H2-blockers, sedatives, certain chemotherapy agents), vitamin deficiency (vitamin B12, vitamin D and folic acid), life circumstances (e.g., grief, bereavement, financial or autonomy losses), substance use, infectious and inflammatory diseases (e.g., HIV encephalopathy, systemic lupus erythematosus) and sleep disorders (in particular, obstructive sleep apnea).

A complete physical examination, cognitive screening, laboratory tests and/or imaging are the first steps in ruling out these differential diagnoses and in assessing for common comorbidities in the elderly. A physician who has good understanding of the patient's personality can identify nonverbal cues and changes in behavior indicating mood problems. In addition, information from family members and caregivers on the patient's mood and behavior is vital for assessing the older person with depression.

WHAT ARE THE RISK FACTORS FOR DEPRESSION?

As in all other aspects of depression, the risk factors for LLD are also better described in a bio-psychosocial model. The main biological risk factors are old age and female sex. In addition, genetic vulnerability also plays an important role, making people with a family history of mood disorders more susceptible to LLD than others. Patients with poor physical health (e.g., multiple comorbidities, sleeping disorders, etc.) and more medication use may also be predisposed to LLD. The notion of frailty affects several domains of functioning, leading to a deterioration in the resilience and capacity for dealing with stressors. Frailty can be defined by the Fried criteria: weight loss, decreased handgrip strength, slowness, exhaustion and low physical activity. Poor nutritional status is also associated with frailty and LLD; therefore, nutritional supplements (vitamins D, B12, folate and protein) could benefit the depressed frail patient. Neurodegenerative disease (e.g., Parkinson or Alzheimer) and mild cognitive impairment (MCI) are also considered possible risk factors for LLD. We know that LLD and dementia frequently co-occur, and depression can be the first sign of dementia. The vascular hypothesis holds that cerebrovascular disease may cause or predispose to LLD and can be explained by reduced cerebral perfusion, altered brain connectivity, and chronic low-grade inflammation.

Psychological factors such as loss of purpose in life or human relationships seem to be associated with LLD. Moreover, lower level of education, being a widower or single, loneliness, lack of social supports, stressful life events and poverty are all valid risk factors for LLD. Decrease or loss of functional status, visual or hearing impairment, poor lifestyle habits, smoking and alcohol use also increase the risk of developing LLD. In addition, the use of sleep medication such as benzodiazepines and sleep disturbance in general are also correlated with increased risk of LLD.

USEFUL TOOLS FOR THE DIAGNOSIS OF DEPRESSION

Use of validated scales/tools in screening, diagnosis and follow-up response to therapy in depression is an important part of providing appropriate care. They can improve diagnostic accuracy, save time, provide more consistent patient care and monitor a patient's complex emotional and behavioral responses to therapy. Two quick questions from Primary Care Evaluation of Mental

Disorders can provide us with a highly sensitive (94%) but not very specific (35%) screening test for depression: 1) Have you been bothered by little interest or pleasure in doing things? 2) Have you been feeling down, depressed or hopeless in the last month?

If a patient responds positively to either of these two questions, we can screen with the other symptom criteria. Other useful self- or physician-rated screening tools are also available. The Hamilton Depression Rating Scale (HAM-D), the oldest, most widely used and validated instrument, has numerous versions, both clinician-rated and self-reported, as well as a computer administered version. Many clinicians prefer to use a patient-rated scale such as the Beck Depression Inventory (BDI). The BDI has high sensitivity and specificity and is valid and reliable in assessing the severity of depressive symptoms. The Geriatric Depression Scale (GDS) is also a self-report measure designed to minimize the impact of somatic symptoms associated with aging and illness. It has good sensitivity and positive predictive values for diagnosis of major depression. The PHQ-9 also offers a severity score for symptoms, and can also be used to follow outcome. If a clinician is concerned about cognitive impairment, the Mini Mental State Exam (MMSE) and/or Montreal Cognitive Assessment (MoCA) are useful additions.

HOW IS THE DIAGNOSIS OF DEPRESSION CONVEYED TO THE PATIENT?

There is no gold standard for discussing depression diagnosis with elderly patients. It is dependent on the physician's method since research on the topic is lacking. It is helpful to engage the patient with the use of the bio-psychosocial model: inform the patient that the illness is an interaction between physiological (e.g., neurotransmitters hypothesis like serotonin), psychological and social factors. Creating a good therapeutic alliance and trust is pivotal for a good outcome.

WHAT ARE THE TREATMENT OPTIONS FOR DEPRESSION?

The very first step in the treatment of depression is to treat the modifiable risk factors including nutritional deficiencies (vitamin B12, D and folic acid), cardiovascular diseases, and any endocrine and electrolyte abnormalities. Risk factors can also be improved by lifestyle changes, physical exercise, healthy diet, sufficient sleep, smoking cessation, discontinuation of alcohol intake as well as optimal treatment for hypertension, hypercholesterolemia, hyperglycemia and any other comorbid medical condition.

The treatment options of MDD are based on the bio-psychosocial model and the administered choice is according to the severity of the illness and patient preference (Figure 42.1). The severity

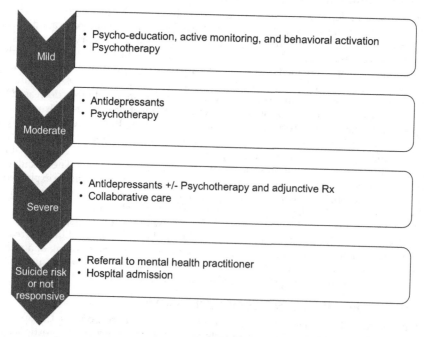

Figure 42.1 Stepped care approach to late-life depression, based on the severity of depression and patient preference

of the illness is defined based on rating scales, functional impairment and clinical impression. Biological treatments include pharmacotherapy with antidepressants, second generation antipsychotics, neuro-modulation approaches like Repetitive Transcranial Magnetic Stimulation (rTMS), electroconvulsive therapy (ECT), light therapy and supplements (Omega 3, vitamin B12). Psychotherapeutic approaches with significant evidence for efficacy include: Supportive Psychotherapy, Cognitive Behavioral Therapy (CBT), Interpersonal Therapy (IPT), Mindfulness-Based Cognitive Therapy (MBCT), Life Review Therapy, Problem-Solving Therapy (PST), Bibliotherapy (mostly based on CBT models), Dynamic Therapy and Existential Therapy. Finally, social interventions play an important role in treatment of depression in the elderly since losses, loneliness, social isolation and a limited support network are very common in this population.

Psycho-Education

The physician's role is to help patient understand depression, to explain therapeutic options, to discuss the bio-psychosocial model of etiology and treatment, to recognize warning signs and to inform and support the family. Moreover, it is important to try to provide a structure in the patient's life and activate the patient through structured and fun activities.

Behavioral Activation

Structured physical activity is recommended for older people with mild or moderate depression who are physically capable.

Psychotherapy

Psychotherapies are the most important type of non-pharmacological treatment and are not inferior to pharmacological treatments in mild to moderate depression. Evidence-based psychotherapeutic treatments of depression in older adults include CBT, IPT, PST, and Life Review Therapy.

Pharmacological Treatment

Geriatric patients have different pharmacodynamics and pharmacokinetics due to age-related physiological changes. Therefore, despite the fact that treatment options and algorithms are the same as for other adults, the medications must be administered at lower doses and slowly titrated while actively monitoring the patient. Increased caution is necessary for drug interactions and polypharmacy. In addition, when choosing a psychotropic drug, keep track of the drug's safety profile since some adverse reactions like falls can lead to increased morbidity and mortality. Selective serotonin reuptake inhibitors (SSRIs), Serotonin-norepinephrine reuptake inhibitors (SNRIs), tricyclic antidepressants (TCAs) and atypical antidepressants are the main pharmacological treatments of choice. Existing evidence unanimously suggests that no one class of antidepressant drugs has been found to be more effective than another in the treatment of LLD. However, newer antidepressants are better tolerated and safer. When choosing an SSRI, slight preference goes to an SSRI with the least known drug interactions such as sertraline. TCAs are as effective as SSRIs for LLD, but are less often used because of side effects. TCAs with lesser anticholinergic side effects, such as nortriptyline, are more recommended. SNRIs are not only effective against depression but also effective in the treatment of peripheral neuropathic pain.

An atypical antidepressant that can be used as an alternative for SSRIs is mirtazapine. The sedative side effects of mirtazapine are used as a treatment for insomnia. In addition, mirtazapine increases the appetite and can be used for the symptom of anorexia. Other atypical antidepressants which are commonly used are bupropion, vortioxetine and trazodone.

HOW DO YOU MANAGE INADEQUATE RESPONSE TO AN ANTIDEPRESSANT?

If a patient has partial or no response to the initial treatment, clinicians should ensure the dose of the medication is optimized to the therapeutic level as much as tolerated (6–8 weeks). There is extensive evidence that shows many patients receive sub-therapeutic doses and/or inadequate duration of treatment.

Evidence shows that switching non-responders to another antidepressant in the same class or another class results in good response and remission rates. However, patients with partial response to the initial antidepressant might benefit from increasing the dose and then the addition of a second medication: adjunctive treatment which means either combination (adding a second antidepressant to the first) or augmentation (adding another medication that is not an antidepressant, e.g., second generation antipsychotics, mood stabilizers like lithium, triiodothyronine).

RESOLUTION OF THE CLINICAL VIGNETTE

Having confirmed the diagnosis of MDD by a comprehensive history and physical exam, a full blood work-up was done that turned out to be negative for other causes or comorbid conditions with MDD as indicated earlier. Mr. D was then started on venlafaxine XR 37.5mg daily. In addition to providing him with psycho-education and support, it was suggested that he restart his physical exercise routine and socialize as much as possible. In the first follow-up visit after 1 week his response to medication and absence of side effects was assessed. His blood pressure and heart rate were monitored and found to be normal. The dose of the medication was increased to 75mg daily. Mr. D returned in 2 weeks with some response to medication but still far from his baseline. The dose of the medication was slowly increased to 150mg daily. After about 6 weeks on the therapeutic dose of venlafaxine, Mr. D still complained of some residual depressed mood, decreased energy and sleep disturbances despite some further improvement. At that point the treatment was augmented by adding quetiapine 50mg at night and the dose very slowly increased to 100mg. When Mr. D was reassessed a few weeks later, he reported that he was completely back to his baseline in terms of mood and interest. He registered in the local community center for yoga classes twice weekly, went swimming with his friends every other day, and traveled to visit his daughter for one week. He was advised to continue the treatment for 9–12 months as this was the first episode of depression and to taper down the treatment under supervision of a physician to avoid withdrawal symptoms and decrease the risk of relapse.

REFERENCES

1. Murri MB, Ekkekakis P, Menchetti M, Neviani F, Trevisani F, Tedeschi S, Latessa PM, Nerozzi E, Ermini G, Zocchi D, Squatrito S, Toni G, Cabassi A, Neri M, Zanetidou S, Amore M. Physical exercise for late-life depression: Effects on symptom dimensions and time course. J Affect Disord. 2018 Apr 1;230:65–70. doi: 10.1016/j.jad.2018.01.004
2. Beyer JL, Johnson KG. Advances in pharmacotherapy of late-life depression. Curr Psychiatry Rep. 2018 Apr 7;20(5):34. doi: 10.1007/s11920-018-0899-6.
3. Van Damme A, Declercq T, Lemey L, Tandt H, Petrovic M. Late-life depression: Issues for the general practitioner. Int J Gen Med. 2018 Mar 29;11:113–120.
4. Knöchel C, Alves G, Friedrichs B, Schneider B, Schmidt-Rechau A, Wenzler S, Schneider A, Prvulovic D, Carvalho AF, Oertel-Knöchel V. Treatment-resistant Late-life depression: Challenges and perspectives. Curr Neuropharmacol. 2015;13(5):577–591.
5. Kennedy SH, Lam RW, McIntyre RS, Tourjman SV, Bhat V, Blier P, Hasnain M, Jollant F, Levitt AJ, MacQueen GM, McInerney SJ, McIntosh D, Milev RV, Müller DJ, Parikh SV, Pearson NL, Ravindran AV, Uher R. Canadian network for mood and anxiety treatments (CANMAT) 2016 clinical guidelines for the management of adults with major depressive disorder: Section 3. Pharmacological Treatments. CANMAT Depression Work Group. Can J Psychiatry. 2016 Sep;61(9):540–560.

43 Assessment of Decision-Making Capacity

Catherine Ferrier, MD

CONTENTS

VIGNETTE

Don is an 83-year-old retired engineer who presents with a one-year history of cognitive symptoms. He forgets people's names and conversations he has had, and loses his keys. He lives with his wife; their two children live in the U.S. He remains independent for all basic and instrumental activities of daily living. He scores 29/30 on the MMSE and 27/30 on the MoCA. Some chronic ischemia is noted on brain CT. Laboratory tests are normal. A diagnosis of mild cognitive impairment is made.

He returns for follow-up 6 months later. His wife reports new spatial disorientation and difficulty understanding the use of electronic devices. He got lost once, so has stopped driving. The MMSE score is 22 and the MoCA 21. A diagnosis of mixed AD/vascular dementia is made and he is started on treatment with donepezil. You assess his capacity to assign a general power of attorney and a protection mandate.

A protection mandate in Quebec allows an individual to name someone or several people to take care of personal needs and property management upon incapacity. It is similar to an Advance Directive in the United States which is governed through different statutes in each state: see Chapter 44, "How Can Older People Be Protected?" In other parts of Canada, documents analogous to a protection mandate may go by other names such as powers of attorney or representation agreement. It is important to consult with a qualified professional, usually an attorney, in the jurisdiction where the individual lives to ensure that documentation is correctly done.

It would appear that a protection mandate can be appointed by an individual in the event of future incapacity which is then determined by the appropriate health care provider. The protection mandate would become effective when homologated by the Court, specifically when a judgment is obtained regarding incapacity. In the United States, an Advance Directive can generally be put in place in order to avoid a Guardianship proceeding.

Don fully understands the concept and content of both documents. He signs them shortly after seeing you, naming his wife as a mandatary, the person appointed to act under the protection mandate. His cognition continues to decline gradually. Two years after the initial visit, he needs help with basic activities of daily living and is occasionally incontinent. He has home care services at home. His wife has taken over financial management, using the power of attorney. She has to watch him constantly as he falls easily, including falling off chairs and falling when he gets up at night to urinate. She rarely has a decent night's sleep. His MMSE score is 15/30.

Six months later, he is admitted to hospital with delirium. His wife says that she can no longer take care of him, and he is discharged to a nursing home, with his consent. His wife would like to sell the house, which is in his name, and move into a small apartment close to the nursing home.

DOI: 10.1201/9781003344476-49

Shortly after discharge, you receive a call from the patient's sister in Boston. She says that his wife should be caring for him at home and had no business sending him to the nursing home. She says she will go to court if necessary to have him sent home.

You see the patient to assess decision-making capacity. The patient believes that he can still drive and care for himself. He is not sure whether he has moved recently. He does not know what his income or expenses are. After a detailed examination you find him incapable of making personal decisions and managing his assets. His wife obtains a psychosocial assessment from their social worker, and their notary (who has a distinct legal role in Quebec) initiates the process to have the protection mandate homologated.

*****

Sound ethics requires that we not examine or treat any patient without having obtained their informed consent to do so. If a patient lacks the capacity to make an informed decision about treatment, a substitute decision-maker must be sought.

The terms *Competency, Decision-making capacity, and Aptitude* are sometimes used interchangeably to reflect the same notion. We will use the term *Capacity* or *Decision-making capacity*, which is used widely in the medical literature.

Decision-making capacity is a person's ability to make, and act on, his or her own decisions.

WHERE DO WE START?

For a long time capacity was decided on the basis of diagnosis. This is sometimes called the *status approach*. A person who had a cognitive or psychiatric disorder was no longer allowed to make decisions. As our collective understanding of brain disorders improved, it became apparent that this black-and-white distinction lacked the necessary subtlety and unjustly categorized people. In the twentieth century, most jurisdictions updated their laws to require individual capacity evaluation before declaring anyone incapable.

It can also be tempting to base our opinion on the reasonableness of the decision being made by the person, typically a refusal of a medical treatment thought necessary: the *outcome approach*. A *"functional approach"* assesses whether a person's knowledge, skills, and abilities allow her/him to make a particular decision in a particular context. Now we commonly use an *integrated approach*, in which a patient's *status* (diagnosis) or foreseen *outcome* (decision-making that is seen as harmful) triggers a *functional* decision-making capacity assessment.

CRITERIA

There is a widely accepted consensus on four criteria to be used to decide whether a patient is capable of decision-making.[1] They can be summarized as follows:

- Ability to *understand* information relevant to decision-making.

- Ability to *appreciate* the significance of that information for one's own situation.

- Ability to *reason* with relevant information so as to engage in a logical process of weighing options.

- Ability to *express a choice.*

Someone who can *understand, appreciate, reason,* and *express a choice* is capable of decision-making. Someone who lacks all these abilities is not. Of course they all admit of degrees, and a person may have lost some abilities but not others, whence the need to look at each pertinent decision in detail in order to fairly judge the patient's capacity.

THE ASSESSMENT

The fact that the determination of a person's capacity cannot be based on a diagnosis alone does not excuse us from knowing the diagnosis, either through our own examination or by information received from another physician. The situation might be very different depending on whether the patient has a possibly transient disorder such as delirium, a progressive disorder such as dementia, an intermittent and potentially treatable disorder such as psychosis or severe depression, or a fixed disorder such as a developmental disorder or head injury.

Prior to the assessment, it is important to have precise information on the reasons it is being requested. If such an assessment is not required for the patient's well-being or the safety of their property, it should not be done. We also need objective and detailed information about the decisions that need to be made and the alleged lack of judgment or reasoning ability. This allows us to evaluate the patient with respect to her own life and needs, rather than using abstract theoretical examples. For financial capacity we need objective information on the patient's financial situation.

We begin with brief cognitive testing. The Mini-Mental State Examination[2] is by no means an instrument to determine capacity, but the score can provide useful information. For example, one study[3] showed that incapacity is more likely in patients with a score below 19, and capacity more likely if the score is over 23. Psychiatric examination is also necessary, to determine if the patient has a mood disorder severe enough to affect decision-making (e.g. causing loss of hope, diminished self-worth), or psychosis relevant to the decision (e.g. "my doctor wants to harm me"). We then proceed to assess the patient's ability to *understand, appreciate, reason*, and *express a choice*, as applied to the type of decision being questioned. We do so by "walking through" the decision with the patient.

CAPACITY TO CONSENT TO MEDICAL TREATMENT

Does the patient understand the nature of the illness, the nature and purpose of the proposed treatment, the benefits and risks of the proposed treatment, and alternative treatment options?

Does the patient appreciate how this information applies to his personal situation? Does he/she acknowledge the presence of the medical condition, and appreciate the expected consequences (to him or herself) of the proposed treatment and of the alternatives, including no treatment? Is the patient able to reason (i.e. engage in a rational process of manipulating the relevant information)? Can the patient express a choice and reasons for the choice? Does the patient consistently express the same choice? If so, the patient is capable of making the decision.

Several tools have been devised to help clinicians assess capacity to make medical decisions. A very helpful one is the *Aid to Capacity Evaluation*, from the University of Toronto.[4] It is essentially a structured interview to help answer these questions.

Law courts across Canada frequently use the *Nova Scotia criteria*:[5]

In determining whether or not a person in a hospital or a psychiatric facility is capable of consenting to treatment, the examining psychiatrist shall consider whether the person understands and appreciates: (a) the condition for which the specific treatment is proposed; (b) the nature and purpose of the specific treatment; (c) the risks and benefits involved in undergoing the specific treatment; and (d) the risks and benefits involved in not undergoing the specific treatment.

CAPACITY TO MAKE PERSONAL DECISIONS (LIVING SITUATION)

Other personal decisions for which patients' capacity may be questioned often are related to their living situation: can they make capable decisions regarding the safety of living in their own home, or a possible need for help or supervision, or to move into a more structured environment? We apply the same criteria to the patient's approach to these decisions:

Does she/he *understand* any change of health status or circumstances that might affect the living situation, potential risks related to the living situation, and possible interventions to reduce the risk (get help, move, etc.)? Can he/she *appreciate* the effect of a change of health status or circumstances on his/her own safety or well-being in a given living situation, and the expected consequences of living with the risks, or of intervening? Is the patient able to *reason* (i.e. engage in a rational process of manipulating the relevant information)? Can the patient *express a choice* and the reasons for the choice? Does the patient consistently express the same choice? If so, the patient is capable of making the decision.

CAPACITY TO MANAGE ONE'S ASSETS AND MAKE FINANCIAL DECISIONS

Managing one's financial affairs requires similar abilities to other decision-making: being able to understand, appreciate, reason, and express a choice. It also requires certain skills.

Does the patient understand her/his financial situation; any problems there might be related to financial management; changes in health or cognition that could make it difficult to manage finances; a possible need for help; and other decisions that need to be made? Can the patient appreciate the expected consequences of continuing as is, having help, having someone take over, understanding a possibly abusive situation? Can the patient appreciate the consequences of the various alternatives, in the case of other decisions? Is the patient able to reason (i.e. engage in a rational process of manipulating the relevant information)? Can the patient express a choice? Express the reasons for the choice? Does the patient consistently express the same choice?

Does the patient possess sufficient functional skills to be able to manage his affairs independently? This might include receiving income and paying bills, banking, and budget management, or more complex skills such as making decisions about investments or other property. Are the patient's memory, ability to calculate, and organizational abilities sufficient to continue carrying out these tasks? We should keep in mind how the patient organized these tasks in the past: has a meticulous record-keeper lost the ability to maintain and balance his/her checkbook? Or was his/her style always haphazard but good enough for his/her needs? A patient who can understand, appreciate, reason, and express choices about financial issues, and has the necessary skills to carry out the financial management required by his own situation, is capable of continuing to do so.

DECISION-MAKING FOR PATIENTS WITH DEMENTIA

A patient with early dementia may retain capacity to make decisions in many spheres. We know, however, that the disease is likely to progress, and that decision-making capacity will be gradually lost. It is thus very important, at the time of diagnosis, to find out whether the patient has made plans for the future, and if not to encourage him/her to do so. This may include making a will, giving a power of attorney or protection mandate, and advance care planning.

When a patient with dementia lives alone, safety hazards may arise, such as fire risk, malnutrition, or the effects of forgetting essential medicines or taking them inappropriately. Many such patients lack insight into the presence of the dementia and assume they have normal cognition. Decisions based on this assumption are not competent decisions, and if the patient refuses interventions to improve his/her safety, steps must be taken to formally assess decision-making capacity and name a substitute decision-maker.

Conversely, some patients with early cognitive symptoms may retain insight and be able to address problems and even to competently accept certain risks in order to maintain their independence, thus entering into conflict with family members who want their safety at all costs.

Even when a person is clearly incapable of decision-making, fundamental respect for the person requires us to continue caring for her or him in keeping with her/his known values and wishes. This might include food preferences and special diets, maintaining his/her appearance and grooming, religious observance, as well as favorite routines and activities. An elder with dementia remains a full member of the human community and should be treated as such.

CAPACITY TO SIGN LEGAL DOCUMENTS
Power of Attorney

"You can give someone a power of attorney to represent you when you cannot do something yourself."[6]

A bank or notary may request a letter from a doctor attesting to an older patient's capacity to give a power of attorney. To be capable, the patient must understand the concept and content of the document and its possible implications, including the approximate value of the assets, the power that is being entrusted, the risk of harm to the assets from poor judgment or dishonesty on the part of the mandatary, and the fact that she/he has the right to revoke the power of attorney at any time.

PROTECTION MANDATE

A protection mandate "is a document that lets you name, in advance, one or several people to look after your well-being and manage your property if you become incapable of doing this yourself."[7] It has no effect while the person who signed it remains capable of decision-making.

To be capable of signing a protection mandate, the patient must possess the same capacities as for a power of attorney. In addition, she/he must understand that the power given only takes effect if in the future she/he becomes incapable of decision-making, and that after that time it can no longer be revoked. She/he must understand that it applies not only to management of property but also to personal decisions such as health care or housing.

TESTAMENTARY CAPACITY

To be capable of making a will, the patient must understand its nature and effect, and recollect approximately what property he/she has and the persons who might expect to inherit from him/

her. He/she must understand the extent of what is being given to each beneficiary, and know if he/she has excluded someone who might have expected to benefit.

PROTECTIVE SUPERVISION

Decision-making capacity only needs to be formally assessed if it is required for the protection of the person or her/his property. Many families continue to care for their loved ones and to manage their affairs without any such assessment. For example, they may continue to manage their assets online or using a power of attorney, and to make personal decisions in consultation with the patient. All adults are presumed capable unless there is evidence to the contrary.

Under the law, the need for protection exists when an incapacitated person must be assisted or represented in the exercise of their civil rights. This need may arise from the person's isolation, the duration of their incapacity, the nature or state of the person's affairs, etc.[8]

We might need to assess capacity, for example, if there is disagreement among family members regarding the needs of the patient, or if major financial transactions are foreseen, such as the sale of a house. In cases of abuse or neglect, a legal decision-maker may be required to protect the person from harm. Finally, if the person refuses interventions essential for his/her safety, or has delusions regarding those caring for him/her, capacity assessment will be needed.

If a person who has become incapable of decision-making has a protection mandate, the family may proceed to have it homologated.[9] This requires a medical assessment and a psychosocial assessment by a social worker. Through a juridical process, the person is declared incapable and the mandatary named. This is usually undertaken by the family with the help of a notary or lawyer.

If there is no protection mandate, the family or another concerned party may apply for private or public curatorship or tutorship. If the person is only partially incapable a tutor is named, who is responsible for some decisions, while the patient retains control of others, as determined by the court. If totally incapable, a curator is named. Wherever possible, the tutor or curator will be a family member or friend of the patient. If no one is available, this role is taken by the Public Curator.[10]

BACK TO THE CASE

When you first saw Don, he had early cognitive symptoms but still independent, and was presumed capable of making decisions. On your advice he put measures into place to authorize his wife to make personal and financial decisions in his name should he lose capacity. She was able to care for him for several years without any formal capacity assessment; it became necessary when a major financial transaction was being contemplated and a family member was challenging her authority to make decisions on his behalf. You found that Don lacked the necessary understanding, appreciation, and ability to reason and express a choice about his personal and financial needs. Protective supervision was put into place.

REFERENCES

1. Applebaum PS, Grisso T. Assessing patients' capacity to consent to treatment. NEJM 1988; 319:1635–1638.
2. https://www.ncbi.nlm.nih.gov/pubmed/1202204
3. https://www.ncbi.nlm.nih.gov/pmc/articles/PMC271553/
4. http://www/jcb.utoronto.ca/tools/documents/documents/ace.pdf
5. Nova Scotia Hospitals Act article 52.sA: https://nslegislature.ca/sites/default/files/legc/statutes/hospital.pdf
6. https://www.educaloi.qc.ca/en/capsules/power-attorney
7. https://www.educaloi.qc.ca/en/capsules/protection-mandates-naming-someone-act-you
8. Ibid.
9. https://www.educaloi.qc.ca/en/capsules/protection-mandates-naming-someone-act-you
10. http://www.curateur.gouv.qc/cura/en/majeur/inaptitude/role/index.html

44 How Can Older People Be Protected?

Randy S. Perskin, Esq., JD

CONTENTS

*Disclaimer: The information contained in this chapter is provided only as general information and not intended as legal advice, nor should it be used as a substitute for complete review of your case by an experienced elder law attorney. All situations differ. By reading this chapter there is no attorney-client relation established between you and Randy S. Perskin, Esq.

VIGNETTE

Mary Smith is a 75-year-old woman with early onset dementia diagnosed by her physician. She is otherwise healthy and is able to perform ADLs (activities of daily living) such as toileting and bathing. She is married, lives with her husband and has two adult children who care for her deeply.

As the dementia progresses Ms. Smith becomes confused and although she speaks clearly she cannot follow conversations or express her concerns. Although mobile, she needs direction for purposes of dressing, bathing, toileting and feeding herself. It is no longer safe for her to perform certain daily tasks unattended such as cooking. She can no longer travel outdoors without company as she will often forget where she is, where she is going or where she lives.

Ms. Smith, when suffering from advanced dementia, is not self-directing. She becomes unable to coordinate her care and needs assistance with all activities of daily living to the extent that she needs reminders to take her medications, bathe and pay her bills. Although she is still physically healthy it is no longer safe for her to be left to her own devices.

DISCUSSION

Considerations in the care and treatment of the elder population focus on personal needs, including but not limited to health care, living situation and property management. This latter includes payment of bills and managing finances. Elder adults who suffer from physical disabilities which do not impact on their ability to handle their needs or who do not suffer from any significant incapacity can continue to manage their needs as they always have. The issues facing elder persons who suffer from disabilities which impact their ability to understand their needs and manage them can be effectively dealt with if the proper safeguards are in place.

Advance Directives can protect the elder population if and when they can no longer care for themselves. Agents can be appointed to effectively stand in the place of the elder person to make decisions on their behalf should they be unable to do so. In the United States, the Health Insurance Portability and Accountability Act of 1996 (HIPAA) restricts the ability of health care providers and insurance companies to provide personal health information (PHI) without consent.[1] Although protecting a patient's privacy is of significant importance, concerns arise when an individual requires the support of others for care, management and treatment. Pursuant to federal law, a health care provider can discuss relevant health information and billing practices if the patient gives consent, or with family members involved with the care, treatment and payment if in the provider's professional judgment the patient would consent.[2] That being said the patient can limit the amount of information given to family members. A HIPAA release can be executed, allowing the health care provider to release information to the named individual. The Family Health Care Decisions Act (FHCDA)[3] establishes the authority for health care providers in general hospitals and health care facilities, notably nursing homes, to speak with family members or close friends in order to make health care decisions should the patient become unable to do so. FHCDA can be applied when the elder person is in an institutional setting and health care decisions need to be made for a patient no longer able to act on their own behalf. However it does not apply to those individuals in the community who may need the assistance of others in making determinations

DOI: 10.1201/9781003344476-50

on their own behalf. A Health Care Proxy can be executed, appointing an agent to act on an individual's behalf for purposes of medical care, including care management, in case of an inability to act.[4] An agent should act in accordance, as much as possible, with the principal's wishes even if they disagree. As such, the principal should have a conversation with their agent as to their wishes and desires regarding health care issues. The Health Care Proxy should indicate that the agent is aware of the principal's wishes in such regard. The preferences can be related orally or in writing. The Health Care Proxy will become effective when it is determined that the principal no longer has the capacity to act for him/herself.

A Living Will is a document that sets forth health care wishes regarding life-prolonging procedures and other end-of-life care. A Living Will can specify the types of treatment desired to prolong life or the measures that the principal wishes to be avoided.

A Do Not Resuscitate Order (DNR), on the other hand, is generally written by doctors in a hospital and specifically instructs health care professionals not to perform CPR or other life-sustaining measures when the heartbeat or breathing stops.

A Power of Attorney is a legal document which appoints an agent to act with regard to financial and legal matters.[5] It can be as broad or as specific as desired and is often used to protect a party who is unable to act on their own behalf with regard to their financial needs. There are three types of Powers of Attorney: Nondurable, Durable and Springing. A Nondurable Power of Attorney usually applies to a specific transaction such as the sale of a home. A Nondurable Power of Attorney is valid until revoked or the principal becomes incapacitated. A Durable Power of Attorney allows an agent to act on behalf of the principal even after incapacity. A Durable Power of Attorney is often used to avoid unnecessary and expensive Guardianships. A Durable Power of Attorney can be revoked and is valid until the death of the principal. A Springing Power of Attorney becomes effective when a named event, such as the incapacity of the principal, arises or after a specified period of time. Generally for incapacity purposes a letter from a physician testifying to that circumstance will work. Powers of Attorney become effective when signed, except for a Springing Power of Attorney. However it is the intent of the Durable Power of Attorney that the agent will act once the principal becomes unable to do so. Effective September 2009 and further amended in September 2010 changes were made to the statutory short-form Power of Attorney to the effect that the Power of Attorney must contain the signatures of both the principal and agent; the agent's authority to make gifts be granted through a separate statutory gifts rider that has the signatures of two witnesses; multiple agents must act together unless otherwise designated; a principal can appoint someone to monitor the actions of the agent: this person has the authority to request records of transactions entered into on behalf of the principal; the principal's rights are stated on the first page in bold faced print; the agent's role, fiduciary obligations and legal limitations are explained; and a signature constitutes acknowledgment. A Power of Attorney in New York can also include language allowing for the release of medical information protected under HIPAA for financial planning purposes, specifically the payment of medical bills. A Power of Attorney drafted prior to 2009, if compliant with the General Obligations Law, can remain in full force and effect. It is possible that a Power of Attorney can be accepted multi-jurisdictionally if drafted in accordance with the General Obligations Law or the law of the state where it was executed. A conversation with an attorney well versed in the law in this regard is recommended.

Agents acting under a Power of Attorney are fiduciaries and should act in the best interests of the principal. Proper record keeping is imperative. Interested parties, such as financial institutions and family members, can bring special proceedings questioning the agent's actions. The appointment of an agent to act under a Power of Attorney is a decision which should not be taken lightly. The agent should be someone who the principal trusts and has an understanding of their financial situation and needs.

Practical issues in dealing with Advance Directives include capacity. It is hoped that proper planning is put into effect prior to the occurrence of incapacity. Capacity for purposes of executing the proper Advance Directives means the ability to understand the nature of the document being signed and the authority being granted. An attorney skilled in the preparation of such documents, either in conjunction with estate planning or separately, can effectively determine if such capacity exists. By interviewing the principal, asking questions about their wishes, explaining the documents and relating the issues therein, a reputable and knowledgeable attorney can make a determination as to the capacity for these purposes. Optimally, an attorney well versed in elder care issues is consulted. Essentially, a person with diagnoses that affect mental capacity, such as early onset dementia, may not be precluded from creating Advance Directives.

Even the most comprehensive Advance Directive will not be properly utilized if its existence is unknown. In this regard copies should be provided to any agents appointed, to medical and health care providers where necessary, to financial institutions and, in the case of Health Care Proxies and Living Wills, kept on hand on the principal's person, as in a wallet. Originals and copies should be kept somewhere safe but not necessarily in a safety deposit box which cannot be accessed by the appropriate parties. Discussions with family members, close personal friends or agents as to the existence of Advance Directives and their locations is important.

Under New York law there are two types of Guardianships that can be established. The Surrogates Court Procedure Act (SCPA) Article 17-A can be used to establish a Guardianship for people who are mentally retarded or developmentally disabled attributable to conditions such as cerebral palsy or neurological imbalances.[6] A Guardianship can be established for elderly persons, trauma victims and, at times, mentally ill or developmentally disabled persons pursuant to Article 81 of the Mental Hygiene Law.[7]

A Guardianship proceeding pursuant to Article 81 of the Mental Hygiene Law (MHL) is commenced by Order to Show Cause and Verified Petition in the county where the Alleged Incapacitated Person (AIP), the person to whom the Guardianship proceeding relates, resides or is physically present. The petitioner can be the AIP, the CEO of a facility in which the AIP is a resident, an adult relative, Adult Protective Services or any other person concerned with the welfare of the AIP. The Order to Show Cause includes identification information for the AIP, such as name and address, as well as the reasons why a Guardianship is being sought. A Verified Petition is more detailed in that in addition to the information given in the Order to Show Cause it will include financial information, a description of the functional level of the AIP including behavior, understanding and appreciation of the nature and consequences of any inability to manage personal needs or property. Factual allegations of actual occurrences, demonstrating that the AIP will suffer harm due to her/his lack of understanding of the consequences of the inability to provide for personal needs or property management, are tailored to relate to the powers being sought, the duration of the powers being sought, and the approximate value and description of the financial assets of the AIP. It is noted whether the AIP is a recipient of public assistance; the nature of any claim, debt or obligation of the AIP; names, addresses and telephone numbers of any presumptive distributes; available resources and an opinion as to the sufficiency of those resources as well as other information which would assist the Court Evaluator in conducting an investigation and writing a report.

There are instances where a Temporary Restraining Order is included in the Order to Show Cause, for example where there is an eviction proceeding pending or where abuse is alleged. Language to the effect that personal medical information may be provided should additionally be included in the Order to Show Cause. An AIP may consent to provide health care information protected by HIPAA, or a Court Evaluator can move to obtain a Court Order to obtain medical records. Additional Orders might be necessary where records from financial institutions are required.

Once the Order to Show Cause is signed by a Judge, a hearing date will be set within 28 days of the date of the Order. The Judge will generally appoint a Court Evaluator who is responsible for explaining the Guardianship proceeding to the AIP, investigating the claims made and writing a report, including recommendations, to be supplied to the Court. The report should also relate any jurisdictional and service issues. The report may also be supplied to the attorney for the AIP and Petitioner with prior Court approval.

The Court Evaluator is an independent individual appointed by the Court to effectively act as the eyes and ears of the Court and does not represent any of the parties in the Guardianship proceeding. The Court Evaluator does not have to be an attorney. An attorney for the AIP can also be appointed for representation in the Guardianship proceeding. The attorney for the AIP acts as an advocate. Personal service of the Order to Show Cause and Petition, as well as the Notice of Proceeding which sets forth the time, date and place of the hearing, is required. Service of the Order to Show Cause, Verified Petition and Notice of Proceeding should also be effectuated on the Court Evaluator and attorney for the AIP. Service of the Order to Show Cause and Notice of Proceeding, not the Verified petition, should additionally be effectuated on other interested parties such as the spouse, adult children, siblings and the person with whom the AIP resides.

The AIP is entitled to be present at the Hearing. The AIP's appearance can be waived if it is determined that they cannot meaningfully participate. Generally, the Court will make every effort to allow for the AIP's participation including adjourning the hearing where necessary or conducting bedside hearings. At the Hearing evidence will be presented via testimony, including that of the Court Evaluator, a psychiatric care provider if a psychological assessment was provided, the AIP, as well as family members and other interested parties if available and relevant. Documentary evidence, such as the Court Evaluator's report, is introduced into the record. After listening to the testimony and reviewing the evidence the judge will make a determination as to the Guardianship.

The Court's determination as to the Guardianship will be set forth in an Order and Judgment. The Court, in making its determination, should consider the least restrictive alternative, thereby giving the AIP the greatest amount of freedom while considering functional limitations that make it difficult to understand or appreciate the nature or consequences of any inability to provide for personal needs or property management. The desires of the AIP are therefore taken into account. The Guardianship can be tailored to the specific needs of the AIP and be broad or narrow. Primary consideration is given to family members; however independent Guardians are often appointed particularly where there are allegations of abuse or neglect, where there is no family member available or where a particular skill set is required to resolve particular issues.

The AIP may be declared an Incapacitated Person, within the scope of Article 81 of the Mental Hygiene Law. It is significant that incapacity in this regard is a legal, not medical, term and limits an individual's ability to enter into contracts or other legal issues that require capacity. However it is not always the case that a person is adjudged incapacitated for purposes of a Guardianship. There are instances where an individual is designated as a Person in Need of a Guardian (PING) usually for specific issues that need to be addressed by a Guardian.

A Guardian can be appointed for personal needs or property management. A Guardian of the Person can be given powers that relate to personal needs such as determining the living situation, health care and placement of aides. A Guardian of the Property can be given powers relating to property management including marshaling and managing assets, paying bills and applying for and maintaining private and public benefits. A Guardianship can be tailored to the specific needs of the AIP. Therefore a Guardian's powers can be limited to a specific issue, such as dealing with an eviction proceeding and relocations issues, stopping abuse or Medicaid planning. Additionally a Guardian of the Property may be appointed but not a Guardian of the Person. A Temporary Guardian may be appointed during the pendency of the proceeding in order to assist with specific issues that need immediate attention. A Guardian, once appointed, will have the powers set forth in the Order and Judgment upon obtaining a commission to act. If an expansion of powers is necessary, an order can be obtained via motion for such purposes. The Guardianship terminates upon the death of the IP or PING or the completion of the duties set forth in the Order and Judgment.

Guardianships are subject to Court oversight. A Guardian is required to submit an Initial Report within 90 days of appointment detailing the ward's current circumstances, and Annual Accounting thereafter. Annual Accountings will be reviewed by a Court Examiner appointed by the Court and a report and proposed order to judicially settle the account will be presented to the Court. Upon the death of the ward, following notice to the Court, a Final Accounting can be presented which can be reviewed by a Referee to Review for purposes of settling the Final Account and discharge. In instances of Temporary or Limited (Special) Guardianships a Report will generally be submitted describing the actions taken to resolve the issues addressed in the Order and Judgment.

Guardianship fees, to the Court Evaluator, Attorney for the AIP and on occasion to the petitioning attorney can be chargeable to the AIP's estate. Additionally, payment to the appointed Guardian is also generally made from the ward's funds. Where limited funds are available fees are often paid by the Department of Social Services to the Court Evaluator or Temporary Guardian and to the attorney for the AIP.

A Guardianship can be transferred to another state pursuant to the Uniform Adult Guardianship and Protective Proceeding Act (UAGPPJA) when adopted by that state. Such a transfer can alleviate the expense and duplicative work required to establish a new Guardianship in a different state. Discussions with an attorney familiar with the UAGPPJA and the states that have adopted it should be entered into when such a transfer may be necessary.

Practical considerations for the aging population include safe living arrangements and financial management. A Geriatric Care Manager, usually a trained nurse or social worker, can assist in determining the specific needs of the elder client and locate housing and other services that are appropriate for care. Various factors need to be considered in determining whether the elder person should remain at home or consider placement in a nursing home or assisted living facility. In determining whether it is safe for an elder adult to live in the community, the condition of the home should be considered, whether assistance is needed to provide for the activities of daily living and whether the individual lives alone or with someone else who can be responsible for their care. Health aides are an invaluable resource to an elder individual who is no longer totally independent but wishes to reside at home. Assisted living facilities and nursing homes are alternatives to a community residence when an elder individual needs more care than can be safely provided in the home. A nursing home generally follows more of a medical model than assisted living facilities do. Assisted living communities therefore provide more of a home atmosphere. Many assisted living facilities in New York do not accept Medicaid or Medicare so financial concerns can come into play.

Financial planning for the elder population includes determining if they are receiving the benefits they need to survive. Long-term care insurance is a private policy that covers the expenses for assistance in the community with the activities of daily living, and health aides. The cost of long-term care insurance depends on the age at which it was purchased. Medicare parts A, hospital, and B, medical, is available to any person in any state upon reaching age 65. Medicare Part D, for prescription drug coverage, can be obtained through any Medicare approved insurance carrier. Supplemental insurance can be used to cover those expenses that Medicare does not, such as copays. Medicaid is a needs-based program for low-income families. The income and asset levels vary from state to state. In New York, community Medicaid can be used to pay for health aides, in addition to health care, and institutional Medicaid can be used to pay for nursing homes. Medicaid rules and qualification issues are complicated and the proper planning should be discussed with an elder law attorney expert in the field. Social Security retirement benefits in New York can be collected at age 62. A Representative Payee is an individual who is determined to be qualified to collect social security benefits for the senior individual. Supplemental Security Income, SSI, is a federal income supplement program designed to help aged blind and disabled people who have little or no income and is used to meet basic needs such as food, shelter and clothing. Social Security Disability, SSD, is a federal program designed to supplement the income of people whose physical disabilities limit their ability to work. The Supplemental Nutrition Assistance Program, SNAP, is a federal income supplement program designed to assist people in obtaining food, previously recognized as food stamps. The Senior Citizens Rent Increase Exemption, SCRIE, freezes the rent of heads of household aged 62 and older who live in rent-regulated apartments in New York City. Death benefits from a spouse, either from Social Security or pensions, should also be explored.

Recognizing the signs of elder abuse in the aged population is a key factor in their care. Elder abuse, which can be physical, financial or psychological, may occur at the hands of a caregiver or other person in a position of trust. See Chapter 40 on Elder Abuse for further information.

Financial exploitation can include the misuse of funds or the taking of property. Financial abuse can be recognized by a financial institution if funds are withdrawn without the consent of the account holder or their representative. Additionally, there have been instances where caretakers take their aged clients to the bank to withdraw cash for them or simply use their bank card. In such instances a financial representative can step in to protect the interests of the elder client. Physical and psychological abuse cannot be as easily identified, especially where the elder person has a disability that prevents them from communicating what is happening. Physical injuries can be the result of abuse. If the injury resulted from someone pushing or hitting the senior it qualifies as abuse. If the elder person lives in an assisted living community or nursing home there are often cameras set up in the hallways and public areas that can give proof positive of abusive behavior. Additionally, such institutions are highly regulated. An incident report should be generated detailing the incident and steps that were taken to prevent it from happening again. Abuse can take the form of neglect, even self-inflicted in the case of an individual who is not properly feeding themselves or obtaining the proper medical treatment. Such incidences can be reported to Adult Protective Services (APS) who can then step in and evaluate whether protection needs to be implemented and the form it should take. The Attorney General of the State of New York has an elder abuse hotline where instances of abuse can be reported. Complaints are investigated and it is then determined whether the incidence rises to the level of a criminal act. The Elder Abuse Education and Outreach Program provides information and advice to elder abuse victims and their caregivers. Even if an act does not rise to the level of elder abuse it still may be negligent, such as in the case where no care or inappropriate care is given for an injury. In such cases a civil action may be brought and discussions with a personal injury attorney can be useful.

It should be noted that all references herein are made to New York law unless otherwise indicated as Federal Law of the United States. Advice of counsel in the jurisdiction of residence should be used to navigate the legal ramifications of the needs of an elderly client.

CONCLUSION

Mrs. Smith's son consulted counsel when his mother was originally diagnosed with dementia. He was asked whether she had any Advance Directives in place. As he was uncertain, he was advised to see if his mother had a Will, as often Advance Directives are put in place when estate planning is performed. Fortunately Mrs. Smith was able to remember the name of the attorney who prepared her Will. It was discovered that Advance Directives, including a Power of Attorney and Health Care Proxy, had been executed and were effectively used to assist Mrs. Smith when she became unable to manage her finances and personal needs. It was fortuitous that Mrs. Smith had a loving family that was able to work together to protect her interests.

REFERENCES

1. HIPAA; PUBL 104–191, 110 flat 1936.
2. 45 CFR 164.510(b)
3. Public Health Law Articles 29-CC & 29-CCC
4. Public Health law Article 29-C
5. General Obligations Law Section 5–1501
6. Surrogates Court Procedures Act Article 17-A
7. Mental Hygiene Law Article 81

45 Financial Guidance for Seniors

Karen C. Altfest, PhD, CFP®

CONTENTS

Many seniors are primarily troubled by three financial issues:

1. Will I have enough to support the lifestyle I desire in retirement?

2. How can I address healthcare issues and costs?

3. How best can I leave my assets to my family, friends, and causes I believe in?

This chapter will address all these issues as they affect seniors and their caregivers in the United States today. It will also offer some tips for physicians caring for older persons who may be losing the cognitive ability to manage their finances on their own.

According to a recent study, only 25% of Americans believe they have prepared adequately for retirement. Reasons include: 1) lack of access to good strategies; 2) poor understanding of the retirement plans that are in place for them; and 3) believing that planning for retirement is just too complicated. For many people, retirement can last almost as long as their work lives. A 30-year retirement period is not uncommon for those who retire in their 60s and live into their 90s. How, they can wonder, can they be secure when the average American retiree has less than $15,000 in retirement savings and they no longer have a regular paycheck?

Of course, the best time to begin preparing for this long period is as early as possible. Savers who begin in their 20s and 30s can end up with enough money to cover costs for decades to come. Those who begin to save in their 40s and 50s may have a greater challenge. Figure 45.1 shows when most Americans begin to save for retirement.

As you can see, some people do begin saving for retirement in their 20s and 30s, while also repaying their education debt, and planning for children and their first home.

Later in life, if they face a retirement gap (that is, greater expenses than savings), many people work into their late 60s and even 70s, sometimes part-time.

The great majority of people living in the United States today would like to continue their current lifestyle after they retire. Few people want to cut back, although their spending may start going for different items, that is, less on travel, but potentially more for healthcare or personal assistance (this can be less true in Canada where medical expenses, shared with the government, are not so great a factor).

A MODERN-DAY CHALLENGE

Financial literacy is low in the United States for a developed country. The United States places 14th in the world in financial literacy, while Canada lands much higher, in fourth place. Even top universities spend little or no time teaching cash management or providing investing courses to students. People are left to pick up financial wisdom on their own, generally through trial and error, or by way of family example. According to *Forbes* magazine, two-thirds of Americans cannot pass a basic financial literacy test.

DOI: 10.1201/9781003344476-51

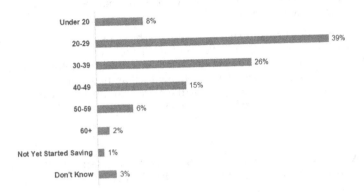

To the best of your memory, at what age did you start saving for retirement?

Of adults who are saving for retirement

- Under 20 — 8%
- 20-29 — 39%
- 30-39 — 26%
- 40-49 — 15%
- 50-59 — 6%
- 60+ — 2%
- Not Yet Started Saving — 1%
- Don't Know — 3%

Figure 45.1 Saving for retirement.

In addition, credit card debt may keep many people from achieving their goals. According to Forbes, the average amount owed on credit cards in the United States is $16,000, which can take 10 years to pay off for those just paying the minimum amount each month.

With that poor showing at financial literacy in mind, here's more on the three most common financial concerns for most older persons.

WILL I HAVE ENOUGH TO SUPPORT THE LIFESTYLE I DESIRE IN RETIREMENT?

Many people are insecure about calculating how long their money will last. Some want to preserve their capital for the next generation, yet hope for growth in their portfolio; others want to help children and grandchildren now, yet have a substantial estate to divide in the future. Some people, not knowing where to turn for professional help, do their own retirement calculations. They often neglect to factor in inflation, which can have a major effect over an extended retirement period, or to use probability analysis, which can run thousands of scenarios showing what will happen when costs rise while earnings decline, or vice versa. Others neglect to account for lifestyle differences over the decades. They may assume that a stagnant plan, developed on costs while they were still at work, can be used as a guide during retirement. But this is not so—a worthwhile retirement plan contains all those elements (such as recognition of inflation and probability analysis results) and more. It should be revisited and updated whenever a person's lifestyle or circumstances change.

COMMON SOURCES OF INCOME IN RETIREMENT

Most people's income comes from a few of these sources in retirement:

1. Employer-sponsored retirement plans—if a company has a defined contribution plan, such as a 401(k), the worker and the employer can both contribute, and the amount a person ends up with varies, according to savings patterns. Qualified plans are built with pretax dollars, and the money being saved is tax-deferred until withdrawal, which is allowed at age 59½, and currently mandated at age 70½. Defined contribution plans, such as 401(k)s, 403(b)s, and individual retirement accounts (IRAs), are fairly common types of tax-qualified plans. The amount a worker can contribute is decided by federal law, and can be changed.

   A Roth 401(k) is a fairly new retirement vehicle, taxed upon contribution to the employer plan, but not later upon withdrawal. In other words, taxes are paid up front, and then money is allowed to grow in the account. Choosing the most useful retirement savings plan is highly important to a person's ultimate financial health.

2. Social Security—the full retirement age at which workers are eligible for coverage under this government program has risen to age 66 (depending on an applicant's year of birth) and likely

will continue to rise as people live longer. By 2050, some estimates project 83.7 million people aged 65 or older living in the United States—nearly twice as many senior citizens as in 2012. In the United States, 10,000 people are turning age 65 every day. Social Security spending on the elderly is greater than income taken out of paychecks to contribute to it for the first time in almost four decades. This should be a reality check for younger generations to take earlier action to protect their own retirement years.

3. Personal savings—this is money that can be kept in a brokerage account or a bank and withdrawn as needed, or left to grow over time. For some people it is their emergency fund—available on very short notice, ready to be put to use for a major and sometimes unexpected need, such as a home repair. There is confidence in knowing that there is a pot of money readily accessible in good times and bad. Simply put, the more a family or individual has saved, the more comfortable they are likely to be in retirement.

HOW CAN A PHYSICIAN DETECT SIGNS THAT AN OLDER PERSON IS NOT FINANCIALLY PREPARED FOR RETIREMENT?

Physicians are often the first to notice signs of stress in the elderly. For example, you may notice that a patient says he or she is fearful of running out of money. Another recurring negative fantasy for some older persons is that they may lose their housing and be homeless. When there is no paycheck coming in, they may worry about how to maintain their current standard of living. They may fear that they could live an overly long life, and worry about how they will support that. The older patient may be afraid to talk to family members about their financial status, worrying that responsibility for financial decisions may be taken away and assumed by an adult child.

One woman whose husband recently died told her doctors she had made plans "to end it all." This brought her to the attention of a psychiatrist, who is now treating her.

WHAT CAN PHYSICIANS AND CAREGIVERS DO TO HELP OLDER PATIENTS?

Physicians may spot financial problems with older patients before others do. Here are some ways physicians can help.

Ask relevant questions of the patient and those close to him or her. Determine if the patient is accurately aware of their financial situation, and if they are fiscally responsible. Refer patients to the appropriate specialist or public agency for help. If the case is less extreme, recommend some groups to join or information to read to address their financial misgivings or changes in cognitive ability. Consider having some relevant reading material in your office. Urge patients to communicate with their spouses, children, and other loved ones about money questions or fears. Encourage them to use the money they've worked long and hard for to live the life they would like. Check on their mental state, or suggest someone who can. Note when a senior is no longer able to handle his or her finances or to make clear decisions. Ask if there is someone with power of attorney for the older person, or someone the patient can reach out to. Look for signs of abuse or scams against the elderly, and notify the family or the caregivers or government agencies if you suspect this is happening. With people living longer, there are more opportunities both for financial fraud to occur, but also to help steer elderly people toward assistance, perhaps to pro bono elder-care legal counsel or a financial planning organization to address their continuing financial needs.

CHECK FOR SCAMS BY STRANGERS

Difficult family situations can arise from aging patients' declining money management abilities, so physicians and caregivers can listen for potential scams when a financial situation seems to take an unusual turn. For example, if a patient mentions giving most of his money away to a younger woman he has just met after the woman promised to marry him, that should raise red flags. A son or daughter could be alerted to obtain a court order to gain access to the patient's finances if the situation is thought to be harmful to the older person. This sometimes involves having an attorney start the process to deem the patient mentally incompetent, or bring him into the adult child's home to live.

LISTEN FOR STORIES OF ABUSE

This can include stealing by family or caregivers. These stories may or may not have basis in fact.

BE ALERT TO YOUR OLDER PATIENTS' SIGNALS

Signs of distress may include:

- A sudden change in behavior.
- Keeping secrets.
- Money missing from accounts.
- Personal items gone.
- An abrupt rise in expenses.
- Sudden new friendships.
- A decline in standard of living or quality of care.
- Extreme worries about money.

PHYSICIANS AND TRAINED OR FAMILY CAREGIVERS CAN WATCH FOR:

- The illness of a partner.
- The death of a spouse.
- Significant or long-lasting stress or signs of depression.
- Separation from family or friends.
- Elder abuse, which is often centered on finances.

Managing Risk

Another aspect of money management to consider is the senior's capacity for, and comfort level with, taking financial risks. There is a saying in financial planning that the most serious risk is one individuals don't know they are taking. Here are some types of risk that financial advisors are aware of and seniors and their caregivers can learn to think about.

Liquidity Risk—An asset may be tied up in an investment and not readily available to the investor, for reasons such as a lockup date, an early withdrawal penalty, a hedge fund redemption date or restrictions arising from private real estate investments. As a result, an investor may only be able to withdraw funds at specified times.

Longevity Risk—A person may live a shorter or longer life than expected. If they die young, they may not have worked long enough to accumulate assets to support their family after they are gone. If they live a very long life, they will need extra assets to cover several years of late-in-life expenses.

Health Risk—In the United States, the possibility of large, unreimbursed medical costs always looms. Healthcare costs have been growing about 4–5% per year in the nation. In 2017, healthcare collectively cost Americans $3.5 trillion, or 17.9% of gross domestic product (GDP). More critically for older persons, medical costs typically more than double between the ages of 70 and 90.

Investment Risk—Assets placed in financial accounts may not perform as expected, and values can decline.

Withdrawal Risk—This comes from withdrawing money at a disadvantageous time, typically from a portfolio when prices are low, particularly early in the retirement period. At that time more shares of an investment may need to be liquidated, leaving fewer shares to continue to grow and finance future costs.

Average Health Spending by Age in the United States

Spending per year based on age group (2016)

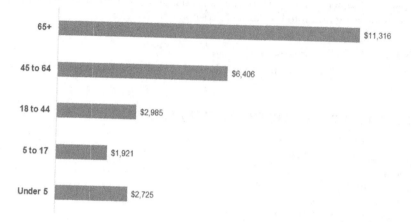

Average health spending by age in the United States

Inflation Risk—If inflation is not considered when planning for expenses in the future, the individual may be hurt when living costs rise.

HOW CAN I ADDRESS HEALTHCARE COSTS AS A SENIOR?

In the United States, it is important to make sure that you have appropriate medical insurance coverage in place, either as an individual or through your workplace.

For the elderly, there are usually greater medical or personal needs costs that exceed insurance coverage. Medicare for seniors in the United States, along with supplemental insurance, can fill this gap.

In addition, some people like to have a long-term-care insurance policy. This coverage can be costly, but it can defray spiraling costs that may come from the need to live in a care facility in the future or to require assistance at home with basic activities of daily living (ADL). The average age to purchase long-term care insurance in the United States is 55–64. But seniors cannot wait too long to obtain this coverage because poor health may disqualify them from purchasing a policy or make it prohibitively expensive.

Medicaid is a program for financially needy people that is paid for in part by states and in part by the federal government. The program pays for medical care administered by medical professionals, and also may cover assisted living costs, dental care, and continuing-care facility costs, if necessary. To find out more, it is best to check with the applicable state Medicaid office on its eligibility rules or with an elder care attorney who is an expert at guiding seniors in Medicaid planning.

WHO WILL TAKE CARE OF THE OLDER PERSON?

Many families in the United States are having fewer children and at older ages, and living greater distances from each other around the country. That can mean that there are fewer offspring able to divide the care of the older person. In many families, caregiving becomes the responsibility of one member of the family.

Baby boomers, now between ages 54 and 72, are entering retirement. Gen X, now between ages 38 and 53, is raising children, concerned about education, coping with the cost of housing, and trying to save for future retirement. They are often in the unenviable and untenable position of having responsibility for two generations other than their own. Millennials are still young, currently ages 22–37, and are newer in the workforce. (Note: all age groups have been recalculated by the Pew Organization, which has recently issued new guidelines.)

People who are concerned about getting proper care for aging parents while simultaneously raising their own children are often referred to as "the sandwich generation," squeezed between the needs of the older person and their own offspring.

As a result of growing longevity, younger elderly people are often caring for parents living into their 90s and beyond. The *New York Times* in mid-2019 published an article titled "When the Older Care for the Oldest," which gave examples of adult children in their 60s and 70s caring for parents in their 90s. For some of these families, the children sacrifice their own finances to pay for parents' needs, sometimes giving up jobs to care for their elders. Others take parents into their own homes. Sometimes the aging children's health is affected.

Because aging generations are working toward their own retirement, and younger generations may not be available to help, some families choose to hire a caregiver or move an older person into a facility. Caregivers often assist with the ADL (activities of daily living) that an older person can no longer handle alone. At times, these caregivers become involved in family and money matters, such as bill-paying. Currently, 43.5 million people in the United States say they have been caregivers. Many say they have given unpaid help, sometimes to children, other times to spouses, and often care to relatives. A major problem, however, is that there is currently a shortage of trained caregivers in the United States. With an aging population, there soon will be many older people without proper care. An equally important challenge to caregiving is high, protracted cost, which can be prohibitive for many families.

IS THERE A DIFFERENT PORTFOLIO FOR OLDER PEOPLE?

To arrive at a suitable investment portfolio, first discuss goals with family members, then create a diversified portfolio that makes sense for the older person's needs. Start by dividing the portfolio into two asset classes, stocks and bonds, depending on the amount of risk or volatility that is tolerable in the portfolio. Then divide each of those categories even further. Do some reading or consult a professional financial advisor to determine the best way to do more (see sample diversification diagram in Figure 45.3). Basically, the investor's age is just one factor in deciding how much risk to assume in a portfolio. Others have to do with investment growth potential, tolerance level for market declines, and assumed length of the retirement period.

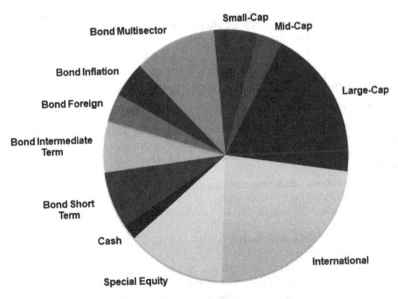

Figure 45.2 Investment management: the role of diversification.

It helps when the older investor is honest about goals, and what they want to happen to the money someday. Are they planning to use it soon, do they have an emergency fund that is not invested in the markets and therefore not subject to fluctuation to see them through unexpected events? Although some older persons wish to take less investment risk as they age, that is a choice, just as it is for all investors. There is no older-investor formula that will suit all people in this age group.

Here is a sample of one way to divide the investment pie.

This chart shows one example of how an investor might diversify his or her portfolio. Note the various bond slices on the left, and the stockholdings on the right, beginning with small-capitalization stocks through special equity, generally investments—such as real estate holdings—that do not act the same way as other stocks and bonds in the portfolio.

Of course, an investor might choose a very different asset allocation from the one presented in Figure 45.3, depending on goals, appetite for risk, and beliefs about the markets and world events. It is best to have an open discussion with family members and investment professionals when forming a portfolio.

FINANCIAL MISTAKES THE ELDERLY COMMONLY MAKE

1. Cashing out investments in declining markets. People may want a sense of security from knowing their cash is readily available, even at the cost of taking losses or earning very little from certificates of deposit (CDs) or money market accounts.

2. Investing too conservatively. Some people have heard that as they age their appetite for risk should drop. But few people really want their money to be gone at their deaths. They would prefer to pass their assets on to younger generations.

3. Subtracting their age from 100 to find a comfortable asset allocation (stock-to-bond ratio). Because many people today live longer than when that "formula" was popularized, it's likely they would have to raise the 100 by 10–25%, or discard this old saw and invest in a way suitable for their goals.

4. Living beyond their means. This is the hardest behavior to modify. Some seniors do not want to leave the family home they raised their children in, or stop entertaining and buying expensive cars and clothes. People tend to believe that what happened before can happen again, so if they were able to support a lavish lifestyle in the past, they may assume there's no reason to change it now.

5. Forgetting where assets are, how they are titled, or even whether they still own an asset. The ability to understand and make clear decisions is key to arriving at good financial choices. If this ability is no longer present, an appropriate person—often an adult child—should assume financial responsibility for the elderly person.

STEPS FOR SENIORS OR THEIR CAREGIVERS TO TAKE

To have a successful and comfortable retirement period, it is worthwhile for people to:

1. Decide how much money they will need to support that lifestyle, and work toward it.
2. Account for all income and expenses now and in the future.
3. Make a plan for when to sell a business, home, or other major assets.
4. Use realistic aging tables.
5. Use probability (known as Monte Carlo) analysis.
6. Determine when extra help is indicated.
7. Decide where to keep the assets, and let loved ones know how to gain access to them when needed.
8. Make sure one's will is up to date; the family and the senior should not do this alone, but with an estate attorney.
9. Name beneficiaries for retirement accounts. Be aware of what passes through a will or trust, and what passes outside the will. (In the United States, all retirement accounts should have named beneficiaries—these will transfer outside whatever is stated in a will.)

10. Give a trusted relative or friend power of attorney so that designate can make personal and financial decisions on behalf of the senior when necessary while they're still living.
11. Leave room for growth in investment portfolios; few people want the assets to "die" when they do, as most people prefer to leave them to the family members. Investor age is a factor but it is not the sole factor in determining asset allocation.
12. Identify the best retirement plans for each situation—if you are a small-business owner, this is particularly important.

HOW BEST CAN I LEAVE MY ASSETS TO MY FAMILY, FRIENDS AND CAUSES I BELIEVE IN?

Many people are reluctant to address their own mortality. But several steps taken now can ease matters at time of death.

It is important for seniors to have an up-to-date will, signed power-of-attorney authorization, a person with healthcare proxy, beneficiaries for retirement accounts, and trusts, if needed.

Meeting with an estate attorney is the best way to accomplish all this preparation. Generally, if a will has gone unchanged for a long period of time, it warrants a fresh look.

Dying intestate (without a will) leaves too much up to others deciding about a person's final wishes.

It helps to have a letter of intent to leave heirs with guidelines for investing or distributing assets after someone is gone.

CONCLUSION

If physicians and caregivers can help older persons address and seek help with their greatest fears about money (Will I have enough? How can I pay for potentially costly healthcare? How can I best leave my assets when I'm gone?), life in the later years can be much more productive and pleasant. A fee-only financial advisor can offer objective help with these problems. As this chapter has outlined, there are many ways to tackle complex money issues faced by seniors, but often, noticing warning signs, speaking frankly about goals with family, and preparing for decline and mortality can be the best prescription for older patients and their finances.

REFERENCES

CFP Board. Morning Consult Survey Retirement Presentation, Apr. 15, 2019. https://www.cfp.net/docs/default-source/news-events—-research-facts-figures/cfp-board-morning-consult-survey-2019.pdf

Pascarella, Dani. "4 Stats That Reveal How Badly America Is Failing at Financial Literacy," Forbes. Apr. 3, 2018. https://www.forbes.com/sites/danipascarella/2018/04/03/4-stats-that-reveal-how-badly-america-is-failing-at-financial-literacy/#54ce96a62bb7

Leatherby, Lauren. "Medical spending among the U.S. elderly," Journalist's Resource, Shorenstein Center on Media, Politics and Public Policy, Harvard Kennedy School. Feb. 22, 2016. https://journalistsresource.org/studies/government/health-care/elderly-medical-spending-medicare/

Bergman, Adam. "Social Security Feels Pinch as Baby Boomers Clock Out for Good," Forbes. June 21, 2018. https://www.forbes.com/sites/greatspeculations/2018/06/21/social-security-feels-pinch-as-baby-boomers-clock-out-for-good/

Kincaid, Ellie. "The Amount Americans Spend On Healthcare Is Still Growing, But More And More Slowly," Forbes. Dec. 6, 2018. https://www.forbes.com/sites/elliekincaid/2018/12/06/the-amount-americans-spend-on-healthcare-is-still-growing-but-more-and-more-slowly/

National Bureau of Economic Research. "Medical Spending of the Elderly" Report Summary, NBER Bulletin on Aging and Health, 2015, No. 2. https://www.nber.org/aginghealth/2015no2/w21270.html

Garland, Susan B. "At 75, Taking Care of Mom, 99: 'We Did Not Think She Would Live This Long'," *The New York Times*, June 27, 2019. https://www.nytimes.com/2019/06/27/business/retirement-parents-aging-living-to-100.html

AARP Public Policy Institute and National Alliance for Caregiving. "Caregiving in the U.S. 2015—Executive Summary, June 2015. https://www.caregiving.org/wp-content/uploads/2015/05/2015_CaregivingintheUS_Executive-Summary-June-4_WEB.pdf

FURTHER READING

1. Altfest, Lewis, *Personal Financial Planning* 2nd edition (McGraw-Hill) July 2007. A comprehensive book on financial planning and investing with case studies.
2. Altfest, Karen C., "Personal Finance: Planning Your Future. How to Save, Invest, and Grow Your Assets," *Medscape* April 25, 2018. An online course for young physicians on all the parts of their financial lives.
3. Altfest, Karen C., "Life After a Loss: 6 Smart Steps for Coping With Widowhood," *AAII Journal*, July 2016. What to do and not to do for widows.
4. Kahneman, Daniel, *Thinking Fast and Slow*, 1st edition (Farrar, Straus and Giroux) April 2013. An introduction to behavioral finance.

RESOURCE ORGANIZATIONS

AAII (American Association of Independent Investors) provides lectures on investment topics, a journal and speakers in many cities. AAII.com.

The Certified Financial Planner™ (CFP®) Board will help you find a financial advisor in many geographic areas.

Letsmakeaplan.org.

NAPFA (the National Association of Personal Financial Advisors) will help you locate a fee-only advisor who works without commissions, on a fee-for-service or investments-under-management basis. Napfa.org/find-an-advisor.

GLOSSARY

Asset

A resource with economic value that an individual, corporation, or country owns or controls with the expectation that it will provide future benefit. For personal finances, it's the amount of goods of value, such as your house, and money you've accumulated.

Beneficiary

In the financial world, a beneficiary typically refers to someone who is eligible to receive distributions (payouts) from a trust, will, life insurance policy or a retirement account. Beneficiaries are either named specifically in these documents or have met the stipulations that make them eligible for whatever distribution is specified.

Capital

Capital is a term for financial assets, such as funds held in deposit accounts, as well as for the physical factors of production; that is, manufacturing equipment. Additionally, capital includes facilities, including buildings used to produce and store manufactured goods. Materials used and consumed as part of the manufacturing process do not qualify as capital.

Defined Benefit Plan

A defined benefit plan, or traditional pension, is an employer-sponsored retirement plan in which employee benefits are computed using a formula that considers several factors, such as length of employment and salary history. The company administers portfolio management and investment risk for the plan. There are also restrictions on when and by what method an employee can withdraw funds without penalties. Benefits paid are typically guaranteed for life and rise slightly to account for increased cost of living.

Diversified Portfolio

Diversified portfolios include investments spread across different asset categories, such as fixed-income, often bonds and cash, equities, commodities, and sometimes derivatives. Further diversification is possible within each asset category, such as growth and value stocks within equities or domestic and international bonds within fixed income. The asset mix of a portfolio depends on an investor's risk tolerance and financial objectives.

Emergency Fund

An emergency fund is an account for funds set aside in case of the event of a personal financial dilemma, such as the loss of a job, a debilitating illness or a major repair to your home. The purpose of the fund is to improve financial security by creating a safety net of funds that can be available to meet emergency expenses.

Financial Literacy

Financial literacy is the education on and understanding of various financial areas including topics related to managing personal finance, money, and investing. This topic focuses on the ability to manage personal finance matters efficiently, and it includes the knowledge of making appropriate decisions about personal finance such as investing, insurance, real estate, paying for college, budgeting, retirement, estate and tax planning.

Inflation

Inflation is a quantitative measure of the rate at which the average price level of a basket of selected goods and services in an economy increases over a period of time. It is the constant rise in the general level of prices that causes a unit of currency to buy less than it did in prior periods. Often expressed as a percentage, inflation indicates a decrease in the purchasing power of a nation's currency.

IRA

A traditional individual retirement account (IRA) allows individuals to direct pretax income toward investments that can grow tax deferred; no capital gains or dividend income is taxed until it is withdrawn. Contributions to a traditional IRA may be tax-deductible, depending on the taxpayer's income, tax-filing status, and other factors.

Qualified Retirement Plans

A qualified retirement plan meets the requirements of Internal Revenue Code Section 401(a) of the Internal Revenue Service (IRS) and is therefore eligible to receive certain tax benefits. Such a retirement plan is established by an employer for the benefit of the company's employees. Qualified retirement plans give employers a tax break for the contributions they make for their employees. Qualified plans that allow employees to defer a portion of their salaries into the plan can also reduce employees' present income-tax liability by reducing taxable income.

Real Estate

Property comprising land and the buildings on it, as well as the natural resources of the land. It can be grouped into three broad categories based on its use: residential, commercial, and industrial.

Roth 401(k)

A Roth 401(k) is an employer-sponsored investment savings account funded with after-tax dollars up to the plan's contribution limit. This type of investment account is well-suited to people who think they will be in a higher tax bracket in retirement than they are in their working years. In contrast, the traditional 401(k) plan is funded with pretax money, which results in a tax on future withdrawals.

Roth IRA

A Roth IRA is a type of qualified individual retirement account (IRA) that accrues gains tax-exempt but uses after-tax money to fund it. This can be contrasted with a traditional IRA, which uses pretax funds and then defers that income tax until the time of withdrawal.

Social Security

Social Security is the term used for the Old-Age, Survivors and Disability Insurance (OASDI) program in the United States, run by the federal Social Security Administration (SSA). While best known for retirement benefits, it can also provide disability income and survivor benefits.

Titling of Assets

In estate planning, the way one titles his or her property determines which method of distribution is used when the estate is settled upon death. There are several asset-titling options that can help ensure heirs receive the assets according to the owner's wishes. An estate attorney can help with decisions in this area.

46 The Role of Religious Belief in the End-of-Life Care of Older Persons

A. Mark Clarfield, MD, FRCPC

CONTENTS

CLINICAL VIGNETTE

An 88-year-old moderately demented woman with coronary artery disease and atrial fibrillation presents with a massive stroke. For several months, she remains unconscious with complete hemiplegia and difficulty swallowing. Her prognosis is bleak and she has no Advance Directive. The patient's family has strong Jewish religious convictions and requests a permanent feeding tube. While this discussion occurs, she becomes febrile and is diagnosed with pneumonia.

Furthermore, the patient's three children insist that the doctor must under no circumstances tell the patient's elderly husband their mother's bleak prognosis, because "the news will surely kill him". For his part, the husband is cognitively intact and keeps asking about his wife's condition.

QUESTIONS

1. Is it appropriate to insert or refuse to insert a feeding tube in this patient?

2. Should her pneumonia be treated?

3. How should one respond to the husband's queries?

INTRODUCTION

Words have meaning. For example, "feeding", "food", "nutrition", "hydration", "hunger", "thirst", "starvation" and "truth" are all terms fraught with meaning, the problem being that they may mean different things to different people, and at different times. Misunderstandings can thus occur. This is especially the case with various ethnic/religious groups, especially when they come into conflict with the majority culture which in Canada and most developed countries today is largely, or at least avowedly, secular. And it behooves us to keep in mind that this has only been the case for a few short decades.

Before we continue, it must be clear that not everyone who is brought up in a particular religious group will necessarily strictly follow their respective credos and rules. For example, while it is clear that for the Jewish (and Muslim) religions, although some people brought up in these traditions will partake, eating pork is clearly forbidden. As well, in these two religions, some forms of birth control (even abortion) will be allowed under somewhat restricted conditions. Yet, according to Catholicism, most forms of birth control and certainly abortion are strictly forbidden, although there are Catholics who do undergo the procedure. That being said, even avowedly secular people are often influenced, consciously or not, by the belief systems in which they have been raised. As such, certain things may appear more or less acceptable (or not) to them by dint of these early and perhaps ongoing influences.

In this chapter, we examine the previous scenario and explore the Jewish approach, with some brief comparisons to Islamic and Catholic belief systems. I choose to discuss Judaism because I am a member of this faith group and as such am more familiar with its credos and rules than those of other faiths. That being said, Judaism is used simply as an example. While exact belief systems may

DOI: 10.1201/9781003344476-52

differ, in this chapter I will try to bring out the principles of how religious belief can influence end-of-life care, especially for older persons. As well, I offer some general guidelines as to how the members of the treating team might best react, especially if there is a conflict between what the formal caregivers think is in the patient's best interests and the beliefs/wishes of the patient or her family.

Whether religious or not, it behooves doctors to have at least some awareness of how patients' and families' belief systems might affect decisions—for themselves and/or for their loved ones. This is especially the case when a conflict in management arises. The more the doctor can understand where the patient is "coming from" religiously, the more empathy expressed (but without need of formal agreement or approval), the easier it will be to manage many ethical conflicts. The doctor need not be a religious expert but should be ready to query the patient/family whether there might be any religious concerns behind a conflicted issue. At times the physician may ask for clarification or even consult with the relevant pastoral authority.

FEEDING TUBE INSERTION

With respect to the first question relating to the clinical scenario, for the Jewish religion (and Islam too) "feeding" (food and water) can never, as may be held by the believing Catholic, be considered "extraordinary". In such a Christian consideration, logic suggests that we thus need not apply "extraordinary" measures in every case. However, according to Jewish law, given that feeding is considered an "ordinary" measure, it can almost never be denied the patient, at least in some form. The analogy of access to air is sometimes used.

That being said, according to Jewish law there is no injunction as to how nor how much feeding is to be given, with the understanding that invasive percutaneous endoscopic gastrectomy (PEG) and forced nasal gastric (NG) feeding need not always be utilized, especially if such use causes disproportionate pain and suffering. Spoon feeding (however expensive and time-consuming) would be allowed as long as the patient did not show any signs of distress from aspiration or from hunger and/or thirst and was not associated with other harms such as recurrent aspiration.

However, many elderly Jewish patients (and their children) will frequently have a long historical memory of outrages such as the Holocaust—during which millions of Jews were worked, gassed and often just starved to death. These fraught memories can make the use of feeding (or its withholding) a charged issue. While one need not be an expert on religious Jewish law nor in the dolorous history of the 20th century, a sensitivity as to where the patient and especially family may be coming from will help in the management of such fraught cases. While Muslim patients will not have the same historical pressures, they will however usually insist in the same way on feeding and hydrating an end-stage patient for similar religious reasons. Furthermore, the general practice in countries from which most Muslim immigrants to Canada come will usually push the family in the same direction as their Jewish counterparts.

USE OF ANTIBIOTICS

With respect to the use of antibiotics when faced with suspected infection in a dying patient, again since both Jewish and Islamic law follow a "Choose Life" approach, the usual religious practice would be to agree to (even to insist upon) the use of antibiotics. This would be the case, even if antibiotic use is judged as medically "futile" by the treating team. However, that being said, in both this scenario and that relating to feeding tubes, Jewish religious law will also recognize that if the intervention causes undue suffering with little clinical benefit, it may be scaled back or even forgone.

Although it may seem illogical and perhaps even hypocritical to the treating team, many families will be satisfied by even a partial approach—for example giving antibiotics orally rather than by IV to cut down on the use of invasive procedures, especially if venous access is difficult to initiate and/or maintain. When distributive justice is invoked as trumping beneficence (for example, "Using an antibiotic in your mother is not only futile but is likely to cause an increase in antibiotic resistance for others"), this claim will hold less water. Jewish law will tend to put more emphasis on the patient in front of the clinician than on a theoretical population.

SHOULD THE SPOUSE BE TOLD THE TRUTH?

In this vignette, the children demand that their elderly father be shielded from the stress of learning the truth about his wife's dire prognosis. In most cases, however odd this might seem, the family's concern is real and the doctor should treat it as such. According to Jewish law (as is the case with both Islam and Catholicism too), truth telling is always the preferred option in most of life's situations. However, Jewish law does allow for "bending" of the rules but *only* in the case when the doctor in his/her professional opinion (not the family) is actually convinced that this is indeed the case.

Of interest is the fact that apart from religious law as a specific rationale, there are many cultures around the world which believe that older persons (in an analogy to children) sometimes need to be protected, usually by the family, from hearing the truth. Practice in Japan is a good example. Again, it is important for members of the treating team to see where the patient and their family are coming from—that is, usually from a sincere desire to protect their loved ones from avoidable travail.

It may be easy for many clinicians nowadays to look down on these requests as "primitive" or "illiberal". However, a little cultural humility and some historical perspective are in order. This author easily recalls that during his own training in Toronto just a few decades back, senior physicians would routinely withhold the truth from patients; again, in an attempt to protect them from bad news. Our clinical frankness is a much more recent development.

HOW TO APPROACH THIS CASE

Simply recognizing that religious law (or the patient's interpretation of same—even when "incorrect") might be an issue is a good first step. Again, while the physician need not be an expert in these belief systems, even a little knowledge can be helpful. For example, for many years and even up to the present day, many observant Jews incorrectly thought that organ transplantation was forbidden by religious law. In fact, this is actually *not* the case and being able to explain this theological fact to a patient, or if they are still skeptical, suggesting that they ask for a rabbinical opinion, will usually reconcile any disagreement.

Specifically, with respect to feeding, it is worth recognizing early on that not offering such sustenance is against Jewish law and insisting on allowing the patient to "starve" will hold no influence on the family who is insisting on such feeding. However, since there is no injunction as to how or how much a patient must be fed, one can suggest that the family (or a surrogate) take the time to spoon feed the patient, explaining that "like a baby" most patients will take just as much as they want. When they "refuse" to take any more, it is unlikely that they are suffering from hunger or thirst and the episode can be stopped until the next mealtime.

However, if this does not work, either due to the family's refusal or inability to cooperate, there is usually no choice but to insert a PEG. However if this form of tube feeding causes complications and the patient is obviously exposed to pain and suffering or risk to life and health, the physician may well be able to convince the family that on balance the goal must be to minimize suffering. In this way, with careful mouth hygiene and occasional top-ups with fluids, preferably in this case via hypodermoclysis, the terminal patient can be left to die in a humane manner and one in which the family can accept. Issues such as feeding should not be considered photographs but rather more like a video—that is, they often will gradually evolve. Most families can, with time, patience and empathy, be helped to find the right balance—whatever their practices and religious beliefs.

With respect to antibiotic therapy, again this issue can be dealt with via careful explanation and the family's opinion may change over the course of illness. This might especially be the case if repeated fevers ensue. In this case, use of IV antibiotics for a few days and switching to p.o. as soon as possible is an option. However, after multiple bouts of fever (source found or, as is often the case, not), families can often be convinced that repeated attempts to find intravenous access with the resultant patient suffering would tip the balance towards a more conservative approach. Again, the metaphor of a video rather than a snapshot is helpful to keep in mind.

TO TELL, OR NOT

Requests to withhold the truth can be dealt with by explaining that in *your* clinical experience, telling the truth (even difficult ones) is extremely unlikely to cause harm to those who seek information. In fact, the case can be made that trying to withhold the facts is usually counterproductive. Almost always, the truth does slip out and then the person from whom it was withheld will with justice feel betrayed. Again, this process may not occur in one episode and sometimes it takes people time to be convinced.

It is true and helpful that in many countries, Canada and USA included, the secular law in fact demands that patients and families be responded to honestly when the team is queried. This fact, when explained gently, can help the family cope with any guilty feelings about letting their father know the facts. When the physician explains to those who may object that he/she really has no legal choice, usually the issue is resolved.

That being said, our thoughts on truth telling have evolved over the past few decades. It is now more widely known that facts can, like a medication, be offered in various doses and gradually (i.e., "start low, go slow"). In this way the physician can answer the patient's and/or family's queries but not feel the need to tell the "whole truth", especially if it is not asked for. A graded and nuanced practice is probably the best approach over these fraught questions.

CONCLUSION

Whatever the treating physicians' own specific religious upbringing or level of religiosity, it is useful to recognize that religious faiths may play a large role with our patients and their families, especially around the difficult issues surrounding death and dying. The more we know or discover about how their belief systems may be influencing decisions, the better the physician can effectively handle the case. Many people do not realize that it is only a small minority of humankind that have no religious belief. Most people around the globe have some and this can often affect their lives, especially in moments of illness and in the situation of death and dying. The more we physicians can know of and empathize with our patients' health belief models, especially as they relate to religious and spiritual beliefs, the better we can care for them and theirs in the hour of need.

ACKNOWLEDGMENTS

I would like to thank Dr. Shimon Glick and Dr. Shabbir Alibhai for their helpful comments on an earlier draft of this manuscript.

REFERENCES

1. Clarfield AM, Gordon M, Markwell H, Alibhai S. Ethical issues in end-of-life geriatric care. The approach of three monotheistic religions: Judaism, Catholicism and Islam. J Amer Geriatr Soc; 2003; 51:1149–1154.
2. Clarfield AM, Monette J, Bergman H, Monette M, Ben-Israel Y, Caine Y, Charles J, Gordon M, Gore B. Enteral feeding in end-stage dementia: a comparison of religious, ethnic and national differences in Canada and Israel. J Gerontol: Med Sci. 2006; 61A(6):621–627.
3. Jotkowitz AB, Clarfield AM, Glick S. The care of patients with dementia: a modern Jewish ethical perspective. J Amer Geriatr Soc 2005; 53:881–884.
4. Marcus EL, Clarfield AM, Moses AE. Ethical issues relating to the use of antimicrobial therapy in older adults. Clin Infect Dis 2001; 33(15 Nov):697–1705.
5. Goldsand G et al. Jewish medical ethics. CMAJ 2001; 164:219–222.
6. Markwell H et al. Catholic medical ethics. CMAJ 2001; 165:189–192.
7. Daar AS et al. Islamic medical ethics. CMAJ 2001; 164:60–63.
8. Horton R. Offline: Medicine and the holocaust—it's time to teach. The Lancet 2019; 394 (10193):105.
9. Baycrest Hospital. Caring for Holocaust Survivors (see http://holocaustsurvivors.baycrest.org/).

PART VII
MEDICAL TERMS

Medical Terms and Their Meaning: Glossary

Ronald M. Caplan, MD, CM, FACS, FACOG, FRCSC

abscopal effect: Radiation given to a targeted tumor causes untreated tumors elsewhere in the body to shrink. https://www.ncbi.nlm.nih.gov/pmc/articles/PMC6775241/

accountable care organization (ACO): Medical provider organization that incentivizes cost and quality control, for example by reducing inpatient utilization and specialist referrals. Includes Medicare Shared Savings Program (MSSP), which sets a target cost of care for patients.

ACE inhibitor: Drug that inhibits the angiotensin-converting enzyme, stopping the formation of angiotensin II which constricts blood vessels. Blood pressure is lowered, because blood vessels are opened up, and blood can flow more freely. http://www.medicinenet.com/ace_inhibitors/article.htm https://www.webmd.com/heart-disease/guide/medicine-ace-inhibitors#1 https://www.bmj.com/content/363/bmj.k4209

acetylcholine: A neurotransmitter. http://www.ncbi.nlm.nih.gov/books/NBK11143/

acne: Chronic skin condition characterized by seborrhea (oily secretion) and blocked follicles (comedomes) including blackheads and whiteheads that may become infected. https://online.epocrates.com/diseases/10111/Acne-vulgaris/Key-Highlights

acrylamide: Chemical that can form during high heat food preparation of high starch foods from the amino acid asparagine in combination with some sugars. Possible carcinogen in high doses. https://www.cancer.gov/about-cancer/causes-prevention/risk/diet/acrylamide-fact-sheet

activities of daily living (ADLs): Include feeding, dressing, bathing, walking. **IALDs:** Instrumental activities of daily living that allow an individual to live independently in the community. https://www.ncbi.nlm.nih.gov/books/NBK470404/ https://www.ncbi.nlm.nih.gov/books/NBK553126/

acute flaccid myelitis: Post-viral neurologic syndrome sometimes seen following COVID-19 infection in young children, largely in the 3- to 6-year-old range https://www.mdlinx.com/news/physicians-issue-warning-about-rare-neurological-condition-expected-to-appear-this-fall/41HVQbOXEV8SDxaEXYnegB?ipost_environment=m3usainc&iqs=9z2z6d5v1f2le52i8k9pvb8c2ksg7hbdc6ovbphnb90&utm_medium=email&utm_campaign=All%

addiction: Physiologic compulsive need for a substance, use of that substance, inability to abstain, development of tolerance to it, and distinctive withdrawal symptoms and signs. See "Opioid". https://www.cdc.gov/drugoverdose/index.html

adhesion: Abnormal union of surfaces, or fibrous tissue bands between structures. https://www.ncbi.nlm.nih.gov/pmc/articles/PMC5295619/

adoptive cell transfer (ACT): Use of **tumor-infiltrating lymphocytes (TILs)** to overcome immunosuppressive signals and eradicate cancer cells. https://www.cancer.gov/about-cancer/treatment/types/immunotherapy

advance directive: Legal document that ensures one's wishes are followed in the event a person cannot make their own decisions. See Chapter 44, "How Can Older People Be Protected?" by Randy S. Perskin. www.careoftheolderperson.com https://ag.ny.gov/sites/default/files/advancedirectives.pdf

aging: Gradual loss of physiological functions accompanied by increasing risk of mortality and decreasing fertility. The Rate of Aging is the ratio between damage accumulation and compensatory mechanisms. Aspects of aging at the cellular level—cellular senescence—include mitochondrial dysfunction, telomere attrition and genomic instability. See Chapter 1, "Introduction" by Jose Morais. www.careoftheolderperson.com http://journal.frontiersin.org/article/10.3389/fgene.2016.00119/full https://www.nature.com/articles/s41551-017-0093?WT.mc_id=EMI_NBME_1707_JULYISSUE_PORTFOLIO&spMailingID=54556746&spUserID=MTc3MDI4ODk5NQS2&spJobID=1203835636&spReportId=MTIwMzgzNTYzNgS2 https://jamanetwork.com/journals/jama/article-abstract/2703112?utm_source=silverchair&utm_medium=email&utm_campaign=article_alert-jama&utm_content=olf&utm_term=091718 https://www.frontiersin.org/

articles/10.3389/fimmu.2019.01614/full?utm_source=F-AAE&utm_medium=EMLF&utm_campaign=MRK_1046250_35_Immuno_20190718_arts_A https://www.ncbi.nlm.nih.gov/pmc/articles/PMC4678010/

agonist: Exogenous substance that goes to a cell receptor and produces a response. https://en.wikipedia.org/wiki/Agonist

AIDS: autoimmune deficiency syndrome: Sexually transmitted infection caused by human immunodeficiency viruses HIV-1 and HIV-2 which compromise the immune system. https://www.aids.gov/ http://www.thelancet.com/journals/lancet/article/PIIS0140-6736(14)60164-1/fulltext https://jamanetwork.com/journals/jama/article-abstract/2703112?utm_source=silverchair&utm_medium=email&utm_campaign=article_alert-jama&utm_content=olf&utm_term=091718 https://jamanetwork.com/journals/jama/article-abstract/2678246?utmsource=silverchair&utmmedium=email&utmcampaign=articlealert-jama&utmcontent=

akathisia: A movement disorder with restlessness that may be a drug side effect. See Chapter 31, "Psycho-Oncology: Living with the Fear of Death" by Norman Straker. https://www.ncbi.nlm.nih.gov/pmc/articles/PMC1123446/

albumin: Water soluble single chain protein synthesized in liver. Present in egg white and blood serum. http://albumin.org/properties-of-human-serum-albumin-and-albumin-atomic-coordinates/

aldosterone: Mineralocorticoid hormone from adrenal cortex. Increases blood pressure. Implication in alopecia. https://en.wikipedia.org/wiki/Aldosterone

algorithm: Set of instructions to perform a specific task. **data-driven algorithm: machine learning** utilized to design algorithm, with data to learn from, and ongoing data collection. https://www.techopedia.com/definition/3739/algorithm https://ieeexplore.ieee.org/stamp/stamp.jsp?arnumber=8290925

alkaline phosphatase: Immune protein enzymes that catalyze the hydrolysis of phosphate groups, freeing inorganic phosphate. http://journal.frontiersin.org/article/10.3389/fimmu.2017.00897/full?utm_source=F-AAE&utm_medium=EMLF&utm_campaign=MRK_352999_35_Immuno_20170808_arts_A

allele: One of the two forms of a gene, derived from either the mother or the father. Genes are carried on chromosomes. Chromosomes are paired, with one chromosome in each pair coming from the father, and one coming from the mother. http://mcat-review.org/genetics.php

allograft: Transplant from human donor to genetically nonidentical human recipient. http://ndt.oxfordjournals.org/content/early/2013/04/25/ndt.gft087.full.pdf

alopecia: Baldness. https://www.ncbi.nlm.nih.gov/pmc/articles/PMC3149477/

Alzheimer's disease (AD): Common form of dementia. One characteristic is amyloid plaque deposition in the brain. See Chapter 6, "Update on Alzheimer's Disease Diagnosis and Management" by Serge Gauthier; Chapter 5, "Doctor, My Spouse Is Getting Forgetful" by Serge Gauthier; Chapter 9, "Why Does My Patient Have Gait And Balance Disorders?" by Olivier Beauchet; Chapter 32, "Incontinence in Older Adults" by Samer Shamout, Lysanne Campeau. www.careoftheolderperson.com http://www.thelancet.com/journals/laneur/article/PIIS1474-4422(16)00062-4/abstract http://www.ncbi.nlm.nih.gov/pubmed/24028956 http://www.nature.com/nature/journal/v537/n7618/full/537036a.html?WT.feed_name=subjects_neuroscience http://www.jwatch.org/na42506/2016/10/06/new-biologic-treatment-dramatically-shrinks-plaques https://www.ncbi.nlm.nih.gov/pubmed/27025652 http://www.nature.com/neuro/multimedia/alzheimers/index.html?WT.mc_id=BAN_NN_1612_Alzheimers www.nature.com/neuro/multimedia/alzheimers/index.html?WT.mc_id=TOC_NN_1216_Alzheimers&spMailingID=540026 25&spUserID=MTc2NTUxNjM5AS2&spJobID=1160 https://pubs.acs.org/doi/10.1021/acschemneuro.8b00160 https://www.nature.com/articles/s41593-018-0101-9?utm_source=Springer_Nature_website&utm_medium=Website_links&utm_content=AngWan-SN-OD-Neuroscience-Global&utm_campaign=SNOR_USG_SFN18 https://www.alzheimersanddementia.com/article/S1552-5260(18)30068-2/fulltext?rss=yes https://www.ncbi.nlm.nih.gov/pmc/articles/PMC6194148/ https://alzres.biomedcentral.com/articles/10.1186/s13195-018-0441-4 https://www.nature.com/articles/s41591-018-0311-4?WT.ec_id=NM-201901&sap-outbound-id=D7CBD8E437538AF66B20183215057C627E43F6DB

https://jamanetwork.com/journals/jamaneurology/fullarticle/2722842?guestAccessKey=
94b79aa8-7c1d-45f8-9e0b-545a2484647a&utm_source=silverchair&utm_campaign=jama_
network&utm_content=weekly_highlights&cmp=1&utm_medium=email https://
www.nature.com/articles/d41586-019-00879-3?WT.ec_id=NATURE-20190321&utm_
source=nature_etoc&utm_medium=email&utm_campaign=20190321&sap-outbound-
id=01A2C014D0D47D9CED5 https://academic.oup.com/brain/advance-article/
doi/10.1093/brain/awz099/5481202 www.nature.com/neuro/multimedia/alzheimers/
index.html?WT.mc_id=TOC_NN_1216_Alzheimers&spMailingID=54002625&spUserID=

amino acids: The building blocks of protein. Some amino acids can be synthesized in the human body. Essential amino acids must be supplied in the diet, as they cannot be synthesized in the human body. http://www.biology.arizona.edu/biochemistry/problem_sets/aa/aa.html

amniotic fluid: The fluid surrounding the developing fetus, contained in the amniotic sac. The thin amniotic membrane is closely applied to the inner walls of the uterus. http://iaimjournal.com/wp-content/uploads/2014/11/9-Amniotic-fluid-derived-stem-cells.pdf

amplified probe technique: Uses PCR (see "polymerase chain reaction") for nucleic acid amplification and high throughput technology (see "Throughput"). Tests for RNA from genes expressed by SARS-CoV-2 virus https://pubmed.ncbi.nlm.nih.gov/8467630/ https://www.uhcprovider.com/content/dam/provider/docs/public/policies/medadv-guidelines/m/molecular-diagnostic-infectious-disease-testing.pdf

amyloid: Beta amyloid. Protein fragments that can clump in amorphous plaques in degenerative disease. https://www.nia.nih.gov/alzheimers/publication/part-2-what-happens-brain-ad/hallmarks-ad http://www.nature.com/nature/journal/v537/n7618/full/nature19323.html

amyotrophic lateral sclerosis: motor neuron disease. Characterized by degeneration of both upper and lower motor neurons leading to muscle weakness and paralysis. https://www.nature.com/articles/550S105a https://www.ncbi.nlm.nih.gov/pubmed/17023659 https://jamanetwork.com/journals/jama/fullarticle/2724169?guestAccessKey=cefb e6c9-c210-49d6-aca6-9ebca2eaaf86&utm_source=silverchair&utm_medium=email&utm_campaign=article_alert-jama&utm

anastomosis: Relinking of a tubular structure so that the lumen is patent. http://plasticsurgery.stanford.edu/education/microsurgery/intraoperative.html

androgen: The "male" sex hormones. Present in women in different amounts than in males. In men, the testicles are the main source of androgens. In women, androgens are mainly derived from the adrenal glands that sit atop the kidneys, and from the ovaries. https://www.britannica.com/science/androgen https://www.frontiersin.org/articles/10.3389/fimmu.2018.00794/full?utmsource=F-AAE&utmmedium=EMLF&utmcampaign=MRK63294735Immuno20180508artsA

androgen receptor antagonists: Drugs that competitively inhibit testosterone from binding to prostate cancer cells. http://www.nejm.org/doi/full/10.1056/NEJMra1701695?query=main_nav_lg http://www.nejm.org/doi/full/10.1056/NEJMoa1715546?query=main_nav_lg

androstenedione: A form of androgen. https://pubchem.ncbi.nlm.nih.gov/compound/androstenedione#section=Top

anemia: Deficiency of red blood cells or hemoglobin. https://www.jwatch.org/na45561/2017/11/29/anemia-elderly-review?query=etoc_jwgenmed&jwd=000012066693&jspc=OBG

aneurysm: Weakening in a blood vessel wall, leading to a bulge. http://stroke.ahajournals.org/content/44/12/3613 https://journals.lww.com/cardiologyinreview/Abstract/2016/03000/Abdominal_Aortic_Aneurysms_and_Risk_Factors_for.5.aspx https://www.jwatch.org/na47426/2018/09/11/natural-history-small-ascending-aortic-aneurysms?query=etoc_jwcard&jwd=000012066693&jspc=OBG

angina (pectoris): Chest pain caused by inadequate oxygenation (ischemia) of, and circulation to heart muscle, secondary to arteriosclerotic disease in the coronary arteries which supply the heart. https://emedicine.medscape.com/article/150215-overview

angiogenesis: New blood vessel formation. http://www.nature.com/nrd/journal/v3/n5/full/nrd1381.html

angiography: Radiologic visualization of blood vessels after injecting them with radiopaque dye. https://emedicine.medscape.com/article/1603072-overview

angioplasty: The opening of a narrowed blood vessel by balloon inflation, along with stent placement to preserve patency. http://www.ncbi.nlm.nih.gov/pubmedhealth/PMH0021296/

angiotensin: A vasoconstricting hormone. Stimulates aldosterone release from the adrenal cortex. http://www.ncbi.nlm.nih.gov/pubmed/8583476

angiotensin receptorblocker (ARB): Drug that blocks the angiotensin receptor. http://www.ncbi.nlm.nih.gov/pmc/artic https://www.bmj.com/content/363/bmj.k4209les/PMC4395832/

anhedonia: Loss of the capacity to experience pleasure. See Chapter 31, "Psycho-Oncology Living with the Fear of Death" by Norman Straker. www.careoftheolderperson.com https://www.medicinenet.com/script/main/art.asp?articlekey=17900

anorexia: Eating disorder with self-starvation and marked weight loss. See Chapter 10, "Could My Patient Be Malnourished?" by Jose Morais. www.careoftheolderperson.com https://jeatdisord.biomedcentral.com/articles/10.1186/s40337-015-0040-8

anosmia: Loss of the sense of smell. Can be a feature of COVID-19. https://www.ncbi.nlm.nih.gov/pmc/articles/PMC7265845/#:~:text=Anosmia%20is%20a%20prominent%20sign,also%20be%20presented%20%5B26%5D.

anthrax: Serious bacterial infection caused by Bacillus Anthracis. Can be acquired cutaneously, and via the respiratory and gastrointestinal tracts. https://www.cdc.gov/anthrax/specificgroups/health-care-providers/index.html

antibiotic: A drug that kills or inactivates bacteria. Often works by binding and disrupting bacterial ribosomes (see "ribosome"). http://www.nature.com/nrmicro/journal/v13/n1/full/nrmicro3380.html http://www.nature.com/ja/journal/v67/n1/full/ja201349a.html https://en.wikipedia.org/wiki/List_of_antibiotics http://mdlinx.pdr.net/pharma-news/news-article.cfm/6885214/antibiotic-resistant-bacteria-star-shaped-peptide

antibody: A substance that reacts with a foreign invader (antigen), inactivating it. https://www.ncbi.nlm.nih.gov/pmc/articles/PMC4284445/ http://www.nature.com/milestones/mileantibodies/timeline/index.html

antibody-drug conjugates: Antibodies linked to a toxic substance, such as radioactive material, bacterial product or chemical. https://www.ncbi.nlm.nih.gov/pubmed/27299281 https://www.ncbi.nlm.nih.gov/pubmed/26589413 https://www.ncbi.nlm.nih.gov/pubmed/24423619

antigen: Foreign invader of the body. http://www.annualreviews.org/doi/abs/10.1146/annurev-immunol-032712-095910

antimetabolite: Substance that interferes with cell metabolism by inhibiting or replacing a normal metabolite. Used as chemotherapeutic agents in cancer. http://www.ncbi.nlm.nih.gov/pubmed/23361267 http://www.slideshare.net/OribaDanLangoya/antimetabolites-in-cancer-chemotherapy-23606975

antimullerian hormone: Produced by ovarian granulosa cells. Prevents the depletion of follicles in the ovary. http://www.ncbi.nlm.nih.gov/pubmed/22646322

antioxidant: Substance that prevents the chemical combination of oxygen with various other substances, such as fats. http://dspace.uni.lodz.pl:8080/xmlui/bitstream/handle/11089/17754/bartosz2.pdf?sequence=1&isAllowed=y

antisense technology: Turning off genes by introducing pieces of the genetic code. http://smart-therapeutics.com/Technology/RNAi-Antisense-Technologyb

anxiety: Feeling of unease that can rise to the level of panic attacks. See Chapter 41, "Late-Life Anxiety" by Jess Friedland, Paulina Bajsarowicz, Philippe Desmarais. www.careoftheolderperson.com http://www.ajgponline.org/article/S1064-7481(16)30147-6/abstract

aorta: The main artery from the heart to other parts of the body. http://teachmeanatomy.info/abdomen/vasculature/arteries/aorta/

apheresis: Removing blood from the body for the purpose of eliminating a specific component, then reintroducing the blood into the body. https://health.ucsd.edu/specialties/apheresis/Documents/2011%20Conventional-apheresis-therapies.pdf

apolipoprotein E: (ApoE). Protein involved in fat metabolism. A variant is a disease risk factor. http://www.ncbi.nlm.nih.gov/pubmed/11882522 http://www.ncbi.nlm.nih.gov/pubmed/16432152

apoptosis: Programmed cell death. http://www.ncbi.nlm.nih.gov/pmc/articles/PMC2117903/ https://www.ncbi.nlm.nih.gov/books/NBK26873/ http://journal.frontiersin.org/article/10.3389/fimmu.2017.00961/full?utm_source=F-AAE&utm_medium=EMLF&utm_campaign=MRK_368025_35_Immuno_20170822_arts_A https://www.frontiersin.org/articles/10.3389/fimmu.2018.00241/full?utm_source=F-AAE&utm_medium=EMLF&utm_campaign=MRK_571163_35_I https://www.frontiersin.org/articles/10.3389/fimmu.2018.02379/full?utm_source=F-AAE&utm_medium=EMLF&utm_campaign=MRK_812127_35_Immuno_20181030_arts_A

appendicitis: Inflammation of the appendix. Can be treated by minimally invasive surgery. Incidence has possibly been lowered with antibiotic use. http://www.bmj.com/content/357/bmj.j1703.full

aptamer: Single-stranded DNA or RNA molecule that can bind to preselected targets. http://www.basepairbio.com/research-and-publications/what-is-an-aptamer-2/

aromatase inhibitors: The enzyme aromatase catalyzes conversion of testosterone to estradiol. Aromatase inhibitors are drugs that prevent this type of estradiol formation. http://www.nature.com/nrc/journal/v15/n5/abs/nrc3920.html http://erc.endocrinology-journals.org/content/20/4/R183.full

arrhythmia: (cardiac) Abnormal beating of the heart. Includes tachycardia (abnormally fast heartbeat), bradycardia (abnormally slow heartbeat) and irregular heartbeats. http://www.clevelandclinicmeded.com/medicalpubs/diseasemanagement/cardiology/cardiac-arrhythmias/

ART: Advanced assisted reproductive technology. Techniques that enhance the ability to conceive children, including ovum and sperm retrieval, and ICSI. http://www.cdc.gov/reproductivehealth/infertility/ http://www.hfea.gov.uk/ICSI.html

arteriosclerosis: Literal meaning is hardening of the arteries. In **atherosclerosis**, a common type, calcified fat deposits build up in the lining of arteries, narrowing and obstructing them. http://www.ncbi.nlm.nih.gov/pubmed/11001066 http://bmcmedicine.biomedcentral.com/articles/10.1186/1741-7015-11-117

artery: A blood vessel that usually carries oxygenated blood from the heart to other areas of the body. Exceptions are the pulmonary artery, which carries blood from the heart to the lungs for oxygenation, and the umbilical arteries in the fetus, which carry blood from the fetus to the placenta for oxygenation. https://training.seer.cancer.gov/anatomy/cardiovascular/blood/classification.html

arthritis: A group of conditions of varying etiology characterized by inflammation in the joints. http://www.rheumatology.org/Practice-Quality/Clinical-Support/Criteria/ACR-Endorsed-Criteria

arthroscopy: Direct visualization into the joints by minimally invasive technique. http://www.arthroscopytechniques.org/ http://www.bmj.com/content/357/bmj.j1982

artificial heart: Mechanical device that replaces the heart. **Mechanical cardiac support** refers to devices that assist the failing heart. https://www.nature.com/articles/d41586-018-07197-0?WT.mc_id=EMX_NJOBS_1103_NATUREJOBSNEWSLETTER_A&WT.ec_id=EXTERNAL&spMailingID=57708268&spUserID=NjYxMzYyNDIyMjIS1&spJobID=1520347411&spReportId=MTUyMDM0NzQxMQS2 http://www.jhltonline.org/article/S1053-2498(14)00976-0/abstract

artificial intelligence: Computer systems able to perform tasks normally attributable to human intelligence. These include visual perception, speech recognition, decision-making and language translation. Ideally, the computer systems would think and act humanly and rationally. Utilizes **machine learning** in which data is fed to a computer and statistical techniques are used to help the computer get better at a task without specifically programming it for that. **Deep learning** is a type of machine learning that runs data inputs through multiple layers of biologically inspired neural network architecture. (See "deep learning", "machine learning".) https://www.lexico.com/definition/artificial_intelligence https://builtin.com/artificial-intelligence **Emotional artificial intelligence (affective computing):** AI subset that measures, understands, simulates and reacts to human emotions. https://mitsloan.mit.edu/ideas-made-to-matter/emotion-ai-explained

asbestos: A mined mineral formerly used for insulation and fireproofing. Fibers can be released into the air which can be responsible for asbestosis, a serious lung disease. http://www.ncbi.nlm.nih.gov/pubmed/25444537

atherosclerosis: See "Arteriosclerosis". http://www.atherosclerosis-journal.com/

ATP: Adenosine triphosphate: A nucleotide involved in intracellular energy transfer. https://pubchem. ncbi.nlm.nih.gov/compound/Adenosine_triphosphate

atrophy: Wasting of body tissue. **Sarcopenia** is the loss of skeletal muscle mass and function. **Cachexia**, which incorporates sarcopenia, is a complex metabolic wasting syndrome associated with underlying disease, characterized by unwanted weight loss, muscle atrophy, fatigue, weakness and loss of appetite. https://www.ncbi.nlm.nih.gov/pubmed/22773188 https://www.ncbi.nlm.nih.gov/pmc/articles/PMC3940510/ https://www.ncbi.nlm. nih.gov/pubmed/20886766 https://www.ncbi.nlm.nih.gov/pmc/articles/PMC4269139/ https://www.ncbi.nlm.nih.gov/pmc/articles/PMC3117995/

aura: A perceptual disturbance. http://www.medicinenet.com/script/main/art.asp?articlekey= 2395

autoantibody: Immune protein (mainly IgM) produced by the immune system that is directed against (targets) an individual's own proteins, tissues or organs. https://www.ncbi. nlm.nih.gov/pmc/articles/PMC2703183/ http://journal.frontiersin.org/article/10.3389/ fimmu.2017.00603/full?utm_source=F-AAE&utm_medium=EMLF&utm_campaign= MRK_294450_35_Immuno_20170608_arts_A

autoimmune diseases: Diseases in which the immune response is inappropriately triggered and attacks the individual's own tissues and organs. Includes systemic lupus erythematosus, rheumatoid arthritis, multiple sclerosis and Sjögren's syndrome. http://www. nature.com/nm/journal/v21/n7/full/nm.3897.html http://journal.frontiersin.org/article/10.3389/fimmu.2016.00587/full?utm_source=newsletter&utm_medium=email&utm_campaign=Immunology-w52-2016 http://www.clevelandclinicmeded.com/medicalpubs/diseasemanagement/rheumatology/laboratory-evaluation-rheumatic-diseases/ https://www.ncbi.nlm.nih.gov/pmc/articles/PMC4122257/

autophagy: Intracellular degradation delivering cytoplasmic constituents to the lysosome. May have implications in anti-aging and starvation adaptation. http://genesdev.cshlp.org/content/21/22/2861.long http://journal.frontiersin.org/article/10.3389/fimmu.2016.00657/full?utm_source=newsletter&utm_medium=email&utm_campaign=Immunology-w1-2017

bacterium: (Plural: bacteria) An old name for a microscopic organism that can be present in, or invade, humans. A pathogenic bacterium or microorganism is one that causes disease. http://www.bode-science-center.com/center/relevant-pathogens-from-a-z.html

bariatric (metabolic) surgery: Weight-loss surgery for selected type 2 diabetics and obese patients. Includes gastric binding, stomach stapling, gastric bypass and stomach shortening sleeve gastrectomy. https://asmbs.org/patients/bariatric-surgery-procedures

basal ganglia: Region at the base of the brain with clusters of neurons including the caudate nucleus, putamen and globus pallidus. http://webspace.ship.edu/cgboer/basalganglia. html https://nba.uth.tmc.edu/neuroscience/m/s3/chapter04.html

base pair: Two (out of four) **nucleic acid bases** on a rung of the spiral ladder of **DNA**. The four nucleic acids involved are adenine (**A**), cytosine (**C**), guanine (**G**) and thymine (**T**). They code the sequences of amino acids that, in turn, make up the proteins. http://www.dictionary.com/browse/base-pair

beta blocker: A drug that lowers blood pressure by taking up the receptor sites that control blood pressure. http://www.medicinenet.com/beta_blockers/article.htm

beta carotene: An antioxidant. Precursor of Vitamin A. http://www.medicalnewstoday.com/articles/252758.php

bile acid sequestrant: Drug that binds bile acids in the intestine, so that they are excreted. http://www.medicinenet.com/bile_acid_sequestrants/article.htm

bioengineering: Rearranging DNA. Manufacturing recombinant DNA. http://www.mdpi.com/journal/bioengineering

biofeedback: Training to acquire voluntary control of a body function, such as heart rate. http://www.ncbi.nlm.nih.gov/pubmedhealth/PMH0070200/

biology: The study of living organisms. Biological Sequence Analysis: Creates probabilistic models of protein and nucleic acid sequences. https://www.well.ox.ac.uk/~wilson/files/

Durbin.pdf Computational Molecular Biology (Bioinformatics): Amalgamates computation, statistics, experimentation and technology to further molecular biology. May utilize **quantum computing**. https://mitpress.mit.edu/books/series/computational-molecular-biology https://www.well.ox.ac.uk/~wilson/files/Durbin.pdfHigh Dimensional Biology: Simultaneous study of DNA variation, transcription (messenger RNA), peptides, proteins and metabolites of a tissue or organ. https://www.ncbi.nlm.nih.gov/pmc/articles/PMC7062297/Molecular Biology: Molecular basis of biologic activity in and between cells. Structure and function of macromolecules (e.g. proteins and nucleic acids). https://plato.stanford.edu/entries/molecular-biology/ Structural Biology: How biological models are built. https://www.nigms.nih.gov/education/fact-sheets/Pages/structural-biology.aspx Synthetic Biology: Giving new abilities to organisms by redesign, engineering. Engineered eRNAi (interference). https://www.genome.gov/about-genomics/policy-issues/Synthetic-Biology https://www.nature.com/articles/d41586-020-00272-5

biorhythm: Cyclic pattern of activity; recurring biologic process. See "circadian rhythm".

biosimilar: Product that is highly similar to an approved biologic product. http://www.fda.gov/Drugs/DevelopmentApprovalProcess/HowDrugsareDevelopedandApproved/ApprovalApplications/TherapeuticBiologicApplications/Biosimilars/default.htm http://jamanetwork.com/journals/jama/fullarticle/2590051 http://jamanetwork.com/journals/jama/article-abstract/2590049

bisphosphonates: Class of drugs that prevent loss of bone mass by inhibiting bone resorption by blocking osteoclasts. http://www.bmj.com/content/351/bmj.h3783

blepharoplasty: Cosmetic eyelid surgery. https://www.ncbi.nlm.nih.gov/pmc/articles/PMC2840922/

blockchain technology in healthcare: Interoperable platform that memorializes every event or step ("block") in a data stream, or chain. Implications in personalized medicine, research and appropriate healthcare data sharing with enhanced security. http://bulletin.facs.org/2017/12/blockchain-technology-in-health-care-a-primer-for-surgeons/#.WIezLK6nHX4

body mass index (BMI): A calculation of body fat. Weight (kilograms) divided by height (meters squared). See Chapter 10, "Could My Patient Be Malnourished?" by Jose Morais. www.careoftheolderperson.com

bone density: Measurement of calcium and other minerals in bone. http://www.ncbi.nlm.nih.gov/pmc/articles/PMC2685234/

bone density scan: Low exposure Xray to measure bone density. https://www.bones.nih.gov/health-info/bone/bone-health/bone-mass-measurement-what-numbers-mean

bone scan (nuclear): Imaging bone after radiotracer uptake to identify tumors, usually metastatic. https://www.ncbi.nlm.nih.gov/pmc/articles/PMC4553252/

Botox: Botulinum toxin type A. Inhibits acetylcholine release. http://www.ncbi.nlm.nih.gov/pmc/articles/PMC2856357/

brain-computer interface (neural control interface): Computer system acquires, analyses brain signals; translates signals into commands; relayed to output devices that carry out actions. https://www.ncbi.nlm.nih.gov/pmc/articles/PMC3497935/

BRCA genes: Breast Cancer Genes 1 and 2. Inherited mutations that predispose to breast and ovarian cancer. BRCA1 may increase risk of endometrial cancer as well. http://oncology.jamanetwork.com/article.aspx?articleid=2531470 https://www.sgo.org/wp-content/uploads/2016/10/2016-SGO-Genetics-Toolkit3.pdf https://jamanetwork.com/journals/jama/fullarticle/2748515?guestAccessKey=99eb27c0-0cd5-45e6-870f-b8251b23d4be&utm_source=silverchair&utm_medium=email&utm_campaign=article_alert&utm_content=etoc&utm_term=082019

breast cancer: Malignant tumor in breast tissue. http://www.jwatch.org/na44519/2017/07/06/asco-2017-report-breast-cancer?query=topic_breastcan&jwd=000012066693&jspc=OBG https://www.acog.org/-/media/Practice-Bulletins/Committee-on-Practice-Bulletins——Gynecology/Public/pb179.pdf?dmc=1&ts=20170710T0228314803 https://tools.bcsc-scc.org/BC5yearRisk/intro.htm https://insights.ovid.com/crossref?an=00006250-201709000-00035 https://www.partnershipagainstcancer.ca/wp-content/uploads/2019/05/

Breast-Cancer-Surgery-Standards-EN-April-2019.pdf http://hormonebalance.org/images/documents/Shyamala%2099%20Progesterone%20differentiation%20Mammary%20gland%20JMGB&N_1311167749.pdf

bronchitis: Inflammation of the bronchial passages. https://www.ncbi.nlm.nih.gov/pubmed/23204254

bulimia: Eating disorder. Food consumption followed by self-induced vomiting. https://www.ncbi.nlm.nih.gov/pmc/articles/PMC2927890/

bundle branch block: Delay in the pathway of electrical impulses to the left or right ventricle of the heart, resulting in a delay of contraction of that ventricle. http://www.acc.org/latest-in-cardiology/journal-scans/2016/08/05/11/45/effect-of-the-antihypertensive-and-lipid-lowering-treatment?w_nav=LC

cancer: Malignant tumor (growth). The hallmark of cancer is its ability to invade normal tissue. Cancer can often metastasize, spreading to distant areas in the body. It is likely to recur even though it has been removed or destroyed at its initial (primary) site. See Chapter 27, "Cancer in Older Adults" by Doreen Wan-Chow-Wah; Chapter 28, "Cancer Screening in the Older Adult" by Catalina Hernandez Torres, Tina Hsu. www.careoftheolderperson.com http://www.cell.com/cell/fulltext/S0092-8674(18)3032-7 http://www.cell.com/pb-assets/consortium/pancanceratlas/pancan/index.html https://www.cancer.gov/about-cancer/treatment/types/targeted-therapies/targeted-therapies-factsheet https://cancerstaging.org/About/news/Pages/-Cancer-Staging-Manual,-Eighth-Edition,-Just-Released-by-American-Joint-Committee-on-Cancer-(AJCC).aspx http://www.jcso-ejournal.com/jcso/november_2016?pg=34#pg34 http://journal.frontiersin.org/article/10.3389/fimmu.2017.00374/full?utm_source=F-AAE&utm_medium=EMLF&utm_campaign=MRK_243180_20170411_arts https://www.nature.com/articles/s41551-017-0067?WT.mc_id=EMI_NBME_1704_APRILISSUE_PORTFOLIO&spMailingID=53957850&spUserID=MTc3MDI4ODk5NQ http://stm.sciencemag.org/content/9/400/eaan2966 http://science.sciencemag.org/content/early/2018/01/17/science.aar3247 https://www.empr.com/home/news/fda-approves-tumor-agnostic-oral-cancer-therapy-vitrakvi/ https://www.nature.com/articles/d41586-018-07602-8?utm_source=briefing-dy&utm_medium=email&utm_campaign=briefing&utm_content=20181206dy&utm_medium=email&utm_campaign=briefing&utm_content=20181206 https://www.frontiersin.org/articles/10.3389/fimmu.2019.00467/full?utm_source=F-AAE&utm_medium=EMLF&utm_campaign=MRK_943967_35_Immuno_20190326_arts_A https://www.frontiersin.org/articles/10.3389/fimmu.2019.00467/full?utm_source=F-AAE&utm_medium=EMLF&utm_campaign=MRK_943967_35_Immuno_20190326_arts_A

cancer marker: Substances produced by tumor cells or by other cells in response to a tumor. See "Tumor Specific Antigen (TSA)". https://www.nature.com/articles/s41551-017-0065?WT.mc_id=EMI_NBME_1704_APRILISSUE_PORTFOLIO&spMailingID=53957850&spUserID=MTc3MDI4ODk5NQS

cannabis: Plant from which cannabinoids are obtained. Tetrahydrocannabinol (THC) is the principal psychoactive compound. https://medicalmarijuana.procon.org/view.resource.php?resourceID=000141 https://www.ncbi.nlm.nih.gov/pubmed/16463612 https://www.frontiersin.org/articles/10.3389/fimmu.2018.02009/full?utm_source=F-AAE&utm_medium=EMLF&utm_campaign=MRK_779779_35_Immuno_20180927_arts_A https://www.empr.com/drugs-in-the-pipeline/cannabidiol-cbd-ischemia-reperfusion-injury-organ-transplantation-revive-therapeutics-orphan-drug/article/813111/?utm_source=newsletter&utm_medium=email&utm_campaign=mpr-dailydose-cp-20181109&cpn=obg https://pubchem.ncbi.nlm.nih.gov/compound/cannabidiol#section=Substances-by-Category https://jamanetwork.com/journals/jamanetworkopen/fullarticle/2716990?utm_source=silverchair&utm_medium=email&utm_campaign=article_alert-jamanetworkopen&utm_content=olf&utm_term=113018 https://www.empr.com/features/medical-marijuana-clinical-practice-geriatric-pain-insomnia-elderly/article/815102/?utm_source=newsletter&utm_medium=email&utm_campaign=mpr-dailydose-cp-201812

cannabis withdrawal syndrome: Can include irritability, hostility, nervousness, anxiety, sleeplessness, restlessness, appetite loss, depression, shakiness, tremors, sweating, fever, headaches. https://www.mailman.columbia.edu/public-health-now/news/more-one-ten-heavy-cannabis-users-experience-withdrawal-after-quitting-cannabis

carbohydrate: Simple and complex sugars that are the energy source for the body. Excess carbohydrate can be converted to fat for storage. http://www.fao.org/docrep/w8079e/w8079e0h.htm

carcinogen: Substance or radiation that predisposes to cancer http://mdlinx.pdr.net/internal-medicine/news-article.cfm/6931990/?utm_source=in-house&utm_medium=message&utm_campaign=mh-im-nov16 https://en.wikipedia.org/wiki/Carcinogen

carpal tunnel syndrome (CTS): Restriction of the median nerve by the transverse carpal ligament at the wrist resulting in compression neuropathy. https://www.ncbi.nlm.nih.gov/pmc/articles/PMC3314870/

CAR-T: Chimeric Antigen Receptor T-Cell therapy: T-cells genetically modified to enhance tumor destruction. https://www.cancer.gov/about-cancer/treatment/research/car-t-cells http://www.nejm.org/doi/full/10.1056/nejmoa1407222#t=article https://jhoonline.biomedcentral.com/articles/10.1186/s13045-017-0423-1www.empr.com/news/first-gene-therapy-antigen-receptor-t-cell-acute-lymphoblastic-leukemia/article/685222/?DCMP=EMC-MPR_DailyDose_cp_20170830&cpn=obgyn_all https://jamanetwork.com/journals/jama/fullarticle/2664338?utm_source=silverchair&utm_medium=email&utm_campaign=article_alert-jama&utm_content=olf&utm_term https://www.frontiersin.org/articles/10.3389/fimmu.2022.817296/full?utm_source=FAAE&utm_medium=EMLF&utm_campaign=MRK_1821768_a0P58000000G0YLEA0_Immuno_20220224_arts_A

catalyst: A substance that facilitates a chemical reaction without being changed by that reaction.

cataract: Clouding, loss of transparency of the lens of the eye. http://www.webmd.com/eye-health/cataracts/extracapsular-surgery-for-cataracts

CAT scan: Computerized Axial Tomography. An advanced, computerized imaging technique that very quickly takes serial Xrays through the body in thin "slices", so that very small abnormalities can be found. With a helical (spiral) three-dimensional CAT scan the Xray tube revolves around the patient. A four-dimensional CAT scan takes multiple images during phases of the breathing cycle, particularly useful in cases of lung tumors that have to be precisely localized and that move with respiration. The fourth dimension is time. https://radiopaedia.org/articles/computed-tomography http://www.jwatch.org/na43480/2017/03/16/radiation-exposure-and-cancer-risk-low-dose-ct-lung-cancer?query=etoc_jwgenmed&jwd=000012066693&jspc=OBG

cautery (electrocautery): Surgical destruction of tissue by direct current heating. **Electrosurgery** utilizes radiofrequency (RF) alternating current to heat tissue. https://en.wikipedia.org/wiki/Electrosurgery

cell: The basic living microscopic structure in the human body. Each cell is surrounded by a cell membrane. Cells generally have a center, the nucleus, which is itself surrounded by a membrane. The nucleus contains the chromosomes, on which rest the genes. https://en.wikipedia.org/wiki/Cell_(biology)

cerebrovascular accident: See "Stroke".

cervical cancer: Cancer of the uterine cervix. Most often caused by specific types of sexually transmitted Human Papillomavirus (**HPV**), which can also cause **carcinoma of the penis**. Largely preventable by **vaccines**. https://www.ncbi.nlm.nih.gov/pubmed/12120445 https://www.cancer.gov/about-cancer/causes-prevention/risk/infectious-agents/hpv-vaccine-fact-sheet https://emedicine.medscape.com/article/2006486-overview

cervix: The mouth, or neck, of the uterus, projecting through the vaginal vault. Its opening is the cervical os. http://www.obgyn.net/gynecological-oncology/identifying-squamous-cancer-colposcopy

checkpoint: T-lymphocyte locus that can shut off T-cell and suppress the immune response. (See "T-lymphocyte".) http://www.cgen.com/focus-areas/immuno-oncology/immune-checkpoints http://journal.frontiersin.org/article/10.3389/fimmu.2017.00692/full?utm_source=F-AAE&utm_medium=EMLF&utm_campaign=MRK_307979_35_Immuno_20170622_arts_A

checkpoint inhibitor (immune checkpoint inhibitor, ICI): Drug that blocks a checkpoint, allowing T-lymphocyte to respond to malignant cell. Ref: Pardoll, Drew: Nature Reviews Cancer 12, 252-264 (April 2012) http://blog.dana-farber.org/insight/2015/09/what-is-a-checkpoint-inhibitor/ http://ascopubs.org/doi/full/10.1200/JCO.2017.74.6065 http://jama-network.com/journals/jama/fullarticle/2653953?amp;utm_source=JAMAPublishAheadofPrint&utm_campaign=08-09-2017 http://ard.bmj.com/content/76/10/1747

chemosis: Swelling of conjunctiva of the eye. https://www.mountsinai.org/health-library/symptoms/chemosis

chimera: A single organism composed of cells from different zygotes. A **chimeric gene** combines portions of different coding sequences to produce a new gene. https://en.wikipedia.org/wiki/Chimeric_gene

CHIP: Clonal Hematopoiesis of Indeterminate Potential: Acquired mutations in hematopoietic stem cells that accumulate in bone marrow, associated with an increased risk of heart attack and stroke. https://www.ncbi.nlm.nih.gov/pmc/articles/PMC4961884/ http://www.nejm.org/doi/full/10.1056/NEJMoa1701719

cholesterol: Normally occurring lipoproteins in the body. If cholesterol levels and levels of low density lipoprotein (LDL) are too high, atherosclerosis can result. http://emedicine.medscape.com/article/121187-overview https://www.ahajournals.org/doi/pdf/10.1161/CIR.0000000000000625 https://www.ahajournals.org/doi/10.1161/CIR.0000000000000625

cholesterol inhibitor: Drug that inhibits the intestine from absorbing cholesterol. http://www.health.harvard.edu/blog/pcsk9-inhibitors-a-major-advance-in-cholesterol-lowering-drug-therapy-201503157801

chorionic villi: Microscopic projections from the placenta in which fetal blood circulates. https://en.wikipedia.org/wiki/Chorionic_villus_sampling

chromatin: The protein (**histone**)/DNA complex in the cell nucleus that forms the chromosome. https://en.wikipedia.org/wiki/Chromatin http://www.nature.com/news/plot-a-course-through-the-genome-1.22553?WT.ec_id=NATURE-20170907&spMailingID=54864391&spUserID=MjA1NjIyNjc4OAS2&spJobID=1244089361&spReportId=MTI0NDA4OTM2MQS2

chromosome: An elongated, stringlike structure in the nucleus of the cell that carries the genes. There are 46 chromosomes in each cell, arranged in 23 pairs. One of each pair is originally derived from the mother, and one from the father. https://www.genome.gov/26524120/chromosomes-fact-sheet/

cilia: Tiny hairlike projections on cells.

circadian rhythm: Biologic process that exhibits endogenous circadian (24 hour, diurnal) cycle. Can be influenced by external factors. https://www.ncbi.nlm.nih.gov/pmc/articles/PMC4353305/ https://en.wikipedia.org/wiki/Circadian_rhythm

cirrhosis: Chronic degeneration of liver cells accompanied by fibrous scarring of the liver. https://www.niddk.nih.gov/health-information/health-topics/liver-disease/cirrhosis/Pages/facts.aspx

claudication: Pain in the legs, or arms, after exercising, usually a symptom of peripheral arterial disease. See "Peripheral Artery Occlusive Disease". https://www.mayoclinic.org/diseases-conditions/claudication/symptoms-causes/syc-20370952

clitoris: The erectile organ above the urethral orifice at the entrance to the vagina. https://www.ncbi.nlm.nih.gov/pubmed/23169570

clone: An exact genetic copy. An identical twin is a clone because the fertilized egg splits in two. A fraternal twin is not a clone because two different eggs, fertilized by two different sperm, develop in the uterus at the same time. https://www.genome.gov/25020028/cloning-fact-sheet/ http://www.cell.com/cell/fulltext/S0092-8674(18)30057-6

cochlear implant: Medical device that replaces the function of the inner ear, sends signals to the brain via the auditory nerve. https://www.nidcd.nih.gov/health/cochlear-implants

codon (triplet): Sequence of three consecutive nucleotides. Part of the genetic code. There are 64 codons. Sixty-one code for specific amino acids. The other three codons are stop signals. See "Nucleotide". https://www.genome.gov/genetics-glossary/Codon?id=36

cognition: Conscious mental activities of thinking, learning, understanding and remembering. https://www.sciencedaily.com/releases/2016/09/160909095045.htm http://psychcentral.

com/lib/in-depth-cognitive-behavioral-therapy/ https://www.mdlinx.com/family-medicine/medical-news-article/2016/12/13/coffee-chlorogenic-acid-vascular-phenolics-flow-mediated-dilatation-fmd-/6965864/?category=last-month&page_id=1 http://journal.frontiersin.org/article/10.3389/fimmu.2017.01101/full?utm_source=F-AAE&utm_medium=EMLF&utm_campaign=MRK_398354_35_Immuno_20170921_arts_A

cognitive impairment: Mild Cognitive Impairment (MCI) is a dysfunction of conscious mental activities with minimal impairment of the instrumental activities of daily life (IADL). In Amnestic MCI memory dysfunction predominates. There can be progression to **Dementia.** See Chapter 5, "Doctor, My Spouse Is Getting Forgetful" by Serge Gauthier; Chapter 15, "Management of Older Patients in the Emergency Department" by Cyrille Launay; Chapter 43, "Assessment of Decision-Making Capacity" by Catherine Ferrier. www.care-oftheolderperson.com http://n.neurology.org/content/90/3/126 http://n.neurology.org/content/90/13/e1158 https://academic.oup.com/brain/article/141/3/877/4818093

colon, colorectal cancer: Cancer of the large intestine and rectum. Detectable at precancerous and early stage by colonoscopy and biopsy. Cancer markers can be used in screening. https://www.ncbi.nlm.nih.gov/pubmed/26151224 https://emedicine.medscape.com/article/1948929-overview https://cancerstaging.org/references-tools/quickreferences/Documents/ColonMedium.pdf https://www.cancer.org/cancer/colon-rectal-cancer/detection-diagnosis-staging/how-diagnosed.html https://gi.org/guideline/colorectal-cancer-screening-recommendations-for-physicians-and-patients-from-the-u-s-multi-society-task-force-on-colorectal-cancer/ https://annals.org/aim/article-abstract/2726664/performance-characteristics-fecal-immunochemical-tests-colorectal-cancer-advanced-adenomatous-polyps https://www.asco.org/practice-guidelines/quality-guidelines/guidelines/resource-stratified#/3494 https://www.asco.org/practice-guidelines/quality-guidelines/guidelines/resource-stratified#/34946

colonoscopy: Direct inspection of the entire large intestine with a flexible fiberoptic instrument called a colonoscope. http://www.asge.org/assets/0/71328/9cf71f1d-ef18-4a34-9259-31f487a6213c.pdf

color flow doppler: Ultrasound with color coding of blood flow velocity and direction. Doppler effect refers to the measurable difference in sound as it moves away. https://123sonography.com/content/1821-principles-color-doppler

coma: Deep, unarousable unconsciousness. https://www.medicinenet.com/script/main/art.asp?articlekey=2803 https://www.ncbi.nlm.nih.gov/pubmed/19001840

concussion: Traumatic injury to the brain. https://www.cdc.gov/headsup/basics/concussion_whatis.html https://www.cdc.gov/traumaticbraininjury/severe.html https://www.fda.gov/NewsEvents/Newsroom/PressAnnouncements/ucm596531.htm

consciousness: Awareness. https://bmcneurosci.biomedcentral.com/articles/10.1186/1471-2202-5-42 https://plato.stanford.edu/entries/consciousness-neuroscience/

cord blood: Fetal blood in the umbilical cord. Can be banked in order to retrieve stem cells. http://www.acog.org/Resources-And-Publications/Committee-Opinions/Committee-on-Genetics/Umbilical-Cord-Blood-Banking

COVID-19: Corona viral disease caused by SARS-CoV-2 virus. Causative RNA virus of global pandemic that emanated from Wuhan, China, in 2019. Affects multiple organ systems. Elders, and people with coexisting medical conditions, especially older persons in nursing homes and similar facilities, are markedly vulnerable to severe sequelae and death. https://www.nejm.org/doi/full/10.1056/NEJMoa2008457 https://www.cdc.gov/coronavirus/2019-ncov/lab/grows-virus-cell-culture.html https://www.uptodate.com/contents/coronaviruses https://www.niaid.nih.gov/diseases-conditions/covid-19 https://www.frontiersin.org/articles/10.3389/fimmu.2020.01880/full?utm_source=F-AAE&utm_medium=EMLF&utm_campaign=MRK_1417202_35_Immuno_202009 https://pubs.acs.org/doi/10.1021/acsnano.0c06726 http://click.engage.frontiersin.com/?qs=c8e442cb-a1e5bb9e7a374260dbbdaae779c281f3bc2efa19a855c2052f4edfa94fba79ec085d0a1cb4ba168d-8bd57c956292c7359e20767bfdec1a47faee676b http://click.engage.frontiersin.com/?qs=c8e-442cba1e5bb9ec13326314edb1e0154b9487f5d5e6e68d3394a1e4f04c5d23d5c106108f0a04b89a0f716fdfe3632efb1cfc34d91d0eadae8663bd6a1b3a1

COX-1 inhibitor: Drugs including aspirin, ibuprofen and Naprosyn are both COX-1 and COX-2 inhibitors, inhibiting cyclooxygenase-I as well as cyclooxygenase 2. http://www.ncbi.nlm.nih.gov/pubmed/11566042

COX-2 inhibitor: Non-steroidal anti-inflammatory drugs (NSAIDs). These drugs target cyclo-oxygenase-2 (COX-2) enzyme that encourages prostaglandin production, leading to inflammation and pain. http://journal.frontiersin.org/article/10.3389/fimmu.2016.00375/full?utm_source=newsletter&utm_medium=email&utm_campaign=Immunology-w40-2016

C-reactive protein (CRP): Plasma protein with increased concentration in the presence of inflammatory disorders. See Chapter 10, "Could My Patient Be Malnourished?" by Jose Morais. www.careoftheolderperson.com https://www.frontiersin.org/articles/10.3389/fimmu.2018.02745/full?utm_source=F-AAE&utm_medium=EMLF&utm_campaign=MRK_838932_35_Immuno_20181129_arts_A.

CRISP R: ClusteredRegularly Interspaced Short Palindromic Repeats: DNA sequences found in genomes of bacteria. Segments of prokaryocytic DNA containing repetitions of base sequences, followed by segments of spacer DNA. Used in **genome editing**. Useful in detecting viral infection. https://www.empr.com/news/vitrakvi-larotrectinib-advanced-solid-tumorsntrk-gene-fusion-approval/article/816725/?utm_source=newsletter&utm_medium=email&utm_campaign=mpr-dailydose-cp-20181129&cpn=obgyn_all,obgyn_md,cambia_august201&hm https://www.nature.com/articles/d41586-019-00601-3?WT.ec_id=NATURE-20190228&utm_source=nature_etoc&utm_medium=email&utm_campaign=20190228&sap-outbound-id=F3F53CF91C70386022609FDF29CEFA2072F7C0D6

crispr-Cas9: Complex of RNA and protein (nucleases): Recognizes sequence of bases in target gene. Cas9 (an enzyme) unwinds double helix. CRISPR RNA sequence binds to target. Cas9 cuts both strands of target DNA. In a modification, DNA sequences are not cut: the Cas9 enzyme carries a molecular switch that turns on target genes. http://www.ncbi.nlm.nih.gov/pmc/articles/PMC4786927/ http://link.springer.com/article/10.1186/s12977-016-0270-0?view=classic https://www.nature.com/articles/d41586-019-01824-0?WT.ec_id=NATURE-201906&sap-outbound-id=D57BDD0F2FB94BAE156838EBF274B4C29D863CA1&mkt-key=005056B0331B1ED782E8AD53A869855D http://www.bloomberg.com/features/2016-how-crispr-will-change-the-world/ http://jamanetwork.com/journals/jama/article-abstract/2600454 https://en.wikipedia.org/wiki/CRISPR http://journal.frontiersin.org/article/10.3389/fimmu.2016.00375/full?utm_source=newsletter&utm_medium=email&utm_campaign=Immunology-w40-2016 https://www.technologyreview.com/s/608350/first-human-embryos-edited-in-us/ http://jamanetwork.com/journals/jama/fullarticle/2646800?utm_medium=alert&utm_source=JAMAPublishAheadofPrint&utm_campaign=10-08-2017 https://www.nature.com/news/crispr-hacks-enable-pinpoint-repairs-to-genome-1.22884?WT.ec_id=NATURE-20171026&spMailingID=55217903&spUserID=MjA1 https://www.ncbi.nlm.nih.gov/pubmed/27052831 http://www.cell.com/cell/fulltext/S0092-8674(17)31247-3 https://www.extremetech.com/extreme/281232-chinese-scientist-reportedly-creates-genetically-engineered-babies-immune-to-hiv https://mail.google.com/mail/u/0/?tab=wm#inbox/FMfcgxvzLrGCZfCRZNMSpDsBnsflHDPC https://www.technologyreview.com/s/612458/exclusive-chinese-scientists-are-creating-crispr-babies/amp/?__twitter_impression=true

cryosurgery: Surgical destruction of tissue by freezing. http://emedicine.medscape.com/article/1125851-overview

cul-de-sac: Rectouterine peritoneal pouch between the posterior wall of the uterus and the rectum. https://en.wikipedia.org/wiki/Recto-uterine_pouch

cybernetics: Control and communication with living tissue, as with a chip implanted in a muscle. http://www.asc-cybernetics.org/foundations/definitions.htm

cyst: A fluid-filled growth (tumor). May be benign or malignant. https://www.ncbi.nlm.nih.gov/pubmed/21845969 http://www.pathologyoutlines.com/topic/ovarytumorwhoclassif.html

cystocele: Bulge of the urinary bladder into the anterior wall of the vagina. https://www.niddk.nih.gov/health-information/health-topics/urologic-disease/cystocele/Pages/facts.aspx

cystoscope: Operating telescope used to visualize the interior of the urinary bladder and the ureteral orifices. See Chapter 32, "Incontinence in Older Adults" by Samer Shamout, Lysanne Campeau. www.careoftheolderperson.com https://www.ncbi.nlm.nih.gov/pmc/articles/PMC4457046/ https://en.wikipedia.org/wiki/Cystoscopy

cytokine: Factor released by a cell that has an effect on other cells. Implications in aging. http://www.ncbi.nlm.nih.gov/pmc/articles/PMC2785020/ http://journal.frontiersin.org/article/10.3389/fimmu.2017.00930/full?utm_source=F-AAE&utm_medium=EMLF&utm_campaign=MRK_352999_35_Immuno_20170808_arts_A https://www.frontiersin.org/articles/10.3389/fimmu.2018.00422/full?utm_source=F-AAE&utm_medium=EMLF&utm_campaign=MRK_571163_35_I https://www.frontiersin.org/articles/10.3389/fimmu.2018.00586/full?utm_source=F-AAE&utm_medium=EMLF&utm_campaign=MRK_608868_35_I https://www.frontiersin.org/articles/10.3389/fimmu.2019.00480/full?utm_source=F-AAE&utm_medium=EMLF&utm_campaign=MRK_943967_35_Immuno_20190326_arts_A

cytoplasm: The contents of a cell outside the nucleus. https://en.wikipedia.org/wiki/Cytoplasm

D-dimer: Fibrin degradation product of blood clot degraded by fibrinolysis that can be detected in blood after a pulmonary embolus (blood clot in the lung). Reference values are adjusted for age. https://www.google.com/search?q=d-dimer+definition+medical&rlz=1C1EJFA_enUS783US783&oq=d-dimer+definition+&aqs=chrome.1.69i57j0l5.64272j0j4&sourceid=chrome&ie=UTF-8

death: Cessation of life. https://jamanetwork.com/journals/jama/fullarticle/2769148?guestAccessKey=c234904b-79e4-4fa8-970e-dbac5739205a&utm_source=silverchair&utm_campaign=jama_network&utm_content=ped_weekly_highlights&cmp=1&utm_medium=email https://jamanetwork.com/journals/jama/fullarticle/2769149?guestAccessKey=002dcb34-be0f-4f21-986ba78ed29ccb96&utm_source=silverchair&utm_campaign=jama_network&utm_content=ped_weekly_highlights&cmp=1&utm_medium=email

deep learning: Deep neural network model. Machine learning technique analyzing large amounts of data, enabling prediction of outcomes (prognosis) when new data is presented. May be used to predict cardiovascular disease risk by observation of the eye retina, and to help clarify psychiatric diagnosis. https://arxiv.org/abs/1708.09843 https://en.wikipedia.org/wiki/Deep_learning https://www.nature.com/articles/s41746-018-0029-1 https://jamanetwork.com/journals/jamapsychiatry/article-abstract/2664960 https://jamanetwork.com/journals/jamapsychiatry/article-abstract/2664960

delirium: Confusional state with altered attention and awareness. See Chapter 8, "How to Diagnose and Manage Delirium" by Haibin Yin. www.careoftheolderperson.com https://www.ncbi.nlm.nih.gov/pubmed/25300023 https://www.uptodate.com/contents/diagnosis-of-delirium-and-confusional-states

delivery: The birth of the baby as it exits the birth canal.

dementia: Loss of cognitive functioning. Frontotemporal dementia refers to a heterogenous group of conditions. See Chapter 5, "Doctor, My Spouse Is Getting Forgetful" by Serge Gauthier; Chapter 44, "How Can Older People Be Protected?" by Randy S. Perskin. www.careoftheolderperson.com http://www.ncbi.nlm.nih.gov/pmc/articles/PMC2211335/ http://www.bmj.com/content/347/bmj.f4827 https://www.jwatch.org/na45523/2017/12/05/healthy-life-healthy-brain-lifestyle-factors-and-dementia?query=etoc_jwneuro&jwd=000012066693&jspc=OBG http://n.neurology.org/content/90/3/126 http://geropsychiatriceducation.vch.ca/docs/edu-downloads/depression/cornell_scale_depression.pdf https://jnnp.bmj.com/content/early/2018/08/26/jnnp-2018-318650 https://www.bmj.com/content/361/bmj.k1315Li https://www.jwatch.org/na48784/2019/04/16/revisiting-plasma-total-tau-levels-dementia-biomarker?query=etoc_jwneuro&jwd=000012066693&jspc=OBG

demography: The study of groups of people and their environment. http://www.pewresearch.org/fact-tank/2016/03/31/10-demographic-trends-that-are-shaping-the-u-s-and-the-world/

depression: A mood disorder marked by prolonged sadness, mood alteration, often with feelings of loss, anger and frustration. See: Chapter 42, "An Overview of Late-Life Depression" by

Artin Mahdanian, Silvia Monti De Flores. www.careoftheolderperson.com http://www.ncbi.nlm.nih.gov/pmc/articles/PMC2922383/ http://geropsychiatriceducation.vch.ca/docs/edu-downloads/depression/cornell_scale_depression.pdf https://ajp.psychiatryon-line.org/doi/10.1176/appi.ajp.2018.17060595

dermabrasion: Surgical procedure to remove skin imperfections by abrading the skin surface. https://ajp.psychiatryonline.org/doi/10.1176/appi.ajp.2018.17060595 http://emedicine.medscape.com/article/1297069-treatment

detrusor muscle: Muscular coat of the urinary bladder. See Chapter 32, "Incontinence in Older Adults", by Samer Shamout, Lysanne Campeau. www.careoftheolderperson.com http://emedicine.medscape.com/article/1949017-overview

DHEA: Dehydroepiandrosterone. Androgenic steroid hormone secreted largely by adrenal cortex. https://en.wikipedia.org/wiki/Dehydroepiandrosterone

diabetes mellitus: Chronic disease characterized by abnormally high blood glucose levels. See Chapter 24, "How to Manage Type 2 Diabetes in Frail Elderly Patients" by Young-Sang Kim, Jose Morais; Chapter 10, "Could My Patient Be Malnourished?" by Jose Morais; Chapter 3, "Frailty" by Sathya Karunananthan, Howard Bergman; Chapter 34, "Polypharmacy and Deprescribing in the Elderly" by Louise Mallet. www.care-oftheolderperson.com http://www.merckmanuals.com/professional/endocrine-and-metabolic-disorders/diabetes-mellitus-and-disorders-of-carbohydrate-metabolism/diabetes-mellitus-dm http://www.onlinejacc.org/content/early/2018/11/23/j.jacc.2018.09.020

diastasis recti: Widening of the linea alba ("white line") with separation of the rectus abdominis muscles. https://www.ncbi.nlm.nih.gov/pmc/articles/PMC5715079/ https://radiopaedia.org/articles/linea-alba https://www.ncbi.nlm.nih.gov/pmc/articles/PMC3649122/

diet: Food intake. See Chapter 10, "Could My Patient Be Malnourished?" by Jose Morais.www.careoftheolderperson.com http://www.pubfacts.com/detail/27465379/Relation-between-mealtime-distribution-of-protein-intake-and-lean-mass-loss-in-free-living-older-adu http://jamanetwork.com/journals/jama/fullarticle/2636710 https://www.nature.com/articles/s41398-018-0293-5

disease: Aberrant state of morphology or pathophysiology. Boudreau, JD, Cassell, EJ, Fuks, A: Physicianship and the Rebirth of Medical Education. Oxford University Press, 2018

diuretic: Drug that causes increased passage of fluid by the kidneys. See Chapter 34, "Polypharmacy and Deprescribing in the Elderly" by Louise Mallet; Chapter 32, "Incontinence in Older Adults" by Samer Shamout, Louise Campeau. www.careoftheol-derperson.com http://emedicine.medscape.com/article/2145340-overview

DNA: Deoxyribonucleic acid. DNA makes up the chromosomes that carry the genes. DNA is arranged in a distinctive double helix, three-dimensional pattern. It resembles a tight spiral staircase, with rungs (steps), each of which holds two (out of four) nucleic acid bases, called **base pairs.** https://www.genome.gov/25520880/deoxyribonucleic-acid-dna-fact-sheet/

DNA microarray: DNA biochip. Collection of microscopic DNA spots on a surface. Used to measure gene expression patterns. https://www.genome.gov/10000533/dna-microarray-technology/

DNA mismatch repair: During DNA replication, erroneous insertion, deletion and misincorpora-tion of bases can occur in the daughter DNA strand. Such errors can also occur during DNA recombination. DNA mismatch repair involves the recognition and correction of these abnormalities. https://en.wikipedia.org/wiki/DNA_mismatch_repair https://jama-network.com/journals/jamasurgery/article-abstract/2647248?utm_medium=alert&utm_source=JAMA+SurgLatestIssue&utm_campaign=15-11-2017 https://www.nature.com/scitable/topicpage/dna-is-constantly-changing-through-the-process-6524876

DNA probe: A highly specific test to detect the DNA of an individual, or a virus. It is used to detect the human papillomavirus (HPV) that is the usual causative organism of cancer of the cervix. The test is used in the criminal investigation of rape, and in identification. An individual male can be identified by the distinctive DNA in his sperm. http://www.nature.com/subjects/dna-probesv

dopamine: A neurotransmitter. http://www.dictionary.com/browse/dopamine

duodenum: First part of the small intestine after the stomach. http://emedicine.medscape.com/article/1948951-overview

dysgeusia: Distorted sense of taste. Can be present in cases of COVID-19. https://www.ncbi.nlm.nih.gov/pmc/articles/PMC7308993/

dyskinesia: Abnormality of voluntary movement. https://en.wikipedia.org/wiki/Dyskinesia

dysmenorrhea: Pain with menses. https://academic.oup.com/epirev/article/36/1/104/566554

dyspareunia: Painful intercourse. See Chapter 35, "After Menopause" by Ronald M. Caplan. www.careoftheolderperson.com https://www.ncbi.nlm.nih.gov/pmc/articles/PMC2671314/

dysplasia: An abnormal, benign, microscopic cell change that can be a precursor of cancer. http://www.cancer.gov/publications/dictionaries/cancer-terms?cdrid=45675

ectopic pregnancy: Pregnancy outside of the normal location in the uterus. Usually in a fallopian tube. https://academic.oup.com/humupd/article/20/2/250/663951

edema: Swelling by accumulation of fluid in tissues. See Chapter 10, "Could My Patient Be Malnourished?" by Jose Morais. www.careoftheolderperson.com http://www.ncbi.nlm.nih.gov/books/NBK53445/

elder abuse: The intentional or neglectful causing of harm to an aging person. See Chapter 40, "Elder Abuse" by Mark J. Yaffe. www.careoftheolderperson.com https://online.epocrates.com/diseases/69735/Elder-abuse/Differential-Diagnosis https://jamanetwork.com/journals/jama/fullarticle/2708121?utm_source=silverchair&utm_medium=email&utm_campaign=article_alert-jama&utm_cont

electrocardiogram: Noninvasive test that measures the electrical activity of the heart. https://www.ncbi.nlm.nih.gov/pmc/articles/PMC1614214/

embolization: Therapeutic introduction of a substance into a blood vessel to occlude it. **Transcatheter arterial chemoembolization (TACE)** combines the introduction of therapeutic substances into a tumor in conjunction with occlusion of the blood vessels of the tumor. http://www.hopkinsmedicine.org/liver_tumor_center/treatments/intraarterial_therapies/tace.html

embolus: Detached thrombus (blood clot) that travels through blood vessels to another site. http://emedicine.medscape.com/article/300901-overview http://emedicine.medscape.com/article/1916852-overview

embryo: The developing baby in the uterus during the fourth to eighth weeks of development, to the end of the second month, by which time all major features of the body are recognizable. All the main organ systems in the body have been laid down by the end of the second month. https://embryology.med.unsw.edu.au/embryology/index.php/Ultrasound https://www.nature.com/articles/d41586-018-07317-w https://www.nature.com/articles/d41586-018-07317-w

emotion: Affective state of consciousness. Feeling. https://www.ncbi.nlm.nih.gov/pmc/articles/PMC3950961/

endocrine glands: Glands that secrete (produce) hormones, including the pituitary gland at the base of the brain, the thyroid gland, the adrenal glands, the ovaries and the testes. https://en.wikipedia.org/wiki/Endocrine_gland

endocytosis: Active transport of molecules into the cell in an energy-using process. https://www.ncbi.nlm.nih.gov/books/NBK9831/

endometrial biopsy: Surgical sampling of the uterine lining. https://academic.oup.com/humupd/article/23/2/232/2632344

endometrial cancer: Cancer of the lining of the uterus. https://www.ncbi.nlm.nih.gov/pmc/articles/PMC5288678/

endometrial hyperplasia: Benign overgrowth condition of the lining of the uterus with crowding of glands. **Atypical (adenomatous) hyperplasia** of the endometrium is considered to be premalignant. https://pdfs.semanticscholar.org/3b81/8cfedf864fca863c378a8028f91e0280b299.pdf

endometriosis: Abnormal deposition of endometrium outside the uterus. http://www.gponline.com/clinical-review-endometriosis/womens-health/endometriosis-fibroids/article/1150448

endometrium: The lining of the uterus.

endorphins: Hormones that affect receptors in the brain. May reduce pain by binding to opioid receptors. http://www.ncbi.nlm.nih.gov/pmc/articles/PMC3104618/

endothelin 1: A vasoconstrictor. http://www.ncbi.nlm.nih.gov/pmc/articles/PMC3005421/

entanglement: In quantum mechanics, the states of two or more objects are described in reference to each other, even though they are spatially separated. https://www.sciencedaily.com/terms/quantum_entanglement.htm

enterocele: True hernia of small bowel covered by peritoneum bulging into the vaginal vault.

entropy: Measurement of molecular disorder or randomness in a system. https://www.britannica.com/science/entropy-physics

enzyme: An organic catalyst. Enzymes facilitate chemical reactions within the human body. https://www.mcat.me/review/bb/enzyme-structure-and-function/

EPF (early pregnancy factor): Pregnancy-specific protein that is present in pregnant woman's serum 48 hours after fertilization. http://www.ncbi.nlm.nih.gov/pubmed/9196793

epidemic: Increase in the number of cases of a disease in a population. https://www.cdc.gov/ophss/csels/dsepd/ss1978/lesson1/section11.html https://www.hhs.gov/opioids/about-the-epidemic/index.html

epigenetic clock: Essentially refers to DNA Methylation Age. DNA methylation: adding a methyl group (CH3) to one of the bases of DNA is an epigenetic mechanism involved in gene regulation. https://www.whatisepigenetics.com/dna-methylation/ http://clinicalepigeneticsjournal.biomedcentral.com/articles/10.1186/s13148-019-0656-7 https://www.ncbi.nlm.nih.gov/pmc/articles/PMC6826138/ https://onlinelibrary.wiley.com/doi/full/10.1111/acel.13028

epigenetics: Study of the processes that regulate the turning on and off genes. http://epi.grants.cancer.gov/i/epigen-lg.jpg https://www.frontiersin.org/articles/10.3389/fimmu.2021.752380/full?utm_source=F-AAE&utm_medium=EMLF&utm_campaign=MRK_1750137_a0P58000000G0YLEA0_Immuno_20211012_arts_A

epigenome: Description of all the chemical modifications to DNA and DNA associated proteins in the cell which alter gene expression. Epigenetic changes can drive aging. Much of the epigenome is reset when the genome is passed to offspring. https://www.genome.gov/27532724/ http://www.nature.com/news/an-epigenetics-gold-rush-new-controls-for-geneexpression-1.21513?WT.ec_id=NATURE-20170223&spMailingID=53480287&spUserID=MjA1NjIyNjc4OA https://www.nature.com/articles/s41467-020-15847-z

epigenomics: Analysis of epigenetic changes. http://anatomyandphysiologyi.com/epithelial-tissue/

epithelium: A microscopic cellular covering of surfaces, including skin and mucous membranes. http://anatomyandphysiologyi.com/epithelial-tissue/

epitope: Antigenic determinant. The part of the antigen molecule that is recognized by the antibody, and to which the antibody attaches. https://www.britannica.com/science/epitope

erectile dysfunction (ED): Difficulty with achieving or maintaining penile erection. See Chapter 35, "After Menopause" by Ronald M. Caplan. www.careoftheolderperson.com http://www.bmj.com/content/348/bmj.g129

erythropoietin: Stimulates the formation of red blood cells. Produced by recombinant DNA technology. https://en.wikipedia.org/wiki/Erythropoietin

estradiol: A form of estrogen produced in the ovaries. https://pubchem.ncbi.nlm.nih.gov/compound/estradiol

estrogen: Female sex hormones, mainly made in the ovary. https://en.wikipedia.org/wiki/Estrogen http://journal.frontiersin.org/article/10.3389/fimmu.2017.00108/full?utm_source=newsletter&utm_medium=email&utm_campaign=Immunology-w7-2017

estrogen replacement therapy (ERT): Treatment of menopausal symptoms, usually in conjunction with progesterone. See Chapter 35, "After Menopause" by Ronald M. Caplan. www.careoftheolderperson.com http://emedicine.medscape.com/article/276104-overview

eukaryote: Any organism whose cells contain a nucleus which contains DNA within chromosomes. http://www.dictionary.com/browse/eukaryote

exercise (aerobic): Generally refers to sustained physical activity designed to promote oxygen utilization. See Chapter 9, "Why Does My Patient Have Gait and Balance Disorders?" by Olivier Beauchet; Chapter 4, "Physical Activity as a Countermeasure to Frailty" by Guy Hajj Boutros, Antony D. Karelis. www.careoftheolderperson.com http://cardiology.jamanetwork.com/article.aspx?articleid=2530563 https://www.frontiersin.org/articles/10.3389/fimmu.2018.02187/full?utm_source=F-AAE&utm_medium=EMLF&utm_campaig https://mail.google.com/mail/u/0/#search/mandsager+k+jama++oct+19+2018++/FMfcgxvzLNXbwjKxFmgDCpgKnVwTXKsz https://jamanetwork.com/journals/jama/fullarticle/2712935?guestAccessKey=c09863bb-66ff-4c16-88c3-06ab0357f57d&utm_source=silverchair&utm_medium=email&utm_campaign=article_alert-jama&utm https://jamanetwork.com/journals/jamainternalmedicine/fullarticle/2714300?guestAccessKey=55c4f5ef-9957-470d-9691-071330b0644d&utm_source=silverchair&utm_campaign=jama_network&utm_content=weekly_highlights&cmp=1&utm_medium=email https://jamanetwork.com/journals/jama/fullarticle/2712935?guestAccessKey=2364bbfc-d62a-4d49-9fdb-9d0114d00fc8&utm_source=silverchair&utm_medium=email&utm_campaign=article_alert-jama&utm_content=etoc&utm_term=112018 https://n.neurology.org/content/92/9/e905 https://jamanetwork.com/journals/jamanetworkopen/fullarticle/2724776?utm_source=silverchair&utm_medium=email&utm_campaign=article_alert-jamanetworkopen&utm_content=etoc&utm_term=030119

exome: All the **exons** in a **genome. Whole exome sequencing:** Identifies variations in the protein-coding region of a gene. Most disease-causing mutations occur in **exons.** https://ghr.nlm.nih.gov/primer/testing/sequencing https://jamanetwork.com/journals/jama/fullarticle/2769138?guestAccessKey=e9f01f60-c67f-4a71-8ee7-a0cbd1f876c0&utm_source=silverchair&utm_campaign=jama_network&utm_content=ped_weekly_highlights&a,p;cmp=1&utm_medium=email

exons: The pieces of DNA that provide instructions for making proteins. https://ghr.nlm.nih.gov/primer/testing/sequencing

exoskeleton (robotic, powered): Wearable robotic unit with computer control that can be used in rehabilitation after spinal cord injury. https://www.ncbi.nlm.nih.gov/pmc/articles/PMC6153133/

exosome: Extracellular vesicle involved in cell communication and immune function. Role in cancer cells. https://www.frontiersin.org/articles/10.3389/fgene.2018.00092/full

extrapyramidal system: Part of the motor system network incorporating the basal ganglia, involved with involuntary actions performed at a subconscious level. Distinguished from the tracts of the motor cortex that travel through the pyramids of the medulla. https://www.sciencedirect.com/topics/neuroscience/extrapyramidal-system

Fabry's disease: Alpha-galactosidase-A deficiency: enzyme utilized in lipid metabolism. Rare X-linked lysosomal storage disease. http://www.ninds.nih.gov/disorders/fabrys/fabrys.htm

fallopian tube: The fine tubular structure arising from each side of the uterus near the fundus, ending in fingerlike projections called fimbria that are close to each ovary, essentially forming the "pickup" mechanism for the egg released at ovulation.

fertility: The ability to conceive children. http://emedicine.medscape.com/article/274143-overview

fertilization: The fusion of the ovum (oocyte, egg) and the spermatozoon (sperm). https://en.wikipedia.org/wiki/Human_fertilization

fetus: The baby developing in the uterus is known as the fetus from the beginning of the third month until the baby is born. The fetal period is the longest period of intrauterine life. http://www.nature.com/news/secrets-of-life-in-a-spoonful-of-blood-1.21430?WT.ec_id=NATURE-20170209&spMailingID=53380605&spUserID=MjA1NjIyNjc4OAS2&spJob

ID=1101425398&spReportId=MTEwMTQyNTM5OAS2 https://www.nature.com/articles/d41586-018-07317-w

FHIT gene: Fragile histidine triad. Aberrant transcripts from this gene are found in some cancers, notably esophageal, stomach and colon cancer. http://www.ncbi.nlm.nih.gov/gene/2272

fiberoptics: Light images sent through fine fibers of glass or plastic. http://www.laserfocusworld.com/articles/2011/01/medical-applications-of-fiber-optics-optical-fiber-sees-growth-as-medical-sensors.html

fibrin: In blood clotting, thrombin causes fibrinogen to polymerize, forming fibrin. Polymerized fibrin and platelets form a hemostatic plug, or clot. https://www.britannica.com/science/fibrin

fibroid: A benign solid tumor of the uterus.

fibroma: A benign solid tumor that can occur in the breast or ovary.

fistula: An abnormal passage from one body cavity to another, or out to the body surface.

follicle (ovarian): The fluid-filled structure surrounding the developing egg (ovum) in the ovary. http://www.embryology.ch/anglais/cgametogen/oogenese02.html

fomite: Inanimate object that can be contaminated and transmit disease (e.g. countertop). https://www.google.com/search?q=fomite+definition&rlz=1C-1CHBF_enUS821US821&oq=fomite&aqs=chrome.1.69i57j0l7.7262j0j4&sourceid=-chrome&ie=UTF-8

frailty syndrome: Weakness, slowness, minimal physical activity, exhaustion and low energy, weight loss. See Chapter 3, "Frailty" by Sathya Karunananthan, Howard Bergman; Chapter 16, "Critical Care of the Older Person" by Astrid F. Pilgrim, Michael R. Pinsky. www.careoftheolderperson.com https://jamanetwork.com/journals/jamasurgery/article-abstract/2656841 http://www.ncbi.nlm.nih.gov/pubmed/17634320 http://annals.org/aim/article-abstract/2668215/effect-physical-activity-frailty-secondary-analysis-randomized-controlled-trial https://documentcloud.adobe.com/link/track?uri=urn%3Aaaid%3Ascds%3AUS%3Af24df018-1e90-454d-af5f-7a345b6d5190 https://jamanetwork.com/journals/jamanetworkopen/fullarticle/2733174?utm_source=silverchair&utm_medium=email&utm_campaign=article_alert-jama https://jamanetwork.com/journals/jamanetworkopen/fullarticle/2740784?utm_source=silverchair&utm_medium=email&utm_campaign=article_alert-jamanetworkopen&utm_content=wklyforyou&utm_term=08022019

free radical: Short-lived uncharged molecule. https://documentcloud.adobe.com/link/track?uri=u https://jamanetwork.com/journals/jamanetworkopen/fullarticle/2733174?utm_source=silverchair&utm_medium=email&utm_campaign=article_alertjaman%3Aaaid%3Ascds%3AUS%3Af24df018-1e90-454d-af5f-7a345b6d5190 http://www.ncbi.nlm.nih.gov/pmc/articles/PMC3249911/

FSH: Follicle stimulating hormone. http://www.ncbi.nlm.nih.gov/pubmed/9741710

GABA: Gamma-aminobutyric acid. A neurotransmitter. http://www.webmd.com/vitamins-supplements/ingredientmono-464-gaba%20gamma-aminobutyric%20acid.aspx?activeingredientid=464&

galactography: Mammography with injection of contrast to image milk ducts.

gamete: A germ (sex) cell: the female ovum, or the male spermatozoon. https://www.khanacademy.org/science/biology/cellular-molecular-biology/meiosis/a/phases-of-meiosis

gene: The determinant of human characteristics and behavior from a cellular level on upwards. Each gene is a section on a DNA molecule and usually resides at a specific point (locus) on a chromosome. Each gene has a counterpart on the other chromosome that makes up the pair. The genes elaborate proteins. http://www.ncbi.nlm.nih.gov/genbank/

gene editing (genome editing): A form of **genetic engineering**. Insertion, deletion or replacement of DNA at a specific site on the genome using engineered nucleases ("molecular scissors") See "CRISPR". https://www.technologyreview.com/s/608350/first-human-embryos-edited-in-us/ https://www.horizondiscovery.com/gene-editing http://jamanetwork.com/journals/jama/fullarticle/2646800?utm_medium=alert&utm_source=JAMAPublishAheadofPrint&utm_campaign=10-08-2017 https://www.technologyreview.com/s/612458/exclusive-chinese-scientists-are-creating-crispr-babies/amp/?__twitter_impression=true

gene expression profiling: Measurement of activity (expression) of thousands of genes, giving a picture of cellular functioning. In breast cancer, for example, identifies distinct molecular entities associated with differential prognoses and response to cytotoxic drugs. http://www.ncbi.nlm.nih.gov/pubmed/11823860 https://www.mdedge.com/hematology-oncology/clinical-edge/summary/breast-cancer/optimizing-gene-expression-profiling-early?utm_source=ClinEdge_OP_cedge_110816&utm_medium=email&utm_content=Gene%20Profiling%20in%20Early%20BC%20|%20CTC%20Clusters%20and%20MBC%20|%20Impact%20of%20Chemo%20Events%20|%20

gene silencing: Regulation of gene expression. siRNA: small interfering RNA potentially can inhibit genes in genetic disease. (See "RNAi".) http://www.ncbi.nlm.nih.gov/probe/docs/applsilencing/ https://jamanetwork.com/journals/jama/fullarticle/2712406?guestAccessKey=22414c3e-162a-4ff0-8b50-5477ff58735b&utm_source=silverchair&utm_campaign=jama_network&utm_content=weekly_highlights&cmp=1&utm_medium=email https://www.ncbi.nlm.nih.gov/pmc/articles/PMC5542916/

gene therapy: Treating a disorder by inserting a gene into cells. http://www.ama-assn.org/ama/pub/physician-resources/medical-science/genetics-molecular-medicine/current-topics/gene-therapy.page? https://www.frontiersin.org/articles/10.3389/fimmu.2018.00554/full?utm_source=F-AAE&utm_medium=EMLF&utm_campaign=MRK_589856_35_Immuno_20180403_arts_A

genetic engineering: Manipulating the genome. http://www.fda.gov/AnimalVeterinary/DevelopmentApprovalProcess/GeneticEngineering/ https://www.frontiersin.org/articles/10.3389/fimmu.2018.00153/full?utm_source=F-AAE&utm_medium=EMLF&utm_campaign=MRK_536191_35

genome: The complete DNA sequence. The human genome project deciphered the complete DNA sequence of humans. **Whole genome sequencing:** Determines the order of all the **nucleotides** in a person's **DNA**. https://ghr.nlm.nih.gov/primer/testing/sequencing http://www.ncbi.nlm.nih.gov/projects/genome/guide/human/ Single-Cell Genomics: Sequencing DNA and RNA in a single cell. https://journals.plos.org/plosgenetics/article?id=10.1371/journal.pgen.1004126 Next Generation Sequencing: Technologies that sample multiple DNA sequences in parallel. https://www.cancer.gov/publications/dictionaries/genetics-dictionary/def/next-generation-sequencing

genotype: The individual genes of each person. The expression of the person's genetic code. **SNP genotyping** refers to variations in single nucleotide polymorphisms between individuals. https://www.niehs.nih.gov/news/assets/docs_p_z/snp_genotyping_508.pdf http://www.nature.com/tpj/journal/v3/n2/full/6500167a.html https://www.britannica.com/science/genotype

GERD: Gastroesophageal reflux disease. https://gi.org/guideline/diagnosis-and-managemen-of-gastroesophageal-reflux-disease/

geriatrics: Medical specialty that focuses on healthcare, diseases, issues of elderly people and the aging process. See Chapter 1, "Introduction" by Jose Morais. www.careoftheolderperson.com http://www.merckmanuals.com/professional/geriatrics/provision-of-care-to-the-elderly/overview-of-geriatric-care http://bulletin.facs.org/2016/12/improving-quality-in-geriatric-surgery-a-blueprint-from-the-american-college-of-surgeons/

gerontology: The multidisciplinary study of aging and its issues in all its aspects. http://biomed-gerontology.oxfordjournals.org/content/59/1/M24.full

geroprotector: Drug that targets the fundamental mechanisms of aging. https://www.nature.com/articles/d41586-018-01668-0?utm_source=briefing-dy&utm_medium=email&utm_campaign=20180215

geroscience: The study of the intersection of aging, biology, chronic disease and health. Covers epigenetics, inflammation, adaptation to stress, proteostasis, stem cells and regeneration, metabolism and macromolecular damage. https://pubmed.ncbi.nlm.nih.gov/25417146/ https://www.nia.nih.gov/research/dab/geroscience-intersection-basic-aging-biology-chronic-disease-and-health

gland: Organ that synthesizes and secretes a substance required by the body. http://www.histology.leeds.ac.uk/glandular/exocr_endocr_properties.php

glaucoma: Condition that causes optic nerve damage and vision loss, often by an increase in intra-ocular pressure. https://www.ncbi.nlm.nih.gov/pubmed/24825645vg

globulins: Include **alpha globulins, beta globulin** and **gamma globulin**, including **(Ig)A, (Ig)G: immunoglobulin G, (Ig)M, (Ig)E and (Ig)D** synthesized by B lymphocytes, important in the immune response. Identified by **serum protein electrophoresis**, which separates the proteins. https://www.aafp.org/afp/2005/0101/p105.html https://www.ncbi.nlm.nih.gov/pmc/articles/PMC2715434/ https://www.reference.com/science/gamma-globulin-2944770f90b33e6c?aq=Gamma+Globulins&qo=cdpArticles

globus pallidus: A subcortical structure in the brain. Part of the basal ganglia. http://webspace.ship.edu/cgboer/basalganglia.html

glomerulonephritis: Lesions of kidney glomeruli (capillary networks that filter blood) resulting from deposition or formation of immune complexes. In the acute phase, hematuria (blood in the urine), proteinuria (protein in the urine) and red blood cell casts in the urine are seen. http://emedicine.medscape.com/article/239278-overview#a4 http://www.sci.utah.edu/~macleod/bioen/be6000/prevnotes/L18-kidney.pdf

GLP-1r: Glucagon-like peptide 1 receptor agonist. Used in treatment of Type 2 (adult onset) Diabetes. http://www.diabetesincontrol.com/newly-updated-glp-1-agonist-medications-chart/

glycoengineering: Altering a cell surface so that infused tumor-specific immunocytes can enter the tumor parenchyma (functional tissue). https://www.frontiersin.org/articles/10.3389/fimmu.2018.03084/full?utm_source=F-AAE&utm_medium=EMLF&utm_campaign=MRK_889258_35_Immuno_20190122_arts_A

GNRH: Gonadotropin-releasing hormone from the hypothalamus. http://emedicine.medscape.com/article/255152-overview

goiter: Enlargement of the thyroid gland. http://www.uptodate.com/contents/clinical-presentation-and-evaluation-of-goiter-in-adults

graft: Healthy tissue taken from one part of the body to replace diseased or damaged tissue in another part. **Xenograft:** graft from a different species. https://www.cancer.gov/publications/dictionaries/cancer-terms/def/xenograft

granulosa cell: A cell in the lining of an ovarian follicle. Granulosa cells manufacture estrogen, and to a lesser extent androgens and progestins. Conversion of androgens to estrogen takes place in granulosa cells. https://embryology.med.unsw.edu.au/embryology/index.php/Granulosa_cell

greenhouse gases: Include carbon dioxide, sulfur dioxide, nitrous oxide, methane. https://www.epa.gov/ghgemissions/overview-greenhouse-gases

growth hormone: Somatotropin. Secreted by the pituitary gland. http://www.ncbi.nlm.nih.gov/pubmed/20020365

HCG (human chorionic gonadotropin): Produced by the placenta. http://www.fda.gov/Drugs/ResourcesForYou/Consumers/BuyingUsingMedicineSafely/MedicationHealthFraud/ucm281834.htm

heart failure: Congestive heart failure. Heart muscle contraction not sufficiently strong to properly circulate blood. Fluid accumulates. http://heartfailure.onlinejacc.org/article.aspx?articleid=1568320

hemorrhage: Excessive bleeding.

HER-2 gene: Human Epidermal Growth Factor Receptor-2. Linked to breast cancer. http://www.cancer.gov/research/progress/discovery/HER2

heredity: Parent-to-child transmission of traits, by inheritance of genes. https://ghr.nlm.nih.gov/primer/inheritance/inheritancepatterns

hernia: Intraabdominal contents enclosed by peritoneum bulging into a weakened wall.

heuristics: Strategies or mental processes used to quickly form judgments, make decisions or find a solution to a complex problem by focusing on the most relevant aspects of the problem. https://en.wikipedia.org/wiki/Heuristics_in_judgment_and_decisionmaking#:~:text=Heuristics%20are%20simple%20strategies%20or,situation%20to%20formulate%20a%20solution.

high density lipoprotein (HDL): Complex of lipids and proteins that transports cholesterol in the blood to the liver. http://www.ncbi.nlm.nih.gov/pmc/articles/PMC3787738/ https://www.jwatch.org/na45882/2018/01/17/continuing-enigma-hdl?query=topic_lipid&jwd=000012066693&jspc=OBG

hippocampus: Area of the brain involved with spatial memory which is important in navigation, and episodic memory (remembering autobiographical events). Located in the medial temporal lobe of the brain. Includes a gray matter ridge on the floor of each lateral ventricle. https://en.wikipedia.org/wiki/Hippocampus https://www.nature.com/nature/journal/vaop/ncurrent/full/nature22067.html https://en.wikipedia.org/wiki/Episodic_memory

hirsutism: Excess hair growth. http://emedicine.medscape.com/article/121038-overview

histocompatibility: Antigenic similarities between tissue donor and recipient so that a transplant is not rejected. https://www.hindawi.com/journals/jtrans/2012/842141/

histone: Protein in chromosomes that binds to DNA, giving shape to the chromosome. Role in controlling gene activity.

HLA (human leukocyte antigen proteins) typing: DNA extracted from cells, genes amplified that encode for HLA peptides using PCR (see "Polymerase Chain Reaction"). Identifies disease markers. Used in matching donors and recipients in transplantation. https://www.ncbi.nlm.nih.gov/pmc/articles/PMC1119473/

HMO: Health maintenance organization. Essentially a health insurance plan.

holography: The scattered light from an object is captured, then illuminated by a beam. Multiple two-dimensional pictures are assembled into a three-dimensional display. http://holocenter.org/what-is-holography

homeostasis: State of balance with constant adjustment among body systems so that body can survive and function correctly. See Chapter 16, "Critical Care of the Older Person" by Astrid F. Pilgrim, Michael R. Pinsky. www.careoftheolderperson.com https://www.cancer.gov/publications/dictionaries/cancer-terms/def/homeostasis#:~:text=homeostasis%20(HOH%2Dmee%2Doh,to%20survive%20and%20function%20correctly.

homeostenosis: Decreased ability to maintain homeostasis under stress; a narrowing (stenosis) of reserve capacity. See Chapter 16, "Critical Care of the Older Person" by Astrid F. Pilgrim, Michael R. Pinsky. www.careoftheolderperson.com https://www.sharecare.com/health/aging-mental-health/whatishomeostenosis#:~:text=As%20people%20get%20older%20or,homeostasis%20(balance)%20under%20stress.

homocysteine: Amino acid derived from the dietary amino acid methionine. Homologue of the amino acid cysteine. http://www.ncbi.nlm.nih.gov/pmc/articles/PMC4146172/

homograft: Transplanted tissue from another human individual. http://bja.oxfordjournals.org/content/108/suppl_1/i29.full

hormone: A substance formed in an endocrine gland and carried by the blood stream to other organs which it affects. Such organs are called end organs. For example, follicle stimulating hormone and luteinizing hormone from the pituitary gland act on the ovary, controlling ovarian secretion of estrogen and progesterone. Estrogen and progesterone act on the endometrium lining the uterus. http://biology.freeoda.com/chemical_composition_of_the_hormones.htm http://www.news-medical.net/health/Hormone-Interactions-with-Receptors.aspx

hormone replacement therapy (HRT): Treatment of menopausal symptoms with estrogen and progesterone. http://press.endocrine.org/doi/abs/10.1210/jc.2015-2236

hot flashes: Sudden onset of a feeling of heat and flushing of short duration. http://theoncologist.alphamedpress.org/content/16/11/1658.long

human connectome project: Mapping the human brain connectivity. http://www.humanconnectomeproject.org/

hyaluronic acid: An anionic nonsulfated glycosaminoglycan. Component of skin. http://www.ncbi.nlm.nih.gov/pmc/articles/PMC3583886/

hydrofluocarbons (HFCs): Several organic compounds. Decreasingly used as refrigerants. https://www.britannica.com/science/hydrofluorocarbon

hyperglycemia: Abnormally increased blood glucose levels. https://ccforum.biomedcentral.com/articles/10.1186/cc12514 http://joe.endocrinology-journals.org/content/204/1/1.full.pdf

hyperplasia: Overgrowth of tissue. Increase in cellular reproduction rate. http://journals.lww.com/jaapa/Fulltext/2016/08000/Benign_prostatic_hyperplasia__A_clinical_review.2.aspx http://emedicine.medscape.com/article/269919-overview

hypertension: High blood pressure. Sometimes defined as 130 mm Hg systolic (pressure during heart muscle contraction), and 80 mm Hg diastolic (pressure during relaxation). http://jaha.ahajournals.org/content/4/12/e002315.full http://www.jwatch.org/na43262/2017/03/02/pharmacologic-treatment-hypertension-older-adults?query=etoc_jwgenmed&jwd=000012066693&jspc=OBG http://hyper.ahajournals.org/content/early/2017/11/10/HYP.0000000000000065 https://jama-network.com/journals/jama/fullarticle/2664350?utm_source=silverchair&utm_medium=email&utm_campaign=article_alert-jama&utm_content=olf&u https://jamanetwork.com/journals/jama/fullarticle/2664350?&utm_source=191323&utm_medium=BulletinHealthCare&utm_term=120217&utm_content=Mornin

hypotension, orthostatic: Low blood pressure on standing. http://www.ncbi.nlm.nih.gov/pubmed/27225359?access_num=27225359&link_type=MED&dopt=Abstract

hypothalamus: Part of the brain below the thalamus. Forms the major portion of the ventral region of the diencephalon. Forms part of the wall of the third ventricle. http://press.endocrine.org/doi/abs/10.1210/jc.2015-2236

hysterectomy: Surgical removal of the uterus.

hysterosalpingogram: Injection of radiopaque dye into the uterus via the cervix to radiologically visualize the uterine cavity, the fallopian tubes and their patency.

hysteroscopy: A minimally invasive surgical technique in which a fiberoptic telescope (hysteroscope) is introduced through the cervical os into the uterine cavity. The endometrial lining of the uterus and the interior openings of the fallopian tubes can be seen.

ICSI: Intracytoplasmic sperm injection. http://americanpregnancy.org/infertility/intracytoplasmic-sperm-injection/

immune system: The system that allows the body to ward off invasion by foreign substances, including infectious agents. Cells including T-lymphocytes that go to infected sites are elaborated in bone marrow and other areas. Antibodies (immunoglobulins) that target specific invaders (antigens) circulate in the bloodstream. Infected areas drain through lymphatic channels to the lymph nodes, where invading organisms are processed. http://emedicine.medscape.com/article/1948753-overview

immunocyte: Leukocyte that induces immune response by antibody production in reaction to an antigen. http://www.feinsteininstitute.org/programs-researchers/immunology/immunocytes-cytokine-biology/

immunoglobulin (ig): Proteins that function as antibodies and bind to antigens. http://www.ebioscience.com/knowledge-center/antigen/immunoglobulin.htm

immunome (cellular): Immune cell subset phenotype and activation/functional status. Used to predict whether a patient will respond to immunotherapy. https://www.frontiersin.org/articles/10.3389/fimmu.2019.01767/full?utm_source=F-AAE&utm_medium=EMLF&utm_campaign=MRK_1064098_35_Immuno_20190808_arts_A

immunosenescence: Age-associated immune change, notably with a reduction in peripheral blood naive cells, and a relative increase of memory cells, along with the inflammatory changes that accompany aging, so-called "inflammaging". https://www.frontiersin.org/articles/10.3389/fimmj.2019.02247/full?utm_source=F-AAE&utm_medium=EMLF&utm_campaign=MRK_1111535_35_Immuno_20191001_arts_A

immunosuppression: Suppression of the immune response. http://emedicine.medscape.com/article/432316-overview

immunotherapy: Prevention or treatment of disease with substances that stimulate the immune response. Blocking the shut-off of the immune response. Anticancer vaccines. https://www.mdanderson.org/treatment-options/immunotherapy.html http://journal.frontiersin.org/article/10.3389/fimmu.2016.00621/

full?utm_source=newsletter&utm_medium=email&utm_campaign=Immunology-w1-2017 http://journal.frontiersin.org/article/10.3389/fimmu.2016.00621/ full?utm_source=newsletter&utm_medium=email&utm_campaign=Immunology-w1-2017 http://www.mdedge.com/jcso/article/135689/gastroenterology/meeting-potential-immunotherapy-new-targets-provide-rational/pdf?channel=213 http://journal.frontiersin.org/article/10.3389/fimmu.2017.00555/full?utm_source=F-AAE&utm_medium=EMLF&utm_campaign=MRK_275249_35_Immuno_20170518_arts_A https://www.frontiersin.org/articles/10.3389/fimmu.2018.00384/full?utm_source=F-AAE&utm_medium=EMLF&utm_campaign=MRK_571163_35_

implantation: The sperm fertilizes (fuses with) the egg (ovum) in the fallopian tube. The fertilized egg then migrates from the fallopian tube into the uterus at a specific time, when the endometrium is most receptive, and attaches to and burrows into the uterine lining.

imprinting (genomic imprinting): The process by which only the copy of a gene from one parent gets switched on in an offspring. https://www.genome.gov/27532724/ https://ghr.nlm.nih.gov/primer/inheritance/updimprinting

induced pluripotent stem cells (IPS): Cells from an adult human that have been reprogrammed into an embryonic-like state. http://stemcells.nih.gov/info/basics/pages/basics10.aspx http://www.nature.com/news/japanese-man-is-first-to-receive-reprogrammed-stem-cells-from-another-person-1.21730?WT.ec_id=NEWS-20170330&spMailingID=53740049&sp https://www.nature.com/articles/d41586-019-00656-2?utm_source=Nature+Briefing&utm_campaign=fb45cec6f6-briefing-dy-20190225&utm_medium=email&utm_term=0_c9dfd39373-fb45cec6f6-42544483

infarct: Cutoff of blood supply causing tissue death, resulting in a scarred area. http://www.omicsonline.org/biomarkers-in-acute-myocardial-infarction-2155-9880.1000222.pdf

infection: Invasion of foreign organisms, such as bacteria or viruses, into the body. http://www.ph.ucla.edu/epi/faculty/detels/epi220/detels_agents.pdf

inflammaging: Increasing chronic, sterile, low-grade inflammation seen as aging progresses. Increased numbers of peripheral immune molecules in older people, with relevance to cognition and age-related disease. https://www.frontiersin.org/articles/10.3389/fimmu.2020.02045/full?utm_source=F-AAE&utm_medium=EMLF&utm_campaign=MRK_1429095_35_Immuno_20200910_arts_A https://www.nature.com/articles/s41574-018-0059-4 https://pubmed.ncbi.nlm.nih.gov/25417146/

inflammation: The body's response to infection or injury, including redness, swelling and heat. The specific responses are geared to killing the infectious agent and repairing the damaged tissue. http://journal.frontiersin.org/article/10.3389/fimmu.2017.00017/full?utm_source=newsletter&utm_medium=email&utm_campaign=Immunology-w4-2017

influenza: Contagious respiratory illness caused by influenza virus. http://journals.lww.com/epidem/Abstract/2015/11000/Review_Article___The_Fraction_of_Influenza_Virus.13.aspx http://www.cdc.gov/mmwr/volumes/65/rr/rr6505a1.htm

information technology (IT): Computerized paperless data keeping, analysis and transmission. http://www.intel.com/content/www/us/en/healthcare-it/collaborative-care.html?cid=sem43700013297809532&intel_term=technology+for+healthcare&gclid=Cj0KEQjw6am-BRCTk4WZhLfd4-oBEiQA3ydA3lK6NZjCN51AIK72GMKucyGNX297Xgy6h66th96XBw-caAhYO8P8HAQ&gclsrc=aw.ds

inhibins: Peptides made in granulosa cells of ovarian follicles that inhibit secretion of follicle stimulating hormone (FSH). http://www.medicinenet.com/script/main/art.asp?articlekey=22571 http://press.endocrine.org/doi/abs/10.1210/endo-124-1-552

insomnia: Sleeplessness.

insulin: Polypeptide hormone, produced by the beta cells of the islets of Langerhans in the pancreas, that regulates blood glucose. http://onlinelibrary.wiley.com/doi/10.1002/bip.20734/full

insulin resistance: Lowered level of response to insulin. http://emedicine.medscape.com/article/122501-overview

integrin: A receptor glycoprotein on a cell surface involved in the adhesion of the cell to other cells such as T-cells. https://www.ncbi.nlm.nih.gov/books/NBK26867/

intelligence: Ability to acquire and apply knowledge and skills. https://www.lexico.com/en/definition/intelligence

interferon: A protein that can inhibit virus replication. https://www.drugs.com/drug-class/interferons.html http://journal.frontiersin.org/article/10.3389/fimmu.2017.00062/full?utm_source=newsletter&utm_medium=email&utm_campaign=Immunology-w7-2017

interstitial cystitis: Painful Bladder Syndrome (PBS). http://emedicine.medscape.com/article/2055505-overview

interstitial space: Small, narrow, fluid containing space between tissues. https://www.ncbi.nlm.nih.gov/pmc/articles/PMC3139075/ https://www.thefreedictionary.com/interstitial+space

interstitium: Fluid-filled interstitial space draining to lymph nodes, supported by a network of collagen bundles. Visualized by laser endomicroscopy in relation to the extrahepatic bile duct, and other tissues that are subject to intermittent compression, including the submucosa of the gastrointestinal tract, and the urinary bladder. https://www.nature.com/articles/s41598-018-23062-6

intrauterine environment: The environment in which the growing fetus lives.

intrauterine growth retardation (IUGR): Fetal growth restriction. http://www.uptodate.com/contents/fetal-growth-restriction-evaluation-and-management

ischemia: Inadequate blood supply to an organ, resulting in inadequate oxygenation.

Kaposi's sarcoma: Malignancy with cutaneous lesions caused by HHV8: human herpesvirus 8. Tends to occur in immunosuppressed individuals, notably those with AIDS (Autoimmune Deficiency Syndrome). http://emedicine.medscape.com/article/279734-overview

keratoplasty: Conductive keratoplasty (CK). Eye surgery utilizing radio frequency energy to change the shape of the cornea.

killer cell: Natural killer (**NK**) cells are derived from hematopoietic stem cells in bone marrow. They kill cancer cells by secreting **perforins** (cytolytic proteins) and **granzymes** (proteases: enzymes that catalyze degradation of protein). https://www.ncbi.nlm.nih.gov/pmc/articles/PMC4346487/ https://en.wikipedia.org/wiki/Granzyme http://medical-dictionary.thefreedictionary.com/perforin http://www.dictionary.com/browse/protease http://journal.frontiersin.org/article/10.3389/fimmu.2016.00492/full http://journal.frontiersin.org/article/10.3389/fimmu.2017.00293/full?utm_source=newsletter&utm_medium=email&utm_campaign=Immunology-w12-2017 http://journal.frontiersin.org/article/10.3389/fimmu.2017.00683/full?utm_source=F-AAE&utm_medium=EMLF&utm_campaign=MRK_307979_35_Immuno_20170622_arts_A http://journal.frontiersin.org/article/10.3389/fimmu.2017.00760/full?utm_source=F-AAE&utm_medium=EMLF&utm_campaign=MRK_320984_35_Immuno_20170706_arts_A http://journal.frontiersin.org/article/10.3389/fimmu.2017.00930/full?utm_source=F-AAE&utm_medium=EMLF&utm_campaign=MRK_352999_35_Immuno_20170808_arts_A http://journal.frontiersin.org/article/10.3389/fimmu.2017.00774/full?utm_source=F-AAE&utm_medium=EMLF&utm_campaign=MRK_333189_35_Immuno_20170720_arts_A http://journal.frontiersin.org/article/10.3389/fimmu.2017.01061/full?utm_source=F-AAE&utm_medium=EMLF&utm_campaign=MRK_398354_35_Immuno_20170921_arts_A

kinase: Enzyme important in the carbohydrate metabolism and energy output of cells. **Protein-Tyrosine Kinases (PTKs)** regulate signaling in the cell. If PTK signaling is disrupted, malignant transformation of the cell can result. http://www.ncbi.nlm.nih.gov/pubmed/10966463 http://www.sciencedirect.com/science/article/pii/S1043661813001771 https://www.empr.com/news/vitrakvi-larotrectinib-advanced-solid-tumors-ntrk-gene-fusion-approval/article/816725/?utm_source=newsletter&utm_medium=email&utm_campaign=mpr-dailydose-cp-20181129&cpn=obgyn_all%2cobgyn_md%2ccambia_august2018&hmS

labor: Period from the onset of regular uterine contractions with dilatation and effacement of the cervix and descent of the fetus through the birth canal culminating in delivery of the baby.

lactic acidosis: Increased plasma lactate. See Chapter 8, "How to Diagnose and Treat Delirium" by Haiban Yin. www.careoftheolderperson.com http://emedicine.medscape.com/article/167027-overview

lactose intolerance: Inability to digest lactose, a disaccharide in milk made up of glucose and galactose. http://emedicine.medscape.com/article/187249-overview

laparoscopy: A minimally invasive surgical technique in which a fiberoptic telescope (laparoscope) is introduced into the abdominal cavity through a small incision near the lower margin of the umbilicus.

laser: Light Amplification by Stimulated Emission of Radiation. A narrow, often powerful, beam of light which does not spread and is monochromatic. This is a directed light beam, not nuclear radiation. http://www.azooptics.com/Article.aspx?ArticleID=44 http://www.nature.com/articles/s41551-016-0008?WT.mc_id=EMI_NBME_1701_LAUNCHISSUE_PORTFOLIO&spMailingID=53217285&spUserID=MTc3MDI4ODk5NQS2&spJobID=1083253126&spReportId=MTA4MzI1MzEyNgS2

leptin: Hormone produced by adipocytes involved in fat storage regulation. Acts on hypothalamus to suppress appetite. http://www.sciencedirect.com/science/article/pii/S0083672905710128

leukemia: Malignant form of white blood cells in the blood stream, commonly arising from the bone marrow. http://www.ncbi.nlm.nih.gov/pmc/articles/PMC3396664/

libido: Sexual drive. See Chapter 35, "After Menopause" by Ronald M. Caplan. www.careoftheolderperson.com https://en.wikipedia.org/wiki/Flibanserin http://www.medscape.com/viewarticle/871481?nlid=110609_2581&src=WNL_mdplsnews_161111_mscpedit_obgy&uac=66536PR&spon=16&impID=1232827&faf=1 https://www.fda.gov/news-events/press-announcements/fda-approves-new-treatment-hypoactive-sexual-desire-disorder-premenopausal-women http://www.addyi.com

life: The capacity to metabolize, grow, reproduce, function and change (adapt). The classic vital functions to assess continuing life are brain activity, respiration and cardiac activity. The **vital organs** without which life cannot be sustained are the brain, heart, lungs, liver and kidneys. https://www.google.com/search?rlz=1C1CHBF_enUS821US821&sxsrf=ALeKk007mA8gEJfS83a8KXD_XDCjMxHuOg%3A1600519500079&ei=TP1lX_2yBK-xytMPyqa7yAo&q=life+definition&oq=+life+definition&gs_lcp=CgZwc3ktYWIQARgAMgwIABCxAxBDEYQ-QEyBggAEAcQHjIGC

life expectancy: The age to which a person or a selected population group might live. See Chapter 1, "Introduction" by Jose Morais. www.careoftheolderperson.com https://www.zionmarketresearch.com/report/home-healthcare-market http://science.sciencemag.org/content/360/6396/1459 http://onlinelibrary.wiley.com/doi/10.1002/sres.2420/full http://www.cdc.gov/nchs/data/hus/2011/022.pdf http://www.statcan.gc.ca/tables-tableaux/sum-som/l01/cst01/health26-eng.htm http://www.cdc.gov/nchs/data/databriefs/db267.pdf http://mdlinx.pdr.net/internal-medicine/news-article.cfm/6986115/?utm_source=in-house&utm_medium=message&utm_campaign=mh-im-dec16 http://journals.plos.org/plosbiology/article?id=10.1371/journal.pbio.2002458#pbio.2002458.ref039 http://science.sciencemag.org/content/360/6396/1459 https://www.cdc.gov/nchs/data/hus/2017/027.pdf https://www.jwatch.org/fw114817/2018/11/30/us-life-expectancy-down-overdose-and-suicide-rates?query=pfwTOC&jwd=000012066693&jspc=OBG

ligand: Molecule or atom that binds to a receptor (receiving protein molecule) See "Receptor Site". https://www.news-medical.net/life-sciences/Ligands-An-Overview.aspx

lipofuscin: Brown-yellow lipid containing residues of lysosomal digestion. Considered to be a "wear and tear" pigment. See Chapter 16, "Critical Care of the Older Person" by Astrid F. Pilgrim, Michael R. Pinsky. https://en.wikipedia.org/wiki/Lipofuscin#:~:text=Lipofuscin%20is%20the%20name%20given,nerve%20cells%2C%20and%20ganglion%20cells.

liposuction: Surgical removal of fat by suction.

liquid biopsy: Blood testing for circulating tumor DNA (ctDNA). Identifies cancer mutations useful as biomarkers, many associated with targeted drug. http://www.ncbi.nlm.nih.gov/pmc/articles/PMC4356857/ http://www.nature.com/nrclinonc/posters/liquidbiopsies/nrclinonc_liquidbiopsies_poster_web.pdf http://www.nature.com/news/liquid-biopsies-success-highlights-power-of-combining-basic-and-clinical-research-1.21883?WT.ec_id=NATURE-20170427&spMailingID=53937339& https://www.nature.com/articles/

s41551-017-0065?WT.mc_id=EMI_NBME_1704_APRILISSUE_PORTFOLIO&spMailingID
=53957850&spUserID=MTc3MDI4ODk5NQS

low density lipoprotein (LDL): Complex of lipids and proteins that transports cholesterol in the blood. Significant factor in the formation of arteriosclerotic plaques. http://www.ncbi. nlm.nih.gov/pubmed/10073963

lung cancer: Malignant tumor in the lung. Major cause of cancer deaths. Predominant type is non–small cell lung cancer (**NSCLC**), strongly linked to tobacco smoking. https:// cancerstaging.org/references-tools/quickreferences/Documents/LungMedium. pdf https://www.ncbi.nlm.nih.gov/pmc/articles/PMC3864624/ https://www.ncbi. nlm.nih.gov/pmc/articles/PMC4367711/ https://www.ncbi.nlm.nih.gov/pmc/ articles/PMC5107578/ http://www.jtcvsonline.org/article/S0022-5223(17)31171-6/ fulltext#sec1.6 https://www.frontiersin.org/articles/10.3389/fimmu.2020.01996/ full?utm_source=F-AAE&utm_medium=EMLF&utm_campaign=MRK_1407965_35_ Immuno_2020082

luteinizing hormone (LH): Secreted by the anterior pituitary, surges prior to ovulation. Acts on the ovary. http://emedicine.medscape.com/article/2089268-overview

lyme disease: Tick-borne illness caused by Borrelia burgdorferi. Other tick-borne illnesses include babesiosis, anaplasmosis, ehrlichiosis, and Rocky Mountain Spotted Fever. http://www. ncbi.nlm.nih.gov/pmc/articles/PMC3542482/

lymph node: Small and bean shaped, lymph nodes are present throughout the body. They are composed of lymphoid tissue, and are connected by lymph channels. The lymphatic system is important in the immune response, in fighting infection. Cancerous cells can enter the lymphatic system and drain to lymph nodes, enlarging them. Cancer surgery often involves the removal of affected lymph nodes, or lymph nodes that are likely to be affected by a cancer. https://www.boundless.com/physiology/textbooks/boundless-anatomy-and-physiology-textbook/lymphatic-system-20/lymph-cells-and-tissues-193/ lymph-nodes-963-3100/

lymphocyte: A form of white blood cell. B cells and T cells are two main types. http://www.ncbi. nlm.nih.gov/pubmedhealth/PMHT0022042/

lymphoma: A solid malignant tumor often composed of cells that resemble lymphocytes. Can arise at various sites within the body and invade the bloodstream. http://www.blood-journal.org/content/125/1/22

Lynch syndrome: Autosomal dominant inherited predisposition for colon and endometrial cancers. https://www.ncbi.nlm.nih.gov/pmc/articles/PMC2933058/ https://www.sgo.org/ wp-content/uploads/2016/10/2016-SGO-Genetics-Toolkit3.pdf

lysosomes: Organelles in the cell containing enzymes that degrade biologic polymers including proteins, carbohydrates and lipids. https://www.ncbi.nlm.nih.gov/books/NBK9953/

machine learning: How computers learn from data. Intersection of statistics and computing algorithms. https://www.ncbi.nlm.nih.gov/pmc/articles/PMC5831252/ https://www.sciencedirect.com/science/article/pii/S0933365717300009X https://www.techemergence.com/ machine-learning-in-pharma-medicine/ https://www.healthcareitnews.com/projects/ ai-and-machine-learning?mkt_tok=eyJpIjoiWVRJNE5qTmpPRE01WmpabSIsInQiOiJCckta VzljSVRpVVpWQ3FYa2lEazc1WHlQSGc5bUV3YXlwTFVtbEdvM2RjSVY

macrophage: A large phagocytic white blood cell. http://www.cell.com/immunity/fulltext/ S1074-7613(14)00235-0

macular degeneration: Deterioration of the macula, the area surrounding the fovea near the center of the retina in the eye. https://www.ncbi.nlm.nih.gov/pmc/articles/PMC3732788/ https://www.nature.com/articles/nbt.4114.epdf?referrer_access_token=8BtrAvy5kx0RIQx VHmwBfNRgN0jAjWeI9jnR3ZoTv0PJSqIFs8CVMGLKXeHOLTvVGIDHNZm

malnutrition: Improper intake and processing of foodstuffs. See Chapter 10, "Could My Patient Be Malnourished?" by José A. Morais. www.careoftheolderperson.com https://www.ncbi. nlm.nih.gov/pubmed/16782522

mammography: Xray breast imaging. http://emedicine.medscape.com/article/346529-overview http:// www.jwatch.org/na42993/2016/12/13/when-stop-surveillance-mammography-older-breast-cancer?query=etoc_jwwomen&jwd=000012066693&jspc=OBG

MAO inhibitors: Monoamine oxidase inhibitors, sometimes still used in the treatment of depression. Monoamine oxidase enzymes catalase oxidation and inactivation of monoamine neurotransmitters, including dopamine, noradrenaline, adrenaline and serotonin. http://www.webmd.com/depression/symptoms-depressed-anxiety-12/antidepressants

mediastinum: Space in the thorax between the pleural sacs, notably containing the heart and its great vessels. https://www.youtube.com/watch?v=2POIlBe2xR4

medulla (oblongata): Part of the brain in the brainstem that controls involuntary activities necessary for life. https://www.neuroscientificallychallenged.com/blog/know-your-brain-medulla-oblongata

meiosis: Cell division resulting in cells (gametes) with a single set of chromosomes, half the number of chromosomes present in the parent cell. https://www.khanacademy.org/science/biology/cellular-molecular-biology/meiosis/a/phases-of-meiosis

melanoma: Tumor of melanin-forming cells. http://www.medicaljournals.se/acta/content/?doi=10.2340/00015555-2035&html=1 https://www.cell.com/cell/fulltext/S0092-8674(17)30952-2

menopause: Cessation of menses. See Chapter 35, "After Menopause" by Ronald M. Caplan. www.careoftheolderperson.com https://www.ncbi.nlm.nih.gov/pmc/articles/PMC3285482/

menstruation: Blood and shedding endometrium from the uterus beginning approximately 14 days after ovulation in a non-pregnant cycle. https://www.ncbi.nlm.nih.gov/pubmed/16160098

MERS (Middle East respiratory syndrome–related coronavirus): First reported in Saudi Arabia in 2012. https://www.niaid.nih.gov/diseases-conditions/covid-19

metabolic acidosis: Increase in plasma acidity. Excess production of acid with inadequate buffer, bicarbonate, to neutralize it. Insufficient renal excretion of acid. http://www.nature.com/nrneph/journal/v6/n5/abs/nrneph.2010.33.html

metabolic syndrome: Central (abdominal) obesity, hypertension and insulin resistance. High levels of triglycerides, low levels of HDL. http://www.ncbi.nlm.nih.gov/pmc/articles/PMC3966331/

metabolism: Molecular chemical reactions within living tissue. http://www.biology-pages.info/C/CellularRespiration.html

metabolite: Substance created, along with energy, by metabolism. https://www.cancer.gov/publications/dictionaries/cancer-terms/def/metabolite

metabolome: All the molecules in a cell that are the result of metabolism (metabolites). https://www.ncbi.nlm.nih.gov/pmc/articles/PMC4850886/ https://www.nature.com/articles/d41586-021-03062-9

metaplasia: A benign cell change. In a common type, glandular epithelium is transformed into squamous epithelium. https://en.wikipedia.org/wiki/Squamous_metaplasia

metastasis: Cancer cells at a distance from the primary tumor. https://www.nature.com/articles/d41586-018-05445-x?utm_source=briefing-dy&utm_medium=email&utm_campaign=briefing&utm_content=20180618 https://www.cancer.gov/publications/dictionaries/cancer-terms/def/metastasis

metformin: Oral anti-hyperglycemic agent used in Type 2 Diabetes. Decreases hepatic glucose production. Implications in other disease states, weight loss and possibly lifespan. https://www.ncbi.nlm.nih.gov/pmc/articles/PMC3398862/ https://pubmed.ncbi.nlm.nih.gov/31405774/ https://www.frontiersin.org/articles/10.3389/fendo.2021.718942/full

microbiome: Bacteria that inhabit the gut. http://jamanetwork.com/journals/jama/fullarticle/2594788

microglia: Immune, phagocytic, central nervous system (brain and spinal cord) cells implicated in Alzheimer's. https://www.frontiersin.org/articles/10.3389/fimmu.2019.00790/full?utm_source=F-AAE&utm_medium=EMLF&utm_campaign=MRK_973135_35_Immuno_20190425_arts_A

microsurgery: Surgery performed with visualization through a microscope, often involving anastomoses of small blood vessels.

migraine: Vascular headaches involving the blood vessels of the brain. http://www.ncbi.nlm.nih.gov/pmc/articles/PMC3663475/ https://www.jwatch.org/fw113584/2017/11/30/migraine-prevention-two-calcitonin-gene-related-peptide?query=pfwTOC&jwd=000012066693&jspc=OBG http://www.pdr.net/drug-summary/Imitrex-Tablets-sumatriptan-succinate-201 https://www.ncbi.nlm.nih.gov/pubmed/29800211 https://www.thelancet.com/journals/lancet/article/PIIS0140-6736(18)32534-0/fulltext https://www.empr.com/ajovy/drug/34876/ https://www.ptcommunity.com/journal/article/full/2018/10/616/emerging-therapies-patients-difficult-treat-migraine?utm_source=PT_NL_2018-10-16_nsp_v9&utm_campaign=PT+NL+18-10-16&utm_medium=email https://www.empr.com/news/ajovy-migraine-prevention-fremanezumab-vfrm-preventative-migraine/article/796090/?utm_source=newsletter&utm_medium=email&utm_campaign=mpr-promo-20181105&c https://jamanetwork.com/journals/jamaneurology/fullarticle/2681442 https://jamanetwork.com/journals/jamaneurology/fullarticle/2681442 https://onlinelibrary.wiley.com/doi/10.1111/head.13456

MIS-C (multisystem inflammatory syndrome in children): Coincident with COVID-19 pandemic. Clinically similar to **Kawasaki disease**, shock syndrome and toxic shock syndrome. Can present with fever, hypotension, gastrointestinal symptoms, rash and myocarditis. https://www.uptodate.com/contents/coronavirus-disease-2019-covid-19-considerations-in-children

mitochondria: Intracellular organelle in which respiration and energy production occur. http://citeseerx.ist.psu.edu/viewdoc/download?doi=10.1.1.572.8830&rep=rep1&type=pdf http://www.cell.com/cell-metabolism/fulltext/S1550-4131(16)30502-2 http://mdlinx.pdr.net/neurology/news-article.cfm/6907659?utm_source=in-house&utm_medium=message&utm_campaign=medhead https://link.springer.com/article/10.1007/s10815-017-1006-3/fulltext.html?wt_mc=alerts.TOCjournals https://www.deepdyve.com/lp/springer-journal/quantitative-and-qualitative-changes-of-mitochondria-in-human-Gh20vR9aBa?key=bioportfolio

mitosis: Cell division resulting in daughter cells identical to the parent cell. https://www.khanacademy.org/science/biology/cellular-molecular-biology/meiosis/a/phases-of-meiosis

mobility: Ability to move freely and easily. See Chapter 9, "Why Does My Patient Have Gait and Balance Disorders?" by Olivier Beauchet. www.careoftheolderperson.com https://www.mayoclinic.org/diseases-conditions/movement-disorders/symptoms-causes/syc-20363893 https://en.oxforddictionaries.com/definition/mobility

mohs surgery: Surgery in which thin layers of cancer-containing skin are stepwise removed and examined microscopically, until only cancer-free tissue remains. http://emedicine.medscape.com/article/2212475-overview

molecular profiling (of cancer patients): The use of Next Generation Sequencing (NGS) gives rise to personalized therapy with selective genome and immune-targeted drugs (see "Precision Medicine", "Next Generation Sequencing (NGS)"). https://www.nature.com/articles/s41591-019-0407-5

monoclonal antibody: An antibody that will go to a specific receptor site. "Monoclonal" refers to the fact that the antibody protein is derived from one clone of cells, all of which are identical. A particular neutralizing IgG1 monoclonal antibody known as bamlanivimab, directed against the spike protein of SARS-CoV-2 virus that causes COVID-19, received an Emergency Use Authorization in the USA from the FDA in 2020. Has not been effective against the omicron variant. http://www.ncbi.nlm.nih.gov/pmc/articles/PMC4491443/

Montreal Cognitive Assessment (MOCA): Test to detect mild cognitive impairment and Alzheimer's disease. See Chapter 5, "Doctor, My Spouse Is Getting Forgetful" by Serge Gauthier. www.careoftheolderperson.com http://dementia.ie/images/uploads/site-images/MoCA-Test-English_7_1.pdf http://www.mocatest.org/ https://www.sciencedirect.com/topics/neuroscience/montreal-cognitive-assessment

motoric cognitive risk syndrome (MCR): Predementia syndrome combining cognitive complaint and slow gait. http://biomedgerontology.oxfordjournals.org/content/71/8/1081

MRI (magnetic resonance imaging): An advanced imaging technique that uses a powerful magnet to alter polarity. https://onlinelibrary.wiley.com/doi/full/10.1002/jmri.23642

MSG: Monosodium glutamate. http://www.mayoclinic.org/healthy-lifestyle/nutrition-and-healthy-eating/expert-answers/monosodium-glutamate/faq-20058196

multiple myeloma: Plasma cell (a type of white blood cell derived from B cell) malignancy. Anemia and osteolytic (bone reabsorbing) skeletal lesions usually present. A monoclonal (M) protein can usually be detected in the blood serum and urine. https://www.mdedge.com/oncologypractice/article/154492/multiple-myeloma/crb-410-update-multiple-myeloma-response-rates?oc_slh=1de3dcf7eb6395af6b796baf8538c https://www.ncbi.nlm.nih.gov/pmc/articles/PMC5223450/ https://www.cancer.gov/publications/dictionaries/cancer-terms?cdrid=46230 https://www.cancer.gov/publications/dictionaries/cancer-terms?cdrid=45810

mutation: Abnormal recombinations of the chromosomes. Permanent alteration in DNA sequence. Alteration in a genome that may or may not be harmful to the individual. http://www.nature.com/scitable/definition/recombination-226 http://www.ncbi.nlm.nih.gov/pubmed/23266571 https://academic.oup.com/annonc/article/29/1/30/4616649

myelin: Insulating sheath around nerve fibers. http://www.news-medical.net/health/Myelin-Function.aspx

myelitis: Inflammation of the spinal cord. https://en.wikipedia.org/wiki/Myelitis#:~:text=Myelitis%20is%20inflammation%20of%20the,as%20paralysis%20and%20sensory%20loss.

myelodysplastic syndrome (MDS): Bone marrow cancer with insufficient presence of normal blood cells, and presence of abnormal blood cells. https://www.cancer.gov/publications/dictionaries/cancer-terms/def/myelodysplastic-syndrome

myeloperoxidase (MPO): Enzyme in neutrophils linked to cardiovascular disease. http://www.ncbi.nlm.nih.gov/gene/4353 http://www.ncbi.nlm.nih.gov/pubmed/26567811/

myocardial infarction: Irreversible injury to heart muscle. http://www.clevelandclinicmeded.com/medicalpubs/diseasemanagement/cardiology/acute-myocardial-infarction/ https://arxiv.org/abs/1708.09843

myocardium: Heart muscle. https://www.boundless.com/physiology/textbooks/boundless-anatomy-and-physiology-textbook/cardiovascular-system-the-heart-18/the-heart-172/myocardial-thickness-and-function-867-10251/

myocyte: Heart muscle cell. https://www.sciencedaily.com/releases/2016/04/160421145756.htm

myomectomy: Surgical removal of fibroids from the uterus.

nanotechnology: Engineering of tiny machines, often for the monitoring, prevention and treatment of disease. http://tedx.tumblr.com/post/35204848311/fight-cancer-with-nanotechnology-sylvain-martel http://iopscience.iop.org/journal/0957-4484;jsessionid=3420F74BB331365A7161E71B24C8121C.c4.iopscience.cld.iop.org http://journal.frontiersin.org/article/10.3389/fimmu.2017.00069/full?utm_source=newsletter&utm_medium=email&utm_campaign=Immunology-w6-2017 https://www.nature.com/articles/s41551-017-0029?WT.mc_id=LDN_NBME_1801_FIRSTANNIVERSARY_PORTFOLIO

narrative medicine: Narrative competence. Listening to and understanding related stories, and appropriately responding. http://www.ncbi.nlm.nih.gov/pmc/articles/PMC3034473/

necrosis: Body tissue death. https://www.ncbi.nlm.nih.gov/books/NBK557627/

nephropathy: Kidney disease or damage. http://www.ncbi.nlm.nih.gov/pmc/articles/PMC3084647/ https://en.wikipedia.org/wiki/Kidney_disease

nephrosis: Generally refers to degenerative disease of the renal (kidney) tubules. http://medical-dictionary.thefreedictionary.com/nephrosis

nephrotic syndrome: Excretion of significant amounts of protein in the urine, along with decreased serum albumin (a protein), and edema (swelling due to fluid accumulation). http://emedicine.medscape.com/article/244631-overview

neural tube defect: Birth defect of brain, spine or spinal cord. http://www.ncbi.nlm.nih.gov/pmc/articles/PMC4023229/

neurodegeneration: Progressive loss of brain function associated with aging. https://www.ncbi.nlm.nih.gov/pubmed/30258237

neurodegenerative diseases: Diseases which cause progressive loss of cognitive and/or motor function. https://www.ncbi.nlm.nih.gov/pubmed/23305823 https://www.ncbi.nlm.nih.gov/pubmed/30258237

neurogenesis: Formation of neurons. https://www.nature.com/articles/nature25975 https://www.nature.com/articles/s41591-019-0375-9?utm_source=nm_etoc&utm_medium=email&utm_campaign=toc_41591_25_4&utm_content=20190405&WT.ec_id=NM-201904&sap-outbound-id=A2CA93DADBF79C1C13E7D04CDCA72468DD68FEE3

neuroimmune communication: Interaction between the nervous and immune systems, influencing each other. http://www.nature.com/ni/journal/v18/n2/full/ni.3676.html http://www.nature.com/neuro/journal/v20/n2/full/nn.4496.html

neuromorphic engineering: Designing hardware and physical models of neural and sensory systems. https://www.frontiersin.org/journals/neuroscience/sections/neuromorphic-engineering http://compneuro.uwaterloo.ca/research/nef/overview-of-the-nef.html

neuron: Specialized nervous system cell that can be stimulated and conducts impulses. http://www.ncbi.nlm.nih.gov/books/NBK21535/ https://www.nature.com/articles/s41593-018-0205-2.epdf?shared_access_token=60bklwIRkphHPPY3R_u069RgN0jAjWel9jn-R3ZoTv0M_ZnMCyHI8KbNyV63mNxsudkNYBmXFIhQDgOHiquMVMmq6S_Ta_jrenQf

neutrophil: A white blood cell containing granules that are enzyme containing sacs. http://jem.rupress.org/content/210/7/1283.full

next generation sequencing (NGS): Rapid (high throughput) DNA sequencing. Used for molecular profiling of tumor samples in order to individualize treatment. https://www.ncbi.nlm.nih.gov/pmc/articles/PMC5808190/ https://www.ncbi.nlm.nih.gov/pmc/articles/PMC4494749/

nicotinamide riboside (NR): A form of Vitamin B3 (nicotinic acid, Niacin). Converts to **NAD**, Nicotinamide Adenine Dinucleotide, a coenzyme in cells that is involved in energy metabolism. http://www.ctl.cornell.edu/events/ctvf12/Sauve.pdf http://jpet.aspetjournals.org/content/324/3/883.full

nitrites: Ester or salt of nitrous acid. Vasodilator. http://circ.ahajournals.org/content/117/16/2151

NNT: Number Needed to Treat. Epidemiological measure of the effectiveness of a medical intervention. The number of patients who need a specific treatment to prevent one additional bad outcome. See Chapter 19, "Stroke Prevention in the Elderly" by Liam Durcan. https://patient.info/doctor/numbers-needed-to-treat#:~:text=The%20number%20needed%20to%20treat,the%20adverse%20outcome%20being%20prevented.

nuclear power: Energy produced by atomic reaction. http://www.nei.org/Knowledge-Center/How-Nuclear-Reactors-Work

nuclear waste: Radioactive byproducts usually from operation of a nuclear reactor. http://www.nrc.gov/reading-rm/doc-collections/fact-sheets/radwaste.html http://www.nrc.gov/reading-rm/doc-collections/fact-sheets/radwaste.html

nuclease: Enzyme that catalyzes the cleavage of phosphodiester bonds between nucleotides. http://www.nature.com/onc/journal/v21/n58/full/1206135a.html?foxtrotcallback=true https://www.ncbi.nlm.nih.gov/pubmed/24690881 https://www.ncbi.nlm.nih.gov/pubmed/24690881

nucleic acid: Substance found in the cytoplasm of cells, as well as in chromosomes, and in viruses. Four specific nucleic acids: adenine (A), cytosine (C), guanine (G) and thymine (T) are arranged in pairs on each rung of the ladder of DNA. They code the sequences of amino acids that make up proteins. http://www.rsc.org/Education/Teachers/Resources/cfb/nucleicacids.htm

nucleoside: Compound found in DNA or RNA made up of a purine or pyrimidine (nitrogenous) base linked to a sugar. Lacks the phosphate group(s) of a nucleotide. Nucleosides used as antiviral and anticancer agents. https://www.google.com/search?sxsrf=ALeKk01w3ybsI878-V5kuWH4SuYetqPYrg:1593538669885&q=Dictionary&stick=H4sIAAAAAAAAAONQesSoyi3w8sc9YSmZ https://www.diffen.com/difference/Nucleoside_vs_Nucleotide

nucleosome: The basic structural unit of chromatin. https://en.wikipedia. org/wiki/Chromatin https://www.nature.com/scitable/topicpage/ dna-packaging-nucleosomes-and-chromatin-310

nucleotide: Building block (subunit) of nucleic acid. Nitrogenous base plus ribose or deoxyribose plus one or more phosphate groups. Malfunction can lead to cancer. https://en.wikipedia. org/wiki/Nucleotide

nucleus: A central structure, surrounded by its own membrane, in the cell. The nucleus contains the chromosomes. https://micro.magnet.fsu.edu/cells/nucleus/nucleus.html https:// micro.magnet.fsu.edu/cells/nucleus/nucleus.html

nursing: Breastfeeding.

obesity: More than 20% above expected body weight; Body Mass Index (BMI) of 30 or more. http://www.ncbi.nlm.nih.gov/pubmed/22171945 https://www.ncbi.nlm.nih.gov/ pubmed/27386756 http://www.cell.com/cell/fulltext/S0092-8674(16)30213-6 https:// www.frontiersin.org/articles/10.3389/fimmu.2017.01745/full?utm_source=F-AAE&utm_ medium=EMLF&utm_campaign=MRK_491010_35_I https://jamanetwork.com/ journals/jama/article-abstract/2685153?utm_source=silverchair&utm_campaign=jama_ network&utm_content=weekly_highlights&cmp=1&utm_medium=email

oncologist: Physician who specializes in the treatment of cancer. http://www.oncologypractice. com/jcso/specialty-focus/lung/single-article-page/genomic-oncology-moving-beyond- the-tip-of-the-iceberg/0a952f61278bdd07e9d7db4e7c6d1fcb.html

ophthalmic nerve: Branch of the trigeminal nerve that gives sensory fibers to the ciliary muscle of the eye, lacrimal gland, eyelids, forehead and mucous membrane of the nose. http:// www.ncbi.nlm.nih.gov/pubmed/11842844

opioid: Naturally occurring and synthetic potentially addictive substances that act on specific (opioid) receptors to produce effects including pain relief. Major cause of drug abuse, addiction and death. https://www.drugabuse.gov/drugs-abuse/opioids https://www. drugabuse.gov/drugs-abuse/opioids/opioid-crisis https://www.fda.gov/Drugs/ DrugSafety/InformationbyDrugClass/ucm337066.htm

osteoblast: Cell that synthesizes bone. www.nature.com/articles/boneres20169

osteoclast: Cell that reabsorbs bone. See Chapter 35, "After Menopause" by Ronald M. Caplan. www.careoftheolderperson.com http://www.ncbi.nlm.nih.gov/pubmed/1873485 https:// www.nature.com/articles/s41413-018-0040-9

osteopenia: Reduced bone mass. Less severe than osteoporosis. medicine.medscape.com/ article/330598-overview

osteoporosis: Reduced bone mass due to depletion of calcium and bone protein. https://www. karger.com/Article/FullText/431091 http://www.thelancet.com/journals/lancet/ article/PIIS0140-6736(17)31613-6/fulltext https://mydigimag.rrd.com/publication/?i=4 70718&ver=html5&p=30&utm_source=PT+eTOC+2018-02+prospect+no+spons&utm_ campaign=PT1802_Digital_Edition_Alert&utm_medium=email#{"page":"30" https:// www.medscape.com/viewarticle/914567?src=WNL_recnl_190722_MSCPEDIT_obgyn&uac= 66536PR&impID=2036955&faf=1

ovarian cancer: Cancer of the ovary. https://www.ncbi.nlm.nih.gov/pmc/articles/PMC5365187/ https://www.uptodate.com/contents/screening-for-ovarian-cancer

ovary: The primary female sex organ. Almond shaped, 3 centimeters long. Two ovaries, one on either side of the uterus in the pelvis. http://emedicine.medscape.com/article/1949171- overview http://www.fertstert.org/article/S0015-0282(17)31879-4/fulltext?elsca1=etoc& amp;elsca2=email&elsca3=0015-0282_201710_108_4_&elsca4=Obstetrics%20 and%20Gyn https://www.fertstert.org/article/S0015-0282(18)31744-8/ fulltext?dgcid=raven_jbs_etoc_email https://www.frontiersin.org/articles/10.3389/ fimmu.2018.02009/full?utm_source=F-AAE&utm_medium=EMLF&utm_campaign= MRK_779779_35_Immuno_20180927_arts_A

ovulation: During the menstrual cycle, several fluid filled follicles, each containing an ovum, develop. One becomes the dominant follicle. The other follicles regress. At midcycle, the dominant follicle ruptures, releasing the egg, which is then picked up by the fimbria of the fallopian tube. https://www.ncbi.nlm.nih.gov/books/NBK279054/

ovum: (plural: ova) The oocyte. The egg. A single cell present in the female ovary that eventually can be fertilized by a single sperm cell from the male. The ovum before fertilization has only 23 chromosomes. These pair with the 23 chromosomes from the spermatozoon to create a genetically new individual with 46 chromosomes. http://www.theodora.com/anatomy/the_ovum.html

palliative care: Team support system of enhanced physical, psychosocial and spiritual quality of life in the face of life-threatening illness. Prevention and relief of suffering and pain. Affirmation of life, and regarding dying as a normal process. http://www.who.int/cancer/palliative/definition/en/ https://www.surgical.theclinics.com/article/S0039-6109(19)30088-X/pdf https://www.sciencedirect.com/science/article/pii/S0039610919300891?dgcid=author

Papanicolaou smear: Cells in cervical mucus examined microscopically. https://www.google.com/search?q=photographs+of+normal+and+ascus+cells&rlz=1C1CHBF_enUS694US694&espv=2&biw=1745&bih=883&tbm=isch&tbo=u&source=univ&sa=X&ved=0ahUKEwittZaMp57PAhUELyYKHeGjBJcQsAQIGw

parathyroid hormone (PTH): Secreted by parathyroid glands. Regulates blood levels of calcium and phosphorus. http://www.ncbi.nlm.nih.gov/pubmed/19395963

parkinsonism: Parkinson's disease. Chronic, progressive debilitating neurologic condition arising in the basal ganglia of the brain. Loss of dopaminergic cells. Decreased dopamine production in substantia nigra. See Chapter 9, "Why Does My Patient Have Gait and Balance Disorders?" by Olivier Beauchet. www.careoftheolderperson.com http://www.neurobiologyofaging.org/article/S0197-4580(16)30060-4/abstract https://www.nature.com/articles/s41531-017-0015-3?WT.mc_id_EMI_PARKD_1708_PMC&WT.ec_id=INTERNAL&spMailingID=54985332&spUserID=MTc3MDI4ODk https://www.frontiersin.org/articles/10.3389/fneur.2018.00809/full https://jamanetwork.com/journals/jamanetworkopen/fullarticle/2723412?utm_source=silverchair&utm_medium=email&utm_campaign=article_alert-jamanetworkopen&utm_content=etoc&utm_term=030119

PARP: A group of enzymes important in DNA repair. Poly Adenosine diphosphate (ADP) Ribose Polymerase. https://www.sciencedirect.com/science/article/pii/S0923753419386478

PARP inhibitors: Used in BRCA associated breast, ovarian and pancreatic cancer, prostate cancer. https://www.nejm.org/doi/pdf/10.1056/NEJMoa1903387#:~:text=This%20article%20was%20published%20on,2019%2C%20at%20NEJM.org.&text=Patients%20with%20a%20germline%20BRCA1,antitumor%20activity%20in%20this%20population. https://www.hematologyandoncology.net/archives/may-2015/parp-inhibitorsin-ovarian-and-other-cancers/ https://www.fda.gov/drugs/resources-information-approved-drugs/fdaapproves-olaparib-germline-brca-mutated-metastatic-breast-cancer https://www.fda.gov/drugs/drug-approvals-and-databases/fda-approvesolaparib-hrr-gene-mutated-metastatic-castration-resistant-prostate-cancer

pathologist: Physician specializing in the diagnosis of disease by inspecting organs and tumors, both by direct vision and microscopically.

patient-generated health data (PGHD): Wearable monitoring devices. https://pages.mobihealthnews.com/WP-Fitbit-Mediashark-2018-10_LP-Multiplying-the-Value-of-Wearables-and-Patient-Generated-Health-Data2.html?topic=analytics%2C%20mobile%2C%20patientengagement&utm_source=epush&utm_medium=email&utm_campa

PCI: Percutaneous coronary intervention. Coronary angioplasty. Stent introduced by catheter and placed in coronary artery. http://emedicine.medscape.com/article/161446-overview http://emedicine.medscape.com/article/161446-technique

peptide: Two or more amino acids linked together. https://www2.chemistry.msu.edu/faculty/reusch/virttxtjml/protein2.htm

perimenopause: The time shortly before menopause.

peripheral artery occlusive disease: Narrowing and blockage of smaller arteries. **claudication:** Thigh pain with exercise is a symptom. http://emedicine.medscape.com/article/460178-overview

personality type: Psychologic classification of individuals. http://mbtitoday.org/carl-jung-psychological-type/

pessary: Device placed in the vagina for support.

PET scan: Positron Emission Tomography. The person being imaged is given sugar, which is tagged by radioactive isotope. Malignant cells tend to metabolize sugar at a higher rate, because they are actively growing and dividing. The increased radioactive uptake measured at a given site in the body infers that there may be a malignant tumor at that site. http://journals.lww.com/thoracicimaging/Fulltext/2013/01000/Overview_of_Positron_Emission_Tomography,_Hybrid.4.aspx

phagocytosis: The engulfing of a cell fragment or foreign body by a cell. http://www.dictionary.com/browse/phagocytosis

phenotype: The observable properties, characteristics and traits of an organism produced by the interaction of the genotype and the environment. https://en.wikipedia.org/wiki/Phenotype

pheromone: Chemical substance released by an individual that stimulates the behavior of other individuals. http://www.scientificamerican.com/article/are-human-pheromones-real/

phlebitis: Inflammation of the walls of a vein. http://emedicine.medscape.com/article/463256-overview

phytoestrogens: Naturally occurring estrogen-like compounds in plants. http://www.ncbi.nlm.nih.gov/pmc/articles/PMC3074428/

pituitary gland: Endocrine gland attached to the base of the brain that secretes hormones that act on other endocrine glands. http://teachmeanatomy.info/neuro/structures/pituitary-gland/

placenta: Disc-shaped organ that forms in pregnancy, nourishes and supports the developing fetus, and secretes hormones. The surface that is in contact with the mother's uterine wall is composed of many tiny villi. The fetal blood circulates within these villi, which are bathed on their outside by maternal blood from arteries in the uterine wall. Exchange between mother and fetus of nutrients, waste products of metabolism, oxygen and carbon dioxide continuously occurs through the external lining of each villus. After the baby is delivered, the placenta detaches from the wall of the uterus, and is itself delivered. https://www.nichd.nih.gov/about/meetings/2014/Documents/BurtonWashington2014.pdf

plasma (blood): Fluid part of the blood that carries the blood cells. https://www.ncbi.nlm.nih.gov/pubmedhealth/PMHT0022021/

plasmid: Circular molecule of DNA found in bacteria. https://www.nature.com/scitable/definition/plasmid-plasmids-28

platelet: Cell fragment in blood involved in blood clotting. https://www.ouhsc.edu/platelets/platelets/platelets%20intro.html

PMDD: Premenstrual dysphoric disorder. Premenstrual mood and behavioral changes.

PMS: Premenstrual syndrome. Various symptoms just prior to, or with the onset of, a period. May include depression, anxiety, bloating, constipation, diarrhea, breast tenderness, weight gain and headache.

pneumonia: Lung inflammation with congestion. https://www.ncbi.nlm.nih.gov/pmc/articles/PMC4072047/ https://www.ncbi.nlm.nih.gov/pmc/articles/PMC4072047/ https://www.ncbi.nlm.nih.gov/pmc/articles/PMC4072047/

polar body: Small cells resulting from two meiotic divisions of the oocyte. Contain the same DNA as the oocyte. http://www.ncbi.nlm.nih.gov/pmc/articles/PMC3164815/

poliomyelitis: Infectious disease caused by the poliovirus that can result in paresthesias, meningitis and paralysis. Widespread use of effective vaccines has largely eliminated this disease from many societies. https://www.cdc.gov/polio/what-is-polio/index.htm#:~:text=Related%20Pages,move%20parts%20of%20the%20body). https://www.ncbi.nlm.nih.gov/pmc/articles/PMC4212416/

pollution: Presence in, or introduction into, the environment of harmful substances.

polygenic risk score: (Genetic Risk Score) Estimating the risk conferred by a number of DNA variants in genes to result in a disease onset or other outcome. https://jamanetwork.com/journals/jama/fullarticle/2730627?guestAccessKey=6579bb87-9479-4cfd-a93c-d39102a0fb5f&utm_source=silverchair&utm_medium=email&utm_campaign=article_alert-jama&utm_

polymerase chain reaction (PCR): Laboratory technique utilizing short DNA sequences to select a portion of the genome to be amplified. DNA replication enzyme acts on the target DNA sequence, making copies. https://www.genome.gov/genetics-glossary/Polymerase-Chain-Reaction https://www.ncbi.nlm.nih.gov/probe/docs/techpcr/

polyp: Benign growth arising from a stalk. Polyps occur in the interior of the uterus and may protrude out the cervical os. Polyps in the large intestine may be malignant. Polyps can grow on the vocal cords, and other areas.

polypharmacy: Simultaneous use of multiple drugs, more than are medically necessary. See Chapter 34, "Polypharmacy and Deprescribing in the Elderly" by Louise Mallet. www.careoftheolderperson.com https://www.ncbi.nlm.nih.gov/pmc/articles/PMC3864987/ https://jamanetwork.com/journals/jama/fullarticle/2714515?guestAccessKey=06cab 41f-eab9-4441-85a3-53b6c4725e5e&utm_source=silverchair&utm_medium=email&utm_ campaign=article_alert-jama&utm

postmenopausal bleeding: Vaginal bleeding occurring after menopause. https://www.ncbi.nlm.nih.gov/pmc/articles/PMC3951032/

precision medicine: Studying how the genomic variation in an individual or their disease (tumor sample) influences drug response. Identification of the specific mutations in a tumor, so that targeted therapy can be brought to bear. See "Next Generation Sequencing (NGS)". http://stm.sciencemag.org/content/7/300/300ps17.full https://academic.oup.com/annonc/article/29/1/30/4616649

prehabilitation: Process of improving the functional capacity of a patient prior to a surgical procedure. See Chapter 39, "Caring for the Older Person Undergoing Plastic Surgery" by Subhas Gupta, Erin O'Rorke"; Chapter 29, "Diagnosis and Management of Bowel Cancer" by Jessica Holland, Barry J. Stein. www.careoftheolderperson.com https://www.facs.org/quality-programs/strong-for-surgery/patients/prehabilitation#:~:text=Prehabilitation%20is%20defined%20as%20a,place%20physically%20before%20an%20operation.

preimplantation genetic diagnosis (PGD): Chromosomal analysis of the polar body (see "Polar Body"), or of a single embryonic cell. http://emedicine.medscape.com/article/273415-overview

preterm infant: Formerly called prematurity. A baby born before 38 weeks of intrauterine life. http://www.adelaide.edu.au/news/news88982.html

prime editing (genome): Overcomes some of the obstacles of **CRISPR-Cas9**. https://e-tarjome.com/storage/panel/fileuploads/2020-04-18/1587192274_E14737-e-tarjome.pdf

probiotics: Microorganisms, usually bacteria, with health benefits. http://www.medicinenet.com/script/main/art.asp?articlekey=11901

progenitor cell: Activated in tissue repair; differentiate to replace damaged tissue. If signal to differentiate not processed, progenitor cells can keep on reproducing, leading to mutations. http://stemcell.childrenshospital.org/about-stem-cells/adult-somatic-stem-cells-101/what-are-progenitor-cells/

progesterone: A female sex hormone, made in the ovary, prominent in the second half of the menstrual cycle. https://en.wikipedia.org/wiki/Progesterone Shyamala, G., Y.-C. Chou, S. G. Louie, R. C. Guzman, G. H. Smith, and S. Nandi. 2002. Cellular expression of estrogen and progesterone receptors in mammary glands: Regulation by hormones, development and aging. J. Steroid Biochem. Mol. Biol. 80:137–148

progestin: A progesterone-like substance.

programmed cell death: See "Apoptosis" for references.

prokaryote: Single-celled organism without a distinct nucleus and no specialized organelles (except ribosomes). Includes bacteria. http://www.dictionary.com/browse/prokaryote

prolactin: Hormone secreted by the anterior pituitary that stimulates lactation. http://www.ncbi.nlm.nih.gov/pubmed/11015620

prolapse: Downward displacement of an organ. http://emedicine.medscape.com/article/276259-overview

prostaglandins: Group of fatty acids that stimulate contractility of uterine and other smooth muscle. http://www.ncbi.nlm.nih.gov/pmc/articles/PMC3081099/

prostate: Gland located below the bladder and surrounding the urethra in males. Prostatic fluid is secreted via ducts that open into the urethra. http://www.ncbi.nlm.nih.gov/pubmed-health/PMH0072475/ http://www.ncbi.nlm.nih.gov/pmc/articles/PMC4633657/ http://jamanetwork.com/journals/jama/fullarticle/2618352?utm_medium=alert&utm_source=J AMAPublishAheadofPrint&utm_campaign=11-04-2017

prostate cancer: Cancer of the prostate gland. https://www.ncbi.nlm.nih.gov/pubmed/28655021 http://www.nejm.org/doi/full/10.1056/NEJMoa1715546?query=main_nav_lg

protein: A specific sequence of amino acids. Specific proteins are elaborated by specific genes. Proteins have vital functions within the body. They make up the structure of various organs and are involved in their function. They make up the hormones and the enzymes which facilitate chemical reactions in the body. They are involved in immune response. A specific protein, the **mTOR protein**, seems to have a role in aging. **Rapamycin** is one drug that is an mTOR inhibitor. **Metformin** inhibits the mTOR protein indirectly. https://en.wikipedia.org/wiki/Proteome https://www.ncbi.nlm.nih.gov/pmc/articles/PMC3398862/ https://www.ncbi.nlm.nih.gov/pmc/articles/PMC3972801/#:~:text=Rapamycin%20forms%20a%20gain%2Dof,)%20complex%201%20(mTORC1).&text=Only%20mTORC1%20is%20acutely%20sensitive%20to%20inhibition%20by%20rapamycin.

proteomics: The study of all the proteins in the body, how they function and interact. http://proteomics.cancer.gov/whatisproteomics

proteostasis: Dysfunction in protein homeostasis that can be seen in aging people. https://www.nature.com/articles/s41580-019-0101-y

proton pump inhibitors: Drugs that inhibit acid secretion by gastric parietal cells. Used in gastroesophageal reflux disease (**GERD**). https://www.ncbi.nlm.nih.gov/pmc/articles/PMC5221858/

PTK: Protein-tyrosine kinase. Regulates signaling in the cell. http://www.ncbi.nlm.nih.gov/pubmed/9393984

pulmonary embolus: PE. Blood clot in the lung. http://emedicine.medscape.com/article/300901-overview

quantum computing: Harnesses quantum mechanics and states including superposition and entanglement to enhance computational function. https://www.ibm.com/quantum-computing/what-is-quantum-computing/ https://www.sciencealert.com/quantum-computers

quantum mechanics: The motion and interaction of subatomic particles. Deals in statistical probability rather than certainty. https://plato.stanford.edu/entries/qm/ https://www.livescience.com/33816-quantum-mechanics-explanation.html

qubit: Basic unit of quantum information. A two-state system (see "Superposition"). https://www.quantum-inspire.com/kbase/what-is-a-qubit/

radiation: Emission of energy as electromagnetic waves or as moving subatomic particles, especially high energy particles that cause ionization. Ionizing radiation has enough energy to remove electrons from the orbit of an atom, causing the atom to be charged (ionized). http://www.who.int/ionizing_radiation/about/what_is_ir/en/

receptor site: Distinctively shaped area on a cell surface, designed to receive a specific substance. http://www.merckmanuals.com/professional/clinical-pharmacology/pharmacodynamics/drug%E2%80%93receptor-interactions https://www.empr.com/news/vitrakvi-larotrectinib-advanced-solid-tumors-ntrk-gene-fusion-approval/article/816725/?utm_source=newsletter&utm_medium=email&utm_campaign=mpr-dailydose-cp-20181129&cpn=obgyn_all,obgyn_md,cambia_august2018&hmS

recombinant DNA technology: Rearranging DNA molecules, manufacturing recombinant DNA. Recombinant DNA molecule constructed from segments obtained from different DNA molecules. https://en.wikipedia.org/wiki/Recombinant_DNA

recombination: Genetic recombination. Interchange of chromosomal parts or genes. Breaking and rejoining DNA strands, forming new DNA molecules. https://en.wikipedia.org/wiki/Genetic_recombination https://www.nature.com/scitable/topicpage/dna-is-constantly-changing-through-the-process-6524876

rectocele: Bulging of the anterior wall of the rectum into the posterior wall of the vagina. https://www.ncbi.nlm.nih.gov/pmc/articles/PMC2967328/

regenerative medicine: Creation of new organs, tissues and body parts from stem cells, which are placed on a dissolvable matrix; tissue engineering, along with self-healing by the body's systems. http://www.nature.com/articles/npjregenmed20167 https://www.nature.com/articles/s41536-017-0008-1?WT.mc_id=EMI_RegMed_1704&spMailingID=53890539&spUserID=MTc3MDI4ODk5NQS2&spJobID=114328 https://www.nature.com/articles/npjregenmed20167?WT.mc_id=EMI_RegMed_1706&spMailingID=54243481&spUserID=MTc3MDI4ODk5NQS2&spJobID=1181517

rejection (host vs. graft): Immunologic response by organ recipient to allograft, damaging it. Immune cells in the transplanted organ can also attack the host: Graft vs. host response. http://emedicine.medscape.com/article/430449-overview#a4

renin: Proteolytic enzyme elaborated by juxtaglomerular cells of the kidneys that acts on angiotensin. https://www.britannica.com/science/renin-angiotensin-system

renin-angiotensin system (RAS): A mechanism of acute renal hypertension. Renal artery compression or occlusion causing ischemia of the renal cortex results in renal juxtaglomerular cells converting prorenin into renin. Renin acts on angiotensinogen in the bloodstream from the liver, converting it to angiotensin I, which is converted to angiotensin II by angiotensin-converting enzyme. Angiotensin II acts on aldosterone producing cells in the adrenal cortex, causing aldosterone production, leading to sodium retention and increased plasma volume. This leads to an increase in blood pressure, and increased blood flow, including to the kidneys, resulting in stretching of renal afferent arterioles, giving negative feedback so that renin secretion tends to return towards normal. Renin-angiotensin systems are present in various other tissues, in addition to the kidneys. http://www.ncbi.nlm.nih.gov/pubmed/17878513

reprogramming (cellular reprogramming): Using the expression of four genes (**Yamanaka factors**) to convert any cell into **induced pluripotent stem cells (iPSCs)**. https://www.salk.edu/news-release/turning-back-time-salk-scientists-reverse-signs-aging/ http://www.cell.com/cell/fulltext/S0092-8674(16)31664-6

resveratrol: Polyphenolic compound in red wine that may be partly responsible for the beneficial cardiovascular effects that have been attributed to red wine. http://lpi.oregonstate.edu/mic/dietary-factors/phytochemicals/resveratrol

reticuloendothelial system, also called mononuclear phagocyte system (mps): Widespread system in reticular (thin banding fibers) connective tissue that forms antibodies to counteract foreign antigens. https://en.wikipedia.org/wiki/Mononuclear_phagocyte_system

retinopathy: Disease of the retina. http://www.ncbi.nlm.nih.gov/pmc/articles/PMC3874488/

Rh isoimmunization: Immune response of Rh negative mother to her Rh positive fetus. First Rh positive child usually not affected. http://emedicine.medscape.com/article/797150-overview

rhytid: Skin wrinkle.

ribosome: The protein manufacturing machine. Complex molecular machine one-millionth of an inch in diameter. Tiny organ (organelle) in the cytoplasm of the cell. Made up of proteins and ribosomal RNA (rRNA)—the active component in protein synthesis. At the ribosome, the genetic code is read and translated into proteins. Amino acids are carried to the ribosome by transfer RNA (tRNA). The genetic code instructions for making a protein are carried to the ribosome by messenger RNA (mRNA) from the DNA in the cell nucleus. At the ribosome, the tRNA recognizes the sequence of the genetic code on the mRNA and lines up the amino acids in the proper order. The ribosome catalyzes the formation of bonds between the amino acids. https://micro.magnet.fsu.edu/cells/ribosomes/ribosomes.html

RNA: Ribonucleic acid. Messenger RNA (mRNA) is essentially a copy of a piece of one strand of DNA. Proteins are not made from the DNA of the gene. A template of RNA is made from the gene DNA. The RNA is then processed. The processing involves splicing of RNA. This spliced RNA, the template upon which the protein is made (protein synthesis), is called messenger RNA (mRNA). mRNA goes to the ribosome in the cell cytoplasm, where it meets the transfer RNA (tRNA) carrying the amino acids. Under the influence of ribosomal RNA (rRNA), the amino acids are bound together to form the protein (see "Ribosome"). http://www.nature.com/scitable/definition/ribonucleic-acid-rna-45 https://jamanetwork.com/journals/jama/fullarticle/2712406?guestAccessKey=22414c3e-162a-4ff0-8b50-5477ff58735b&utm_source=silverchair&utm_campaign=jama_network&utm_content=weekly_highlights&cmp=1&utm_medium=email

RNA editing: Making discrete changes to nucleotide sequences. (See "Nucleotide".) Can change proteins without making permanent changes to DNA. https://www.google.com/search?q=rna+editing+definition&rlz=1C1CHBF_enUS821US821&sxsrf=ALeKk00BTRIVfqmQj4UbehB8M429Om-0aA:1604597416317&tbm=isch&source=iu&ictx=1&fir=e1WL4n9BGtSUIM%252CCUK3YbinpbKiNM%252C%252Fm%252F0855vy&vet=1&usg= https://translational-medicine.biomedcentral.com/articles/10.1186/s12967-019-2071-4 https://www.nature.com/articles/d41586-020-00272-5

RNA interference (RNAi): Pathway that regulates gene expression https://jamanetwork.com/journals/jama/fullarticle/2712406?guestAccessKey=22414c3e-162a-4ff0-8b50-5477ff58735b&utm_source=silverchair&utm_campaign=jama_network&utm_content=weekly_highlights&cmp=1&utm_medium=email https://www.ncbi.nlm.nih.gov/probe/docs/techrnai/ https://www.nature.com/nrg/multimedia/rnai/animation/index.html https://www.ncbi.nlm.nih.gov/pmc/articles/PMC5542916/ https://www.nature.com/articles/d41586-018-05867-7?WT.ec_id=NATURE-20180816&utm_source=nature_etoc&utm_medium=email&utm_campaign=20180816&spMailingID=57190125&spUserID=MjA1NjIyNjc4OAS2&spJobID=1462154550&spReportId=MTQ2MjE1

robotics: A robot is a machine capable of automatically carrying out complex actions, programmable by computer. https://jamanetwork.com/journals/jama/fullarticle/2712406?guestAccessKey=22414c3e-162a-4ff0-8b50-5477ff58735b&utm_source=silverchair&utm_campaign=jama_network&utm_content=weekly_highlights&cmp=1&utm_medium=emailt

robotic surgery: Surgery carried out via robotic telemanipulation. The surgeon's movements at a console are translated to surgical instruments previously placed into the patient by minimally invasive technique. http://allaboutroboticsurgery.com/surgicalrobots.html

sarcoma: A virulent form of malignant, solid tumor. http://sarcomahelp.org/reviews/who-classification-sarcomas.html

SARS: Severe acute respiratory syndrome. SARS-CoV caused by a corona virus. First traced to Asia 2002. http://www.cdc.gov/sars/about/fs-sars.html https://www.niaid.nih.gov/diseases-conditions/covid-19 https://www.frontiersin.org/articles/10.3389/fimmu.2020.01880/full?utm_source=F-AAE&utm_medium=EMLF&utm_campaign=MRK_1417202_35_Immuno_202009

scar: Cicatrix. Connective tissue in which fibroblasts form granulation tissue. Older scars are composed of dense collagenous tissue.

scurvy: Disease caused by lack of Vitamin C (ascorbic acid). http://www.medicalnewstoday.com/articles/155758.php

self-destruct genes: Genes that cause cell death (apoptosis). http://www.nature.com/mt/journal/v23/n9/full/mt2015139a.html

senolytics: Drugs that kill **senescent**, non-dividing cells that accumulate in aging organs. https://www.nature.com/news/to-stay-young-kill-zombie-cells-1.22872?WT.ec_id=NEWS-20171026&spMailingID=55224149&spUserID=MTc2NjY4OTM5NgS2&s http://www.cell.com/cell/fulltext/S0092-8674(17)30246-5 https://www.ncbi.nlm.nih.gov/pubmed/22048312 https://www.ncbi.nlm.nih.gov/labs/journals/j-am-geriatr-soc/new/2017-09-05/ http://onlinelibrary.wiley.com/wol1/doi/10.1111/jgs.14969/full

sensitivity: (in medical testing) Probability that a test result will be positive when the disease is present. https://www.medcalc.org/calc/diagnostic_test.php

sepsis: Systemic inflammatory response to infection. http://www.ncbi.nlm.nih.gov/pmc/articles/PMC3684427/

SERM: Specific estrogen receptor modulator. A class of drugs used during menopause to prevent osteoporosis. Some drugs in this class are protective against the formation of breast cancer. http://www.ncbi.nlm.nih.gov/pmc/articles/PMC3624793/

serotonin: 5HT. 5-hydroxytryptamine. A monoamine neurotransmitter derived from tryptophan. https://en.wikipedia.org/wiki/Serotonin

serotonin/norepinephrine reuptake inhibitors: SNRIs. Medications used in depression. See Chapter 42, "An Overview of Late-Life Depression" by Artin Mahdanian, Silvia Monti De Flores. www.careoftheolderperson.com http://pharmacologycorner.com/serotonin-5ht-receptors-agonists-antagonist/#serotonin%20agonists

shaken baby syndrome: Abusive head trauma. Brain tissue injury, as well as hemorrhage and edema, may result. https://emedicine.medscape.com/article/1176849-overview

SHBG: Sex hormone binding globulin. Protein elaborated in the liver that binds and transports testosterone, dihydrotestosterone (DHT) and estradiol as inactive forms in blood. https://en.wikipedia.org/wiki/Sex_hormone-binding_globulin

shingles: Delayed cutaneous manifestation by **Herpes Zoster** (Varicella: chicken pox) virus. Preventive vaccine available. http://annals.org/aim/fullarticle/2671913/recommended-immunization-schedule-adults-aged-19-years-older-united-states http://bmjopen.bmj.com/content/4/6/e004833

sialomucin: Mucopolysaccharide containing sialic acid. Component of lung airway secretion. http://www.ncbi.nlm.nih.gov/gene/8763

sickness (illness): Inability of individuals to pursue their goals and purposes because of impairments in function considered to be in the domain of medicine. Boudreau, JD, Cassell, EJ, Fuks, A: Physicianship and the Rebirth of Medical Education. Oxford University Press 2018

signal transduction (cell signaling): Transmission of molecular signals from cell surface receptors to the cell interior. https://www.tocris.com/pharmacologicalBrowser.php?ItemId=187888#.V8hjh7ZTFwE

single cell biology: The study of the individual cell. https://genomebiology.biomedcentral.com/articles/10.1186/s13059-016-0941-0 http://www.nature.com/news/single-cell-biology-1.22241 https://www.frontiersin.org/articles/10.3389/fimmu.2018.02425/full?utm_source=F-AAE&utm_medium=EMLF&utm_campaign=MRK_812127_35_Immuno_20181030_arts_A

sirtuin genes: Genes that exert anti-aging effect in yeast. Increased sirtuin activity may be related to the mechanism by which caloric restriction extends life span. https://www.ncbi.nlm.nih.gov/pubmed/18419308

somatic cell nuclear transfer: Therapeutic cloning. Nucleus is taken from an adult cell and placed into an ovum whose own nucleus has been removed. These embryonic stem cells are induced to form specialized cells needed by the adult from whom the adult cell nucleus was taken. http://www.hhmi.org/biointeractive/somatic-cell-nuclear-transfer-animation

spatiotemporal analysis: Computational techniques used to determine patterns of disease; possibly predict where and when a disease may appear in the future. https://www.publichealth.columbia.edu/research/population-health-methods/spatiotemporal-analysis

specificity: (in medical testing) Probability that a test result will be negative when the disease is not present. https://www.medcalc.org/calc/diagnostic_test.php

spermatozoon: The male germ (sex) cell, derived from the testicle. It has a head, body and tail, and is motile. The spermatozoon swims up the female reproductive tract, eventually fertilizing (fusing with) the egg (ovum) in the fallopian tube. https://www.

boundless.com/physiology/textbooks/boundless-anatomy-and-physiology-textbook/
the-reproductive-system-27/physiology-of-the-male-reproductive-system-253/
spermatogenesis-1234-9350/

spindle nuclear transfer: Removal of the nuclear spindle from a maternal oocyte and transferring that spindle to a donor oocyte from which the spindle has been removed, in order to obviate a mitochondrial mutation. The donor oocyte containing the maternal nuclear spindle is then fertilized. https://www.ncbi.nlm.nih.gov/pmc/articles/PMC4005382/ https://www.sciencenews.org/blog/science-ticker/first-%E2%80%98three-parent-baby%E2%80%99-born-nuclear-transfer

splicing: The reattaching of the two ends of a stringlike material, after a piece has been removed. In **gene splicing**, DNA is cut and a gene inserted. http://www.premierbiosoft.com/tech_notes/gene-splicing.html

SSRI: Selective Serotonin Reuptake inhibitor: Medications used in depression. Inhibit reuptake of serotonin, so increase serotonin activity. See Chapter 42, "An Overview of Late-Life Depression" by Artin Mahdanian, Silvia Monti De Flores. www.careoftheolderperson.com http://www.rxlist.com/the_comprehensive_list_of_antidepressants-page2/drugs-condition.htm#ssris https://www.ncbi.nlm.nih.gov/books/NBK554406/#:~:text=Mechanism%20of%20Action&text=As%20the%20name%20suggests%2C%20SSRIs,such%20as%20dopamine%20or%20norepinephrine.

statins: Drugs that reduce circulating LDL (low density lipoprotein) by encouraging the LDL receptor to increase uptake. Decreased production of LDL-C (low density lipoprotein cholesterol) results. https://www.drugs.com/drug-class/hmg-coa-reductase-inhibitors.html

stem cell: An undifferentiated cell that has the potential to become a specialized cell with a specific function, such as a blood cell or a muscle cell. http://stemcells.nih.gov/info/basics/1.htm http://fhs.mcmaster.ca/main/news/news_2016/life_saving_blood_stem_cells.html https://www.nature.com/collections/bhegaaeifa?sap-outbound-id=6C58DC9E6593DB1764AD822FEFE8EBA0A8220E8F&utm_source=hybris-campaign&utm_medium=email&utm_campaign=000_NJN2936_0000016915_Nature%20Outlook%3A%20Stem%20cells&utm_content=EN_internal_32499_20211005&mkt-key=42010A0550671EEA9B9F5C23E82FAC65

stem cell transplant: Injection of stem cells into the body to replace damaged or diseased tissue, blood. http://www.cancer.gov/about-cancer/treatment/types/stem-cell-transplant http://journal.frontiersin.org/article/10.3389/fimmu.2016.00470/full

stent: Self-expanding tube placed in a blood vessel to keep that vessel patent. May be drug-eluting. https://www.sciencedaily.com/releases/2015/03/150316135610.htm

stereotactic radiosurgery (SRS): Precisely focused radiation to scar and close the blood vessels of an arteriovenous malformation (AVM) in the brain. http://www.irsa.org/radiosurgery.html

stereotaxis: Method in neurosurgery for locating points within the brain using an external three-dimensional frame.

stress: Response to physical, mental or emotional pressure. https://www.cancer.gov/publications/dictionaries/cancer-terms/def/stress

stroke: Cerebrovascular accident. Damage to the brain by a blood clot in a vessel supplying the brain, or by hemorrhage into the brain. http://www.neurology.org/content/early/2016/09/16/WNL.0000000000003238.abstract http://www.empr.com/news/repatha-heart-attack-stroke-prevention-pcsk9-inhibitor/article/711332/?DCMP=EMC-MPR_DailyDose_cp_20171204&cpn=obgyn_all&hmSubId=&hmEmail=hIe6FnTBLUDNqAesd8d7sd9Sz-y1cfMN0&NID=1538223656&c_id=&dl=0&spMailingID=18599771&spUserID=MTgxMDk3OTQyMDM0S0&spJobID=1160335565&spReportId=MTE2MDMzNTU2NQS2 http://www.acc.org/latest-in-cardiology/ten-points-to-remember/2018/01/29/12/45/2018-guidelines-for-the-early-management-of-stroke https://www.nature.com/articles/s41746-017-0015-z?utm_source=Springer_Nature_website&utm_medium=Website_links&utm_content=AngWan-SN-OD-Neuroscience-Global&utm_campaign=SNOR_USG_SFN18ttp

subunit: Ribosomal nucleic acid (rRNA) molecules (see "Ribosome"). http://www.microbe.net/simple-guides/fact-sheet-ribosomal-rna-rrna-the-details/

sudden infant deathsyndrome (SIDS): Unexplained death during sleep of a seemingly healthy baby. http://emedicine.medscape.com/article/804412-overview

suicide: Intentional, voluntary taking of own life. Contributory factor influencing average lifespan. http://healthjournalism.org/blog/2014/04/exploring-risk-factors-rates-of-suicide-in-seniors/

superager: Person 80 years or older with episodic memory ability at least as good as an average middle-age adult. Significantly thicker brain cortex than same-age peers. http://jamanetwork.com/journals/jama/article-abstract/2614177

superposition: In quantum mechanics, the state of a particle is not defined for certain until it is measured. https://www.researchgate.net/publication/258566887_The_Superposition_Principle_in_Quantum_Mechanics_-_did_the_rock_enter_the_foundation_surreptitiously

TALENs: Transcription Activator-Like Effector Nucleases. Utilized to alter genes. See "Transcription", "Nuclease". https://www.ncbi.nlm.nih.gov/pmc/articles/PMC3547402/

targeted area correction sequencing: Detection of mutations and rearrangements indicative of cancer in cell-free plasma DNA. https://www.ncbi.nlm.nih.gov/pmc/articles/PMC4755822/ http://journals.plos.org/plosgenetics/article?id=10.1371/journal.pgen.1005816 http://journals.plos.org/plosone/article?id=10.1371/journal.pone.0064271 http://journals.plos.org/plosgenetics/article?id=10.1371/journal.pgen.1005816

targeted therapy: Drug designed to reverse the effects of a specific mutation. http://www.ncbi.nlm.nih.gov/pubmed/23470539

telomerase: Enzyme that maintains and repairs the telomere. http://study.com/academy/lesson/what-is-telomerase-definition-function-structure.html

telomere: The end of a chromosome. It is made up of DNA. The telomere gives stability to the end of the chromosome, preventing abnormal recombinations (mutations). See Chapter 1, "Introduction" by Jose Morais. www.careoftheolderperson.com https://en.wikipedia.org/wiki/Telomere https://link.springer.com/article/10.1007/s10815-017-0967-6/fulltext.html?wt_mc=alerts.TOCjournals

template: The pattern from which copies are made. https://engineering.ucsb.edu/~shell/che170/DNA-notes.pdf

testis: The male gonad. http://emedicine.medscape.com/article/1949259-overview

testosterone: The prominent androgen in the male. Male sex hormone. Present in lesser amounts in women. http://www.livescience.com/38963-testosterone.html

thallium stress test: Radioisotope uptake monitoring and myocardial perfusion assessment while patient is on a treadmill. http://pubs.rsna.org/doi/full/10.1148/rg.317115090

thrombophlebitis: Inflammation of the wall of a vein in conjunction with thrombosis.

thrombosis: Blood clotting in a blood vessel.

throughput: Number of units of information a system can process in a given time. https://www.techtarget.com/searchnetworking/definition/throughput **High Throughput Technology:** simultaneous examination of thousands of genes. https://www.igi-global.com/dictionary/bioinformatics-clouds-for-high-throughput-technologies/39084#:~:text=1.,of%20genes%2C%20proteins%20and%20metabolites https://academic.oup.com/femspd/article/78/8/ftaa061/5919476

thymus gland: Lymphoid gland of the immune system located in the neck that produces T-cells. http://biology.about.com/od/anatomy/ss/thymus.htm

TIA: Transient ischemic arteriospasm. Constriction of blood vessels in the brain with no permanent damage.

tissue engineering: Combining cells, scaffolds and biologically active molecules to create new tissue. https://www.nibib.nih.gov/science-education/science-topics/tissue-engineering-and-regenerative-medicine

tissue typing: Tissue antigens of prospective organ donor and recipient compared for histocompatibility. HLA (human leukocyte antigen) typing. http://www.encyclopedia.com/topic/Tissue_Typing.aspx

T-lymphocyte (T-cell): White blood cell that is immunologically competent. Responsible for cell-mediated immunity. Can attack surface antigens on malignant cells, if activated by prior presentation of the antigen. https://en.wikipedia.org/wiki/T_cell; https://www.frontiersin.org/articles/10.3389/fimmu.2018.00233/full?utm_source=F-AAE&utm_medium=EMLF&utm_campaign=MRK_554072_35_Immuno_20180227_arts_A

totipotentiality: Capability of a cell to differentiate into unlimited number of cell types. http://medical-dictionary.thefreedictionary.com/totipotential+cell

toxemia: The hypertensive disorders of pregnancy.

TPA: Tissue plasminogen activator. Protein involved in the breakdown of blood clots. http://pharmacologycorner.com/thrombolytic-agents-mechanism-of-action-indications-contraindications-and-side-effects/ http://atvb.ahajournals.org/content/29/8/1151.full

trabecula: Supporting structures of connective tissue.

transcription: Transfer of genetic code information between nucleic acids. The process by which the genetic code on the DNA gets into the mRNA template (see DNA, RNA). http://www.vcbio.science.ru.nl/en/virtuallessons/cellcycle/trans/

transcriptome: Gene readouts (transcripts) of all the DNA in a cell by RNA. https://www.genome.gov/13014330/transcriptome-fact-sheet/**Epitranscriptome:** All the modifications in RNA after transcription. https://www.nature.com/articles/s41576-020-00295-8

transformation zone: The outer cervix is lined by squamous cells, much like the vaginal lining. The inner canal of the cervix is lined by tall cylindrical cells. Where these two layers meet, there is an area of microscopic activity where the cylindrical columnar cells are being transformed, or over-ridden, by squamous cells. This is a benign process called **squamous metaplasia.** This area is called the transformation zone. It is in this area of cell activity that cancer of the cervix most commonly arises.

transgenesis: Exogenous or modified gene introduced into an organism of the same or different species. https://www.google.com/search?q=transgenesis+definition&rlz=1C1CHBF_enUS821US821&oq=transgenesis&aqs=chrome.1.69i57j0i20i263i512j0i512l3j0i10i512j0i512l2j0i20i263i512j0i512.26552j0j9&sourceid=chrome&ie=UTF-8

translation: The process by which the genetic code of mRNA becomes proteins. https://bioweb.uwlax.edu/GenWeb/Molecular/Theory/Translation/translation.htm

translational medicine: Mechanisms by which new drugs and tests get from the laboratory into the hands of physicians for administration to patients, and the mechanisms for ensuring that patients get necessary services. https://www.ncbi.nlm.nih.gov/pmc/articles/PMC2829707/ http://www.medscape.com/viewarticle/871305nlid=110427_2581&src=WNL_mdplsnews_161104_mscpedit_obgy&uac=66536PR&spon=16&impID=1228473&faf=1

transplantation: Transfer of organ or tissue from one individual to another. http://www.ajog.org/article/0002-9378(70)90382-0/abstract?cc=y= http://www.who.int/transplantation/organ/en/**Autologous (stem cell) transplant:** Stem cells collected, stored, then given back to same individual. https://www.mskcc.org/cancer-care/diagnosis-treatment/cancer-treatments/blood-stem-cell-transplantation/autologous

trigeminal nerve: The fifth cranial nerve. http://emedicine.medscape.com/article/1873373-overview

triglyceride: Ester formed from glycerol and three molecules of fatty acids. https://en.wikipedia.org/wiki/Triglyceride

triptans: Serotonin (5HT) receptor agonists. Medications that constrict blood vessels in the brain and are used in the treatment of migraine. http://archneur.jamanetwork.com/article.aspx?articleid=782346

trophoblast: Outer ring of cells around the blastocyst cavity that becomes the placenta. http://discovery.lifemapsc.com/in-vivo-development/trophoblast/trophoblast

troponins: Proteins released when heart muscle is damaged. Can be detected in blood circulation and be used to predict cardiovascular disease (CVD) risk. https://www.ahajournals.org/doi/pdf/10.1161/CIRCULATIONAHA.118.038772

tuberculosis: Infectious disease especially affecting the lungs caused by mycobacterium tuberculosis. http://www.thelancet.com/journals/lanres/article/PIIS2213-2600(15)00063-6/abstract

tumor: Abnormal growth. May be benign or malignant.

tumor grade: Appearance, abnormality of malignant tumor cells. https://www.cancer.gov/about-cancer/diagnosis-staging/prognosis/tumor-grade-fact-sheet

tumor infiltrating lymphocyte (TIL): Immune cell from a patient's blood that has moved into a tumor to attack it. TILs can be removed from the tumor, activated, then given back to the patient. https://www.cancer.gov/publications/dictionaries/cancer-terms/def/tumor-infiltrating-lymphocyte

tumor necrosis factor (TNF): Multifunctional cytokine secreted by inflammatory cells. https://www.ncbi.nlm.nih.gov/pmc/articles/PMC2631033/#:~:text=Tumor%20necrosis%20factor%20(TNF)%20is,involved%20in%20inflammation%2Dassociated%20carcinogenesis.

tumor specific antigen (TSA): Protein or other molecule produced in tumor cells that sets off an immune response in the host. Used as tumor markers to identify tumor cells in the body. Used in the immunologic treatment of cancer. Also, **Tumor Associated Antigens (TAA)** that are significantly more abundant in cancer cells than in other tissue. CEA Antigen, Prostate-Specific Antigen, CA125, CA19-9. https://www.researchgate.net/publication/9314460_Demonstration_of_TumorSpecific_Antigens_in_Human_Colonic_Carcinomata_by_Immunological_Tolerance_and_Absorption_Techniques https://www.researchgate.net/publication/12453745_Self_recognition_in_the_Ig_superfamily_Identification_of_precise_subdomains_in_carcinoembryonic_antigen_required_for_intercellular_adhesion

tumor stage: Extent of the malignant tumor: its size and spread. https://www.cancer.gov/about-cancer/diagnosis-staging/staging

tumor suppressor gene (antioncogene): Genes, such as the TP59 gene, that elaborate tumor suppressor proteins that control cell growth. Mutations (DNA changes) in these genes are associated with cancer. Tumor Protein 53 (TP53) that also has a role in germ cell survival, is another example. https://www.cancer.gov/publications/dictionaries/cancer-terms?cdrid=46657 https://www.nature.com/articles/d41586-017-07291-9?WT.ec_id=NEWSDAILY-20171123&utm_source=briefing&utm_medium=email&utm_campaig http://www.fertstert.org/article/S0015-0282(17)32096-4/fulltext?elsca1=etoc&elsca2=email&elsca3=0015-0282_201801_109_1_&elsca4=Obstetrics%20and%20Gyn

turbinates: Shelves of bone covered by thick mucous membrane that project into the nasal passages. http://emedicine.medscape.com/article/874771-overview

ubiquitin-proteasome system: A protein clearance mechanism with implications in aging and age-related diseases. https://link.springer.com/article/10.1007/s10815-016-0842-x?wt_mc=alerts.TOCjournals http://www.nature.com/ncomms/2014/141208/ncomms6659/fig_tab/ncomms6659_F1.html

ultrasonography: Imaging by reflecting high energy "sound" waves off objects. The waves have higher frequency than sound that can be heard by humans. Four-dimensional sonography refers to images being seen in real time. https://www.ncbi.nlm.nih.gov/pubmed/20541656 http://medical-dictionary.thefreedictionary.com/ultrasonography

ultraviolet rays (UV): Short wavelength solar rays that are invisible to the human eye. http://medical-dictionary.thefreedictionary.com/ultraviolet+rays

umbilical cord: The cord that connects the developing fetus to the placenta. Blood circulates in the cord via two arteries and one vein: the umbilical vein carrying nutrients and oxygen from the placenta to the fetus, and the umbilical arteries carrying waste products of metabolism and carbon dioxide away from the fetus, back to the placenta. https://www.ncbi.nlm.nih.gov/books/NBK53254/

umbilical cord blood: Fetal blood that circulates via the umbilical cord. http://www.webmd.com/parenting/baby/features/banking-your-babys-cord-blood#1 http://journal.frontiersin.org/article/10.3389/fimmu.2017.00087/full?utm_source=newsletter&utm_medium=email&utm_campaign=Immunology-w6-2017 https://www.nature.com/nature/journal/vaop/ncurrent/full/nature22067.html

urethra: The passage from the urinary bladder to the vulva in the female, and to the penile meatus in the male.

urethrocele: Bulging of the urethra into the anterior vaginal wall.

urinary incontinence: Involuntary loss of urine. Stress incontinence, urgency incontinence and neurogenic incontinence are types. See Chapter 32, "Incontinence in Older Adults" by Samer Shamout, Lysanne Campeau. www.careoftheolderperson.com http://jamanetwork.com/journals/jama/article-abstract/2595508

uterus: The womb. Its endometrial lining undergoes decidual change to receive the implanting fertilized egg (zygote). During labor, muscular rhythmic contractions of the uterine wall gradually send the fetus through the birth canal.

vaccine: A killed or attenuated (variant) virus given by mouth or injection to activate the body's immune system against the actual dangerous virus. In the case of COVID-19, mRNA vaccines are being used. If a vaccinated person comes in contact with the actual virus, the person's activated immune system kills the virus before it can cause harm. Anticancer vaccines that target malignant cells are now being developed and are in use. See Chapter 14, "Are the Immunizations of My Patient up to Date?" by Dominique Tessier. www.careoftheolderperson.com https://www.jci.org/articles/view/80009 http://journal.frontiersin.org/article/10.3389/fimmu.2017.00800/full?utm_source=F-AAE&utm_medium=EMLF&utm_campaign=MRK_333189_35_Immuno_20170720_arts_A https://jamanetwork.com/journals/jama/fullarticle/2714651?guestAccessKey=1f4ca6ea-c69b-48ab-909f-713499b43cf8&utm_source=silverchair&utm_medium=email&utm_campaign=article_alert-jama&utm_content=etoc&utm_term=120518 https://jamanetwork.com/journals/jama/fullarticle/2714651?guestAccessKey=1f4ca6ea-c69b-48ab-909f-713499b43cf8&utm_source=silverchair&utm_medium=email&utm_campaign=article_alert-jama&utm_content=etoc&utm_term=1205181 https://jamanetwork.com/journals/jama/fullarticle/2770485?guestAccessKey=c95ea2e7-ea01-40d0-90fbe95cd2a1ba7e&utm_source=silverchair&utm_medium=email&utm_campaign=article_alert-jama&utm_content=olf&utm_term=090320 https://www.nap.edu/catalog/25917/framework-for-equitable-allocation-ofcovid-19-vaccine https://www.nature.com/articles/d41586-020-02856-7?utm_source=Nature+Briefing&utm_campaign=7f2b123fc5-briefing-dy-20201014&utm_medium=email&utm_term=0_c9dfd39373-7f2b123fc5-42544483 https://www.ncbi.nlm.nih.gov/pmc/articles/PMC7218962/ https://www.cdc.gov/vaccines/covid-19/hcp/mrna-vaccine-basics.html#:~:text=mRNA%20vaccines%20take%20advantage%20of,virus%20that%20causes%20COVID%2D19.

vagina: The female genital tract extending inwards from the vulva. Closed at rest with the anterior wall resting on the posterior wall. Its muscular, elastic wall is lined by a mucous membrane that has a normal secretion. The cervix protrudes into the inner end, the vaginal vault.

value-based medical care: Quality of care relative to its cost. Quality is assessed in the areas of outcomes, safety and service. Outcomes includes measurement of mortality rates, complications and resultant functional status of patients. Safety includes attention to infection rates, accidental falls and medication errors. Service assesses patient satisfaction, wait times, access to treatment and procedures, and affordability. https://wire.ama-assn.org/education/value-based-care-elusive-concept-enters-curriculum?&utm_source=BHClistID&utm_medium=BulletinHealthCare&utm_term=120616&utm_content=MorningRounds&utm_campaign=BHCMessageID http://jamanetwork.com/journals/jama/fullarticle/2594716

varicose veins: Veins that bulge out due to damage to their valves. http://emedicine.medscape.com/article/462579-treatment

vasopressin: Antidiuretic hormone (ADH). Formed in the hypothalamus and released from the posterior pituitary. Acts on renal collecting system, increasing water permeability and decreasing urine formation. Acts on vascular smooth muscle, causing vasoconstriction. http://www.cvphysiology.com/Blood%20Pressure/BP016

vegetative symptoms: Disturbances of functions necessary to maintain life: See Chapter 42, "An Overview of Late-Life Depression" by Artin Mahdanian, Silvia Monti De Flores. www.careoftheolderperson.com https://en.wikipedia.org/wiki/Vegetative_symptoms

VEGF: Vascular Endothelial Growth Factor. Angiogenic factor that promotes growth in vascular endothelial cells. Has a role in tumor angiogenesis. http://www.nature.com/nrc/journal/v8/n8/full/nrc2403.html http://perspectivesinmedicine.cshlp.org/content/2/10/a006577.full

vein: A blood vessel that carries blood from the body towards the heart, usually transporting carbon dioxide and waste products of metabolism. Exceptions include the pulmonary vein, which carries oxygenated blood from the lungs to the heart for redistribution throughout the body, and the umbilical vein in the fetus, which carries oxygenated blood from the placenta to the fetal heart for redistribution throughout the fetal body.

villus: A tiny projection from a surface.

virus: An infecting agent so small that it cannot be seen under a light microscope. Viruses are made up of DNA or RNA. They can only replicate (divide) by invading into a host cell and causing that cell to manufacture more virus. http://www.ncbi.nlm.nih.gov/books/NBK21523/

vital organ: Organ necessary for life, including the heart, lungs, brain, kidneys and liver.

vitamin: A substance that in small amounts is essential to metabolism, that naturally occurs in food. See Chapter 10, "Could My Patient Be Malnourished?" by Jose Morais. www.careoftheolderperson.com http://annals.org/article.aspx?articleid=1767855

vulva: The female external genitalia. Includes: labia majora, labia minora, clitoris, vestibule, urethral orifice, mons pubis.

West Nile virus: A mosquito borne flavivirus that can cause encephalitis and meningitis. http://www.cdc.gov/westnile/symptoms/

xenobot: Tiny robot constructed from living (frog) cells with the aid of artificial intelligence (AI). https://www.smithsonianmag.com/innovation/scientists-assemble-frog-stemcells-first-living-machines-180973947/

xerostomia: Dry mouth. https://www.mayoclinic.org/diseases-conditions/dry-mouth/symptoms-causes/syc-2035604 Wiseman, Michael, Dental care in older persons, The Care of the Older Person, Fifth Edition RMC Publishing LLC 2022

Yamanaka factors: Four genes that are important in cellular reprogramming to pluripotent stem cells. https://www.ncbi.nlm.nih.gov/pubmed/19030024

zika virus: Mosquito borne. The fetuses of infected pregnant women have an increased incidence of microcephaly. There is an increased incidence of Guillain-Barre Syndrome with flaccid paralysis. Ref: Yale School of Medicine News, 08/26/2016 http://www.bloomberg.com/news/articles/2016-08-19/zika-may-cause-brain-damage-in-adults-too http://www.contagionlive.com/news/zika-research-reveals-virus-may-negatively-impact-adult-neural-stem-cells?utm_source=Informz&utm_medium=Contagion+Live&utm_campaign=Contagion_Live_Trending_News_9-5-16 http://jamanetwork.com/journals/jama/fullarticle/2593701 https://www.mdlinx.com/obstetrics-gynecology/top-medical-news/article/2017/01/02/3?utm_source=in-house&utm_medium=message&utm_campaign=in-the-news-jan17

zona pellucida: The glycoprotein outer envelope of the ovum. http://www.ncbi.nlm.nih.gov/pubmed/10497324

zygote: Fertilization (fusion of ovum and spermatozoon) results in a new cell: the zygote, which has 46 chromosomes including either an X or Y chromosome from the spermatozoon, and an X chromosome from the ovum. The zygote is therefore either XX (female) or XY (male). The zygote develops to a blastocyst stage with an inner cell mass that becomes the embryo, a fluid-filled blastocyst cavity, and an outer ring of cells around the blastocyst cavity called the trophoblast, which becomes the placenta. http://www.biology-online.org/dictionary/Zygote

Bibliography and Supplemental Bibliography

End of Each Chapter
The links under entries in the Glossary
And see www.rcaplanmd.com

Index

Note: Page numbers in *italics* indicate figures and in **bold** indicate tables on the corresponding pages.

ted in the United States
Baker & Taylor Publisher Services